LOVE, FEAR, AND HEALTH

How Our Attachments to Others Shape Health and Health Care

Can the way in which we relate to others seriously affect our health? Can understanding those attachments help health care providers treat us better? In *Love, Fear, and Health*, psychiatrists Robert Maunder and Jonathan Hunter draw on evidence from neuroscience, stress physiology, social psychology, and evolutionary biology to explain how understanding attachment – the ways in which people seek security in their close relationships – can transform patient outcomes.

Using attachment theory, Maunder and Hunter provide a practical, clinically focused introduction to the influence of attachment styles on an individual's risk of disease and the effectiveness of their interactions with health care providers. Drawing on more than fifty years of combined experience as health care providers, teachers, and researchers, they explain in clear language how health care workers in all disciplines can use this knowledge to meet their patients' needs better and to improve their health.

ROBERT MAUNDER is a professor in the Department of Psychiatry at the University of Toronto and the head of research in the Department of Psychiatry at Mount Sinai Hospital.

JONATHAN HUNTER is an associate professor in the Department of Psychiatry at the University of Toronto and the head of the consultation-liaison division in the Department of Psychiatry at Mount Sinai Hospital and the University of Toronto.

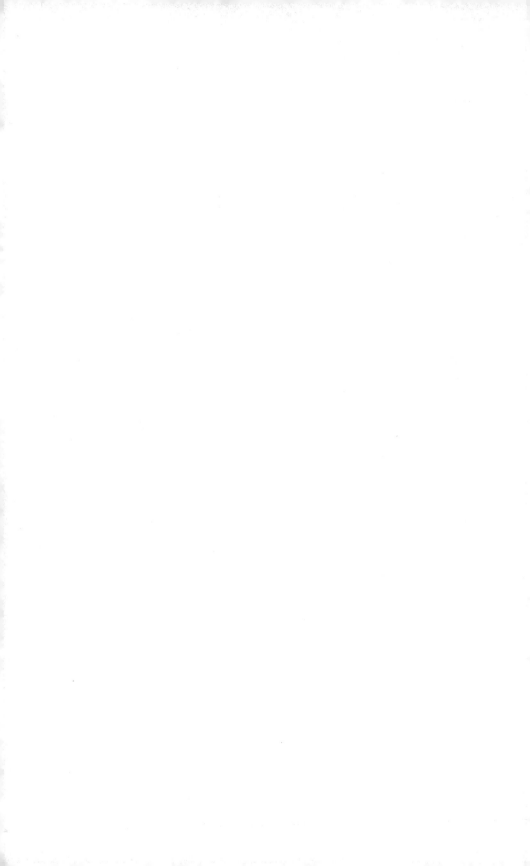

Love, Fear, and Health

How Our Attachments to Others Shape Health and Health Care

ROBERT MAUNDER AND
JONATHAN HUNTER

UNIVERSITY OF TORONTO PRESS
Toronto Buffalo London

ISBN 978-1-4426-4751-0 (cloth)   ISBN 978-1-4426-1560-1 (paper)

Library and Archives Canada Cataloguing in Publication

Maunder, Bob (Bob G.), author
Love, fear, and health : how our attachments to others shape health
and health care / Robert Maunder and Jonathan Hunter.

Includes bibliographical references and index.
ISBN 978-1-4426-4751-0 (bound).   ISBN 978-1-4426-1560-1 (paperback)

1. Attachment behavior.   2. Interpersonal relations – Health aspects.
3. Health.   4. Medical care.   I. Hunter, Jonathan, 1958–, author   II. Title.

RC455.4.A84M39 2015   613   C2015-903100-1

This book has been published with the help of a grant from the Federation
for the Humanities and Social Sciences, through the Awards to Scholarly
Publications Program, using funds provided by the Social Sciences and
Humanities Research Council of Canada.

University of Toronto Press acknowledges the financial assistance to its
publishing program of the Canada Council for the Arts and the Ontario Arts
Council, an agency of the Government of Ontario.

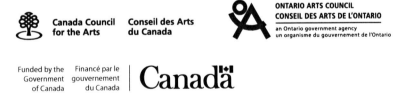

Canada Council   Conseil des Arts
for the Arts   du Canada

ONTARIO ARTS COUNCIL
CONSEIL DES ARTS DE L'ONTARIO
an Ontario government agency
un organisme du gouvernement de l'Ontario

Funded by the   Financé par le
Government   gouvernement
of Canada   du Canada

Canada

Bob
Without music, life would be a mistake.
Friedrich Nietzsche
For Lynn, who is my music.

Jon
I have seen a medicine
That's able to breathe life into a stone,
Quicken a rock, and make you dance...
William Shakespeare
For Nance, who is my medicine.

Contents

Acknowledgments

This book has been written several times. We can't take full credit for its final form because we were pretty happy with the first draft, but it has certainly improved because of a lot of thoughtful criticism and direction about how to think about, and teach, attachment. We are in great debt to the colleagues and especially the students who sat through our lectures and workshops and then asked hard questions. Each time we were stumped, we learned something.

Many people have also read portions of this book and its ancestors and given us thoughtful feedback and advice (sometimes beyond our ability to reconcile – "Leave the jokes out!" "Without the jokes it would be very boring!"). These readers have included Louise Balfour, Leo Chagoya, Lynn Fisher, Janice Halpern, Jeremy Holmes, Elizabeth Knoll, Nancy MacKenzie, Kathleen Maunder, Susan Rabiner, Albert Wong, and some anonymous peer reviewers whom we wish we could thank. We have also had a hundred conversations with colleagues and collaborators who have shaped our thinking and writing over the years. Among these are Ken Adams, Christina Maar Andersen, Leslie Atkinson, Anna Buchheim, Paul Ciechanowski, Carol George, Susan Goldberg, Chris Hinnen, Gary Kraemer, Bill Lancee, Karen Le, Molyn Leszcz, Clare Pain, Paula Ravitz, Gary Rodin, Peter Shapiro, Graeme Taylor, and Malcolm West.

Along the way, we have learned much from our collaborators, students, peer reviewers, friends, patients, and mentors. As authors, we have had weekly conversations about this stuff for so many years that neither of us can remember any longer who contributed what to our shared understanding. It is appropriate to its subject matter that, in the end, this is a book that emerges from conversations. In spite of the many who have contributed to the book's virtues, only we can take responsibility for its errors and shortcomings; we hope that not too many have survived.

We thank Eric Carlson, Lisa Jemison, and the staff at University of Toronto Press for shepherding the book through to publication. Dawn Hunter provided exceptionally constructive copy editing, and Celia Braves built an index with passion and meticulous skill. We are grateful to be able to reproduce Robert Pope's painting *Hug* on the front cover and thank the Robert Pope Foundation for their permission. Robert Pope was a Nova Scotia artist who died of Hodgkin's disease at age 36. The interpersonal perspective on health that is the subject of this book resonates through much of his work.

LOVE, FEAR, AND HEALTH

How Our Attachments to Others Shape Health
and Health Care

Introduction

As I (Bob) drive to work through slow traffic for an hour or so, my mood shifts lazily between contemplation and irritation. I listen to the radio and think about the day ahead. I don't usually weep. So it was peculiar on this grey October morning to be wiping tears from my face as I navigated the last few blocks to the hospital.

In my boredom I had switched from music to a public affairs show just as a documentary started to play. *Breathing with Sandra* described a remarkable friendship between Natalia Ritchie, a young mother with cystic fibrosis, and two women about her age, sisters Michelle Kennedy and Jessica Remington.[1] Their friendship helped to sustain Natalia through her recovery from the double lung transplant that saved her life – just when she had almost lost hope that donor lungs would become available. The extraordinary part of the story, however, was how they met; Michelle and Jessica were the daughters of the woman who donated Natalia's new lungs.

Their mother, Sandra, dying in the intensive care unit, had wanted to be taken off life support and to donate her organs. When Sandra was beyond making choices for herself, it was up to Michelle and Jessica to honour her wishes, which they did – a task that is too difficult for some families. As the lungs were removed, a police car sat outside the hospital, waiting to escort them to the transplant surgeons in another hospital 90 minutes away. Michelle saw the police as she left the hospital and stopped to tell them, "That's my mom. Turn your lights on. Beep your horn real loud."

Natalia cries as she recalls waking up from the surgery. "I wake up in a tiny hospital room ... and I am so lost. I have no idea what's been happening and my dad is the first one I saw. He said 'you got your lungs' and then my husband came up to me and he kissed me and he said 'you got your lungs.'"

Although in Canada donor and recipient families are never introduced and are supposed to remain unknown to each other, Michelle and Natalia came into contact within a few days of the operation. They connected through social media, first tentatively and then enthusiastically, driven by one woman's wish to thank the family of the person who had given her the biggest gift she has ever received and by the sisters' need to soothe their grief with the knowledge that their mother had been "resuscitated."

The parts that got to me, as I drove to work that morning, were Natalia speaking of her gratitude and determination to honour Sandra's gift and Michelle's observations as she attended the baptism of Natalia's daughter: "This is part of my mom ... Those are the lungs that I watched take their last breath. They're still breathing."

The story of Sandra, Jessica, Michelle, Natalia, and Natalia's father, husband, and daughter embodies one of the two central messages of this book: health happens between people. Consider the implications of their story. Natalia would not be alive except for Sandra's generosity in choosing to donate her organs and Jessica and Michelle being brave enough to accept their mother's fate and honour her wishes. Natalia's recovery depended in part on their friendship: "That was such a big factor. Now I know these people and they are counting on me to do well." Then the effects ripple out across relationships and over generations. If not for Sandra's gift, Natalia's daughter would have grown up without a mother – a surprisingly substantial risk factor for poor health throughout her life. Natalia's widowed husband and grieving father would have faced not only emotional loss but also health risks of their own as a result. This book will show how the same principle affects almost everyone's life – health and illness depend far more on the relationships that we share than we realize.

As psychiatrists for people who are physically ill, we have worked to understand how personal relationships shape health. Most often, the interpersonal forces that make us healthier or push us towards illness are subtle, albeit hiding in plain sight. They are driven by the second core principle of this book: human beings do whatever it takes to feel safe and secure. If what it takes to feel secure is good for our health, that's great because we are experts at obtaining that feeling. But if what it takes to feel secure is bad for our health – such as whopping doses of alcohol – then screw health, because we value an immediate sense of safety far more than our long-term well-being.

And when we are sick, our insecurities about trusting and depending on others are laid bare. Illness makes relationships matter more than normal, and the stakes often feel too high for comfort. In reacting to illness, one person becomes preoccupied with being a burden or worries about depending on others too much; another becomes fixated on living as if she is not sick at all, to the extent that she cannot accept the help that others lovingly offer. We organize our lives, whether we are aware of it or not, around a ceaseless quest to feel safe and avoid fear. All too often, the ways that we have organized our lives with others, patterns that have served us well for many years, no longer do the job when we are sick. Then we must search for a workable way to be ill.

A second story, also told from Bob's perspective, illustrates how the necessity of feeling as secure as possible at times when our well-being is at stake shapes the experience of being ill.

Dr Sam Golden just wanted to turn back the clock to feel normal again. When he met me for the first time, he was wearing a casual, unrumpled plaid shirt and khaki pants, the typical uniform of a doctor at the veteran's hospital where he worked, friendly but professional. He looked fit for a man in his fifties, balding yet trim. He extended his hand to shake mine as he walked into my office.

Sam had never had the slightest inclination to speak to a psychiatrist about himself, and so he had no idea who to call when he started to get worried one month after his heart attack. His friend, the head of my department, put him in touch with me. We met after his clinic closed for the day. He was already easing back into his normal work routine, right on schedule. He was polite and funny in a slightly self-conscious way as he told me what was going on, but he didn't waste any time.

"I think I'm becoming a hypochondriac."

"You told me on the phone about your heart attack last month. Is that where the trouble started?" He nodded yes. "Okay, can you start there and walk me through what happened?"

"On March 5 I had some back pain that started when I was at my office, but I didn't think it was anything serious. The next day, Saturday, it was much worse – right between the shoulder blades. I woke up with it and it didn't get any better so I went to the emergency department. It turned out it was an MI."

"That's not a typical presentation for a myocardial infarction."[2]

"Yeah. There was no sweating, no nausea, no shortness of breath, no chest pain, nothing in my arms. Just the back pain."

"How long were you in hospital?"

"Five days. They put in a stent."[3]

"How big was the infarction?"

"The cardiologist said it was 'not small.' A patch of heart muscle is dead, probably forever, but it could have been worse." Sam's manner was matter-of-fact. These are the sorts of details he deals with every day in his job.

"It had been going on for a while before it was diagnosed because of the unusual symptoms, I guess?"

"Yeah. So that's the problem. Now every little twinge, especially in the back or the shoulder or chest, makes me think I'm going to die."

"It makes sense to be vigilant after you have had a scare like that. Why do you call that hypochondriasis?"

"Last week I had a pain in my shoulder. Not a bad pain but it was out of the ordinary. I was worried and then my arm started to hurt, so I called 911. By the time the ambulance came a few minutes later, I was really scared. I was in a sweat and breathing fast and the paramedics were really working to help me calm down. It all got better during the ambulance ride, so I was fine by the time I got to the hospital, and obviously they didn't find any sign of anything wrong with my heart."

"It's obvious now, but it wasn't at the time."

"I know that it was a panic attack."

"Have you ever had one before?"

"No. I was stunned by how real it all was. The physical experience was extremely frightening."

"You've never been a person to panic about things?"

Sam smiled. "I've been a person who *doesn't approve* of panicking about things."

"So how did you feel about that experience afterward?"

"Embarrassed ... pathetic. And now I'm talking to you. I probably shouldn't even be here. You see people with real problems, right?"

"It's pretty common to become a 'hypochondriac' in the sense that you are talking about after a heart attack. It may be the norm. It makes sense, since the stakes are so high and early detection is so critical to a good outcome."

"But I don't want to be the guy who always thinks he is about to die."

"It gets better over time. You need to build up some experience with minor sensations that turn out to be benign so that you can learn to tolerate those twinges. That will be harder for you to do because the symptoms of your MI were so hard to interpret in the first place. Your experience is that the signs of a heart attack may be subtle. What does your cardiologist say?"

"She says that the main threat right now is not subtle. It is the massive infarction that would occur if the stent failed."

"Okay. That's helpful for sorting out your best response to mild symptoms, but it is also a pretty frightening message."

"Yeah. My sons couldn't get along without me. My wife needs me ... although, they would probably disagree."

"Okay, so we need to talk about dying and about your family depending on you. Can we spend a couple more minutes on how to interpret these symptoms first?"

"That would be good."

"The panic you experienced was pretty typical. Those symptoms will usually resolve on their own in about 15 or 20 minutes, if you just ride it out. They may recur since this is a frightening time for you. Since your cardiologist doesn't think that those kinds of symptoms are the big danger at this point, would it make sense to set for yourself a rule of thumb – that mild symptoms get the benefit of the doubt for 30 minutes before you start to react?"

"I could probably fake that I'm not terrified for 30 minutes. But I'll be thinking about it the whole time."

"That would be a good start."

"We can't just make it go away?"

"Your fear?"

"I know you can only do so much, and I don't want drugs and the whole nine yards, but I'm not happy with this."

"So tell me more about that."

Sam is typical of many people who are well and then have a very serious change of health. His heart attack pushed him into unfamiliar emotional territory. It seemed that fear and worry had not had a big place in his life, and he had a strong preference to keep it that way. Since he told me that he thought it was pathetic to be afraid, I was feeling cautious about pushing too hard. This would not be a helpful conversation if he walked away in the end feeling humiliated.

"I'm not the one who asks for help. I'm the one who provides it."

"You mean with your work?"

"And the rest of my life. My wife, Jen, has rheumatoid arthritis. It is not severe and she handles it herself for the most part, but I think of myself as her support. If she couldn't work anymore, I would still be there for the family."

"You're her emotional support?"

"She might say I'm not. I'm not always that good at it. But I don't complain about my health to her. She's the sick one."

"And your sons ..."

"They're at university. They are not as self-sufficient as we were at that age."

"You were self-sufficient by the time you were at university?"

"A decade before that. I was looking after my mother and father."

"Why?"

"God. We're really going to talk about my mother and father? You guys really do that?"

I smiled at Sam's gentle resistance, his teasing tone effectively reducing me to a character in a *New Yorker* cartoon. "If it matters."

"Okay. Well, what you need to know is that my parents were Holocaust survivors. When they moved here after the war, they didn't speak any English. We lived in the Jewish part of town; there were lots of others who had immigrated from Poland and Germany. My father found work as a grocer. He didn't really need to learn the language if he stayed in our neighbourhood. So my brother, Isaac, and I had to manage the house, talk to the school, write the cheques. We were the assimilated ones."

"You assumed an adult role when you were very young."

"Before I was 10."

"And you ended up studying to be a doctor."

"That was what my parents wanted from very early on. I didn't fight it. I liked the idea."

"I can see why thinking of yourself as a sick person is such a shock to your system. You have been the strong one, the one who other people count on right from the start."

"Not my father so much. But my mother was really not capable of looking after herself."

"What do you mean?"

"She was a real hypochondriac. Migraines, 'spells,' whatever. It seemed like every other day there was an ambulance in the driveway when I came home from school. It was dramatic. Everything was a catastrophe."

"She lived in fear. How did your father react to her troubles?"

"He was at the store. But even if he was at home, he was a very distant, quiet guy. Reassuring my mother and calling off the ambulances fell to my brother and me. The ambulance guys all knew her anyway. It was not a big deal after a while."

"Sounds like a big deal."

"My brother and I have a saying, a joke I suppose. No matter what kind of problems we have, we just say 'It's not Auschwitz.'"

"Nothing compares."

"Of course not. But it's a joke. There were lots of kids in our neighbourhood in the same position. So we took it seriously, but still it's a joke."

"I can see that. Black humour works. But I'm also thinking that you grew up in a house where, you know, you couldn't complain. And you went into a line of work where you hear the complaints, not make them yourself. And then when Jen got sick ... well your health concerns aren't rheumatoid arthritis."

"It's not Auschwitz."

"Right. But then you had a heart attack."

"Yeah. Well, that's true. It's not nothing."

"And you are scared of dying."

"Actually more scared of becoming a cardiac cripple. I'm not supposed to lift anything heavy right now. No sports allowed yet, not that I did any before. I imagine becoming one of those people who is afraid to do anything."

"Yeah. This is a major health event, and you are the guy who never needs anybody else's concern."

"Well, what I want ..." Sam paused for several seconds and looked at the floor. "I want ... this is stupid and embarrassing."

"You are in the right place to say something you wouldn't want to say anywhere else."

"What I want is some sympathy. I know it's childish. I want people to have some sense that this is a big thing for me, to feel sorry for me, really, and worried for me."

"Would anyone else know that you want that?"

"I want it without asking for it."

"It doesn't count if you have to ask for it?"

"Something like that."

"The half-life of sympathy is often pretty short, so disappointments may be inevitable. But you are not too likely to get any sympathy at all if you look like you don't need it."

"I doubt I would get it even if I asked. People don't expect that from me and they have their own problems."

"And it's not Auschwitz."

"Right."

"Why do you think it is so important to you to look like you are strong, even when you are feeling like you want some sympathy?"

"I don't want to be pathetic."

"Is that how you feel about other people when they are frightened and needing support?" People almost always answer "no" to this question. My intent was to turn the tables and allow Sam to take a more forgiving stance towards his own emotional needs. But he surprised me.

"I do actually, if I am truthful. I try not to look like that is what I feel. I think most people think that I am pretty empathic. But truly, I think that complaining too much is weak."

"You're not going to like this, because I am about to say something that is just like what you would expect a psychiatrist to say."

Sam smiled. "Let me have it."

"I think you don't want to be a histrionic complainer like your mother, who was always dying. That's what would be pathetic."

"Yeah. I hadn't thought about that, but I wouldn't want to be like that. I'm more like my father anyway."

"Really? He sounds like he was pretty aloof."

"I'm more of a people person than him, but we have a lot in common. We're both hard to rattle."

"Is he still alive?"

"No. He died over 20 years ago of an MI. While I was on the phone with him, actually."

"What happened?"

"He said he wasn't feeling well and then he started to sound confused and then he fell. I hung up the phone and called 911. Then I called my brother to go over because he lived closer."

"And he died."

"Vital signs absent when the ambulance arrived."

"You handled that like a professional."

"I am a professional. I didn't feel all that much at the time. He was 82. He'd had angina for years, and it was not his first MI. I wasn't surprised. It was only at the funeral that I had stronger feelings. Really strong feelings actually – it caught me by surprise."

"And your mother?"

"Died a few years before Dad. Very quickly after she was diagnosed with lung cancer. That was much harder for me. I was very upset. I get a bit choked up even now remembering her."

"Your mother's death was quite different for you than your father's was."

"Yeah. Different people. And, you know, mothers ..."

"You loved her."

"For sure. I hope I didn't give you the sense that I didn't. She was a handful, a pain in the ass really, but I always loved her."

"You've told me a lot, Sam. I can't pretend to know you well, but I want to give you a sense of what I'm thinking so far."

"Okay. Shoot."

"It seems to me that you are having some perfectly normal and expectable feelings – the fear that comes when you get a funny feeling in your chest or your back – but that you don't tolerate them very well because they don't fit your image of yourself and your preferred way of doing things. You have had a very frightening experience and are watchful for signs of another one – I don't think that makes you a hypochondriac. It isn't a psychological problem to be scared of dying or of disability after having a heart attack – who wouldn't be? However, I do think that being a hypochondriac is almost the worst outcome you can imagine because so much of your self-image is wrapped up in being self-sufficient and rational. Which puts you in a bind. You want to feel strong like you used to, but you are afraid and you want other people to feel concerned about you, but you don't want to give them any signal of that – because you don't want to act like your mother."

We talked about this for a little while and decided that it might help to meet a few times over the next few months to see how things were going. I sent a letter to Sam's family doctor as I always do after seeing someone in consultation, describing my understanding of the situation and our plan. A month later when we next met, I was surprised to hear Sam tell me that he had read the letter over in his doctor's office and asked for a copy to take home. "I wanted my sons to read it," he offered quietly.

"Why is that?"

"I wanted them to know that side of me. They don't know me the way you described me."

"What side?"

"That I am afraid for one thing. You put in the letter what I told you about feeling afraid at night, imagining a future as a cardiac cripple.

That is not something I share with them. But also about growing up with Isaac and my parents – the pressure we were under to keep the house together, how we didn't really have any choice but to take control, being there for my crazy mother when my dad wasn't around ..."

"I don't think I said 'crazy.'" I smiled.

"You're not allowed to but I can ... anyway, I wanted them to know there was another side of me."

"Do you think something will change if they know another side of you?"

"I don't know. I was just thinking about all those years. How Isaac and I keep our troubles to ourselves, 'It's not Auschwitz' and all that. I thought it might be helpful to me for others to know me as something more than the guy who never gets rattled."

"Maybe the fear won't be as difficult to tolerate if you feel more comfortable with all sides of yourself."

"We'll see. I'm not saying that I'm comfortable with it. But I wanted them to read the letter."

Sam's story is typical in many ways. His medical situation is serious, but the emotional adjustment to having a heart attack has been harder for him than the medical treatment or the physical effects of his condition. Understanding what is bothering him requires understanding what makes him feel secure – in his case, being calmly in control without having to depend on anyone else is what makes him feel secure – and now his health situation is interfering with that. Thinking about feeling secure and how that arises out of important relationships in his life brings a new perspective to understanding his situation that isn't otherwise available.

Where that understanding will take Sam is another question. Maybe Sam will use his new perspective to make some more changes in how he acts – being more direct in asking for others' support or more willing to let others see his vulnerabilities. Maybe he will adjust his own image of himself, to become more accepting of normal anxieties. Maybe he will want to make that adjustment easier by reducing the anxiety – for example, by learning relaxation skills. Or, as is often the case, maybe it will be enough just to have a new way of understanding himself that makes sense and is more forgiving than the intolerance of weakness that comes to him automatically. Any of these paths may lead to greater peace of mind. And just as importantly, if he can get some help with his anxiety, it will help his heart as well as his mind.

Wherever Sam's new understanding leads him, the road will be lit by two core principles. The first, as Bob was reminded when he listened to *Breathing with Sandra*, is that health happens between people. The second is that to understand what happens between people, look for what they are doing to feel safe and secure.

In this book we use attachment theory to understand how close relationships affect health. Attachment theory is a psychological theory that describes what goes on in our closest relationships – the bonds between parents and their children. It was developed first by John Bowlby over 50 years ago.[4] Although Bowlby was a psychoanalyst, his theory was a major departure from the psychoanalytic orthodoxy that was influential at the time. For one thing, attachment theory incorporated insights from several sources: studies of the behaviour of parents and offspring of other species (especially observations made by Konrad Lorenz and Harry Harlow), systems theory, and direct observations of human infants interacting with their parents.[5] In time, the theory would also incorporate emerging knowledge of brain physiology.

Today, attachment theory is one of the most robustly supported psychological theories that we have. It has spurred on a new tradition of learning about child development by watching infants, children, and their parents scientifically, which has been enormously productive.[6] Attachment theory has also grown over time to generate a theory of *adult* attachment – which describes how romantic partners (and other adults who are very close) interact in ways that make each member of the partnership feel more or less secure.[7] It wasn't until the 1990s, however, that much work was done to understand health in the context of attachment. From the start, Bowlby recognized that being sick is experienced as a threat to feeling secure and typically leads to *attachment behaviour* (e.g., trying to get close to the person who can make you feel safe and secure). However, it was only after good models of adult attachment were developed (with tools to measure security and insecurity in adults) that there were empirical tests of the idea that attachment is relevant to health.

In the 1990s, we were working in the hospital wards as consultation-liaison psychiatrists, trying to figure out the best ways to respond to the interpersonal difficulties between patients and professionals that often lead surgeons, internists, and nurses to ask a psychiatrist to join the team. The phenomenon that we were grappling with was always referred to as "the difficult patient," as if all the trouble came from one side of the interaction. Beyond responding effectively to this challenge, we were also trying to figure out how to then teach these skills. We found that wise observations and advice had been published but very little useful theory.[8] We settled on attachment theory as a practical way to describe what happens between a patient and a health care provider when one member of the pair is feeling sick and scared and the other is trying to provide care and protection – and why those interactions sometimes go wrong.

We were certainly not the first to use attachment theory to understand health. A seminal review of the effects of social phenomena, such as isolation and the quality of relationships, on health had been published in 1988.[9] Judith Feeney had published important papers in the early 1990s looking at the role of adult attachment in choosing behaviours that put health at risk and in the experience of being sick.[10] At the same time, Brooke Feeney (no relation) was starting to explore how attachment was related to the physiology of stress.[11] The seeds of an understanding of health in terms of attachment bonds were already growing when we wandered into the field.

Our enthusiasm for the idea was reinforced when we had the luck to meet up with Paul Ciechanowski, who was as excited as we were about the possibilities of understanding health and health care in terms of close relationships. In 2001, we (Bob and Jon) published our model of the paths by which insecurity in attachment relationships could contribute to illness and a complementary description of how attachment theory illuminates the behaviour of people who are ill.[12] These are the two sides of the story of attachment and health: how relationships contribute to our getting sick and how our responses to being ill play out within relationships. Paul published groundbreaking research in 2001 linking attachment insecurity to control of diabetes and in 2002 explaining his model of the role of attachment in somatization and health care use.[13] The foundations were set for the decade-plus of exploration and clarification of the role of human attachment relationships in health that has followed.[14]

Today, the field of human attachment and health has legs. Peer-reviewed journal articles on the topic are now common. It is part of the curriculum for psychiatry residents at some universities. A book has been written, Gregory Fricchione's *Compassion and Healing in Medicine and Society: On the Nature and Use of Attachment Solutions to Separation Challenges*, as have several chapters in edited books.[15] This idea is no longer on the fringe. What is lacking – the need that we are trying to address with this book – is a practical, clinically focused introduction to the topic for practitioners of the helping professions who are not experts in psychology.

This book addresses very common phenomena in health care: symptoms that are poorly explained; chronic diseases that don't get better; interactions that leave patients and professionals frustrated and unsatisfied; patients who overuse health care resources or who neglect their health; all of us who eat too much, exercise too little, smoke, or drink to excess. We have come to understand that these very common problems – which are often viewed as annoying impediments to providing health care – actually lie at the core of what health care is all about. We use attachment theory to understand these vexing problems and to illuminate new possibilities for their management – strategies that vary across people according to their interpersonal style. Attachment theory gives insights that allow front-line health care professionals to individualize care, providing each patient with what works for him or her – a personalized form of health care that starts with understanding each patient as a whole person, inextricably bonded to the other persons in his or her life.

We have written this book for our colleagues. The reader we imagine as we write is – broadly speaking – almost anyone we might meet in the hallways of the places where health care occurs, practitioners of the helping professions. Health care is so complex that a list of its professionals will inevitably be incomplete, but the list includes, at least, nurses, doctors, social workers, psychologists, occupational therapists, physiotherapists, respiratory therapists, midwives, chiropractors, counsellors, chaplains, patient advocates, and students of those fields. Each discipline has its own expertise and its own domains of special interest, but all of us grapple with how to manage the part of our work for which so few of us feel well prepared: interacting with people who are sick, scared, and vulnerable and who do not seem to be acting in their own best interests. Since we don't assume that our readers have any familiarity with our subject, and since our subject is of universal relevance, general readers may also enjoy this book, but the reader we address is a colleague.

A few notes about format, words, and people. We know that some readers will want to follow up on original sources and to explore the academic asides that we find interesting or important but that are not critical to understanding our main points. We have used endnotes liberally for those readers.

We refer to *patients* rather than *clients* or other terms for people who are seeking or receiving health care (and put our rationale for this choice in an endnote). On the other side of health care transactions, we usually refer to the professionals who provide care as *health care providers*, *health care professionals*, or *clinicians*. We use these labels interchangeably, for the sake of variety, and intend these terms to be inclusive of the many professional disciplines that compose our intended audience. We prefer to speak of *health care* than of *medicine* because the latter has a physician-centric connotation, while our intent is more inclusive. An exception occurs at the start of Chapter 1, where we discuss cultural prototypes and definitions of medicine, which are linked to that word.

The gender of the persons we are discussing is usually irrelevant. We have opted for the phrases *he or she* and *his or her* in some passages, but in many others this construction would have become clumsy, and so we have chosen a gender indiscriminately, with the intention that the male and female characters will balance out in the end. In describing interactions between two people, we have usually made them of opposite genders, primarily because it allows for a useful economy of language (attachment has little to do with sex).

When our examples are clearly from the perspective of only one of us, we indicate which one. Otherwise you can correctly assume from the use of *we* as our preferred first-person pronoun that we (Bob and Jon) share a great deal of professional experience and largely agree on how we understand that experience. We generally speak with one voice.

Finally, this book includes many descriptions of individuals who serve as case examples. In some instances the individuals whose experience we are drawing on are patients. In others they are family, friends, or ourselves. We have changed some details for the sake of privacy, and if the descriptions are substantial and the persons we have modelled them on are still alive, we have obtained their permission. In other cases, the persons who we describe are an amalgam of several people. Even in these cases, the spirit of the persons we describe and some of the details of their lives are real.

SECTION ONE

Vexing Health Care

1 What Is Health Care?

Health care is not what it seems. Consider a few popular prototypes of medicine.[1]

The *House* version: Medicine is a detective exercise in which only logic, instinct, and high-tech investigation stand between health care providers and the identification of the problem.

The *ER* version: Medicine consists of a series of life or death crises that demand swift and dramatic professional intervention.

The *Scientific American* version: Medicine consists of the application of dazzling scientific breakthroughs to improving health.

The *Conspiracy Theory* version: Medicine is a shell game in which mega-corporations exploit human suffering for profit.

The *Marcus Welby* version: Medicine is the way that wise and kindly doctors who know best help patients to get better.

The *Money Pit* version: Medicine is an unstoppable force pushing Western economies to the brink of bankruptcy.

None of these versions is dead wrong. But none is completely right.

Even the *Oxford English Dictionary* falls short. The *OED* defines medicine as "the science or practice of the diagnosis, treatment, and prevention of disease," which excludes medical attention to normal life events (as occurs in obstetrics, which is usually not focused on disease). Worse, if medicine consists only of the diagnosis, treatment, and prevention of disease, then most of the time, most health care providers are not practising medicine. Instead, we spend our time reassuring patients that they have no disease, or helping them to manage suffering that will never be adequately explained by a disease, or supporting them in the disability that results from the very limited power of treatment and prevention. If this seems incorrect, or simply too bleak, read on. Health care can be a very powerful endeavour, but first we have to see things as they actually are.

We can try to determine the main activities of health care in two ways. We can measure where we, as a society, spend our health care money, or we can measure how health care providers and patients spend their time. In either case, the evidence leads us away from *House*, *ER*, and *Scientific American*. If we use money as our standard, the primary business of health care in developed countries undoubtedly is treating chronic disease. This emphasis arises because chronic disease is so common – diabetes, cancer, cardiovascular diseases, and respiratory diseases kill 36 million people a year, which amounts to 63% of all deaths worldwide.[2] The largest costs to society, however, do not result from people dying of chronic diseases but from people living with them. In the United States, chronic diseases are projected to cost $47 trillion over the next 20 years,[3] which offers some credence to the *Money Pit* version of health care. Among the *OED*-endorsed triumvirate of diagnosis, treatment, and prevention, the majority of this money will be spent on treatment, so "treating chronic disease" is one evidence-based definition of the main business of health care.

Prevention, on the other hand, *should* be where the money goes. The World Health Organization estimates that up to 80% of heart disease, stroke, and type 2 diabetes, and over 30% of cancers could be prevented by reducing tobacco use, improving diets, increasing physical activity, and reducing the harmful use of alcohol.[4] The problem is that we don't know how to do those things very effectively. Habitual behaviour is notoriously resistant to change. Worse, we spend a tremendous amount of effort and money on things that don't work. Although it is difficult to quantify such things, it seems that when it comes to budgeting prevention dollars, the first instinct is always to bet on the same two losing horses: the naive assumption that educating people about what is harmful will change their behaviour and the related belief that well-informed people tend to act in their own self-interest. Very little evidence shows that these ideas are true, at least when it comes to health.

Experience suggests that self-interest and information are very weak forces for change. Let's look at a case example of the common phenomenon of managing diet, exercise, and weight. Will is a clinical nutritionist, an expert in healthy consumption. Have a look at the graph that illustrates the fluctuations in Will's weight over six years (Figure 1.1). The record starts with a weight of 197 pounds in May 2006. Will had just been diagnosed with mild hypertension (high blood pressure) and decided to try to lose weight to help keep his blood pressure under control. The 197 pounds on Will's frame equalled a body mass index (BMI) of 30, which is considered high enough to pose a long-term health risk. Motivated by the knowledge that a BMI of 30 and hypertension are both cardiac risk factors, Will started recording his weight and adjusting his diet.

Interventions to help people to lose weight fail about 80% of the time (more often than that if you keep track for more than a year). This failure happens not because most people doubt the health risks that come with obesity or are unaware of them. Certainly in Will's case, there was no knowledge gap to overcome. However, Will did have to think about what to change and how to maintain the change. The best evidence about weight-loss programs says that the ones that work share some common features: a low-fat diet, some degree of increased activity, and a record or diary of food intake.[5] Since the program advocated by

Figure 1.1 Will's weight over six years

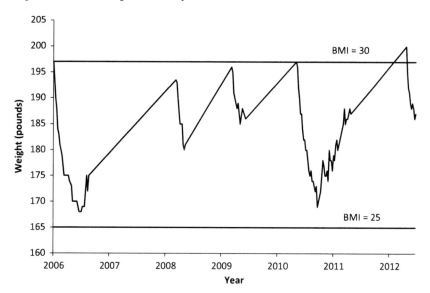

Weight Watchers meets that description, Will joined. He also told his family doctor, his wife, and a couple of friends and family members what he was doing, to help him to keep on track.

Scanning the graph shows us that Will succeeded for a while, then quit trying for a while, then tried again, and repeated the pattern four more times. The graph also illustrates some other things. The long straight-line ascent from one period of lower weight to the next peak represents many months when he was not even weighing himself; he had abandoned the entire project. Also, notice that each peak of weight is a little higher than the last. This pattern is typical for weight loss and gain in someone who is overweight – it says less about Will than it does about the phenomenon of trying to reverse habitual behaviour. In particular the weight curve illustrates how difficult it is to reverse a pleasurable behaviour when change requires effort and the behaviour's adverse consequences are far in the future. Will's knowledge that he would be healthier if he weighed less is a minor part of the forces determining the shape of Figure 1.1.

For examples of more successful behaviour change in the service of public health, consider the relatively recent increase in seat belt use and decrease in smoking. Increasing the use of seat belts took decades and was largely driven by legislation. Fines for flouting the law were not very effective; it took the addition of driver's licence demerit points, the threat of curtailing freedom, to accomplish the change. The prevalence of smoking has been reduced from over 40% in 1955 to about 20% now, through an extensive, multifaceted effort that has included not only public education but also changes in public policy, pricing, and the availability of effective individual treatments to support smoking cessation.[6] After all these measures, however, the prevalence of smoking has been more or less constant for the past decade.[7] We seem to have run out of ideas.

These are the first vexing aspects of health care. It is rarely a sprint and much more often a seemingly perpetual marathon – which is to say that health care is not usually about identifying and curing acute diseases but rather about managing the impact of chronic ones.[8] Beyond that, we are much better at treating chronic diseases (which almost never means "curing") than we are at preventing them. It makes perfect sense to prevent the diseases that show every sign of being preventable and of crippling our future economy – we just don't know how.

If we put aside the question of where society spends its health care dollars and instead look at how health care providers and patients spend their time, chronic disease remains prominent, but the discussion gets more complicated. Take the providers in the department where we work, for example. Not too long ago, in an effort to increase access to treatment for people who were being underserved, we decided to look at the data regarding patients' visits to see how we were spending our time. Most of us were quite surprised to discover that as a group we spend almost 70% of our time seeing 13% of our patients. That is a lot of effort and expertise being directed towards a relatively small group of people. The people in that 13% have chronic diseases, to be sure, but so do most of the other 87%. Disease alone isn't what drives this pattern of intense use of health care workers' time by relatively few people. Something else is going on.

Because we work in a department of psychiatry, it could be that our practice is not representative of our colleagues' practices in other areas of health care, but it turns out that our situation is, in fact, the norm. High health care use is one of the forces that the Institute of Medicine has identified as creating a "quality chasm" in contemporary health care.[9] Even in emergency departments, which would seem on the surface to be geared towards the care of acute medical needs rather than chronic concerns, heavy users or, colloquially, "frequent flyers," are recognized as a major drain on resources that are best suited to acute care.[10]

In business, this result is called the 80/20 rule: around 80% of sales come from 20% of clients. In health care, however, our goal is not to "increase business" but to distribute a limited resource for the maximal benefit of all. What is it about the 20% of patients that accounts for the disparity in their use of health care resources? First, it is worth dismissing some possible explanations that often come up before people look at the data. The 20% are *not* highly privileged in their access to health care services. Neither does disease severity account for high use; it *isn't* simply that we spend a lot of attention and resources on the people who are the sickest. Instead, when we examine the data about high use of medical resources what we find are that high users are consistently characterized by two things: health care providers find interactions with them to be "difficult," and these patients are likely to have some form of mental illness, most often depression or anxiety.[11] Some other characteristics vary a little between health care settings. In primary care settings, high users are very likely to have multiple physical symptoms that can't be explained by physical disease processes. In emergency departments, heavy users are often struggling with addictions. In specialists' offices high users are usually either people suffering from the symptoms that are the currency of that specialty but without the expected underlying biological disease (e.g., non-cardiac chest pain in the office of a cardiologist or irritable bowel syndrome in the office of a gastroenterologist), or people with identifiable disease processes who are experiencing anxiety about their disease that is out of proportion to its severity. We will soon see that these apparently different situations are all just variations on a theme.

That difficult interpersonal encounters are a consistent marker of patients with high use is one of the more direct indications that the forces underlying vexing health care are often relational. The difficulty lies *between* the patient and the provider. A "difficult patient" is one that a health care provider walks away from feeling something that she finds hard to tolerate – like anger, fear, helplessness, or hopelessness.[12] And the frustration is usually mutual.

So, another vexing truth about contemporary health care is that most health care providers do not feel well trained or confident in managing difficult interpersonal problems, and yet the evidence suggests that doing this is how we spend a large part of our time.

As much as high use drains fiscal and human resources, underuse is also a problem. In this case, the trouble is that people who avoid medical interactions excessively, or who lack access to health care, do not receive prompt attention to health concerns when they arise. The usual assumption (which has not been tested as thoroughly as one would hope) is that attending to problems early prevents them from getting worse and that ignoring them leads to bad outcomes and complex, expensive care. The example that comes to mind is of discovering a lump and dealing with it promptly rather than letting it grow into an untreatable cancer.

A second way in which underuse increases the burden of disease for individuals and its cost to society occurs when a person who is managing his or her health in isolation has a chronic disease. This situation may be the most expensive form of underuse.[13] A couple of examples paint the picture. First, think of a person with high blood pressure. Treating hypertension is fairly easy and not very expensive compared with the treatment of other medical conditions. At the same time, high blood pressure is usually invisible – it has no symptoms – and so it is an easy problem to *avoid* treating. Unfortunately, the cost of untreated hypertension can be quite high over the long run. A person who is not monitoring and treating her high blood pressure is at risk for problems that have a very large impact on quality of life and health care costs, especially stroke and heart attack.[14]

As another example, diabetes is a chronic disease that often requires high maintenance to keep it under control. Making lifestyle changes, monitoring food intake and exercise carefully, monitoring blood glucose, and, for some, adjusting insulin doses in response to these variables is a complex and demanding regimen. Collaborative cooperation between patients, their families, and health care professionals helps to manage the complexity. On the other hand, a person who ignores signs of illness and prefers not to see health care professionals (let alone follow their instructions) is at a disadvantage. From an interpersonal perspective, a person who takes self-reliance to an extreme while also avoiding collaborating with or depending on others will find it harder to manage diabetes effectively. Evidence supports this notion; people with this interpersonal style have significantly worse control of their diabetes.[15] This result is further evidence of one of the core theses of this book: understanding patterns of interpersonal relationship style shines a new light on the problems of vexing health care.

We have sketched out an image of Western health care that is frustrating, to say the least. Put bluntly, the costliest parts of medicine involve the chronic treatment of preventable diseases that we don't know how to prevent; much of health care providers' time is dedicated to interactions that are unsatisfying to both providers and patients; the common reasons for which patients need intensive management go beyond the diseases that providers feel they are experts in treating; and access to effective, affordable, and timely care is compromised by both extraordinarily high and low users of health care resources. Finally, and worst of all, many health care providers don't seem to notice or acknowledge that this is what it is like to practise their craft. The "quality chasm" of vexing health care cannot be rectified if providers and patients treat each frustrating impasse as an anomaly that is due to individual deficits, such as difficult patients or bad clinicians. Making changes requires changing peoples' behaviour, providers and patients alike. And there we hit another roadblock – we can't change behaviour if we start from the premise that our best tools will be logic and information. To find a solution, we need a new way of understanding the problem.

To build a new approach to vexing health care, we want to find a way to *adapt health care to the relational needs of individual people.* We want people who are experiencing intense and unmet needs for support and reassurance to feel supported and reassured. We want health care providers who feel as if they cannot exercise their expertise when they are caught in a frustrating no-win interaction to feel skilled not only at "diagnosing, treating, and preventing disease" but also at relating to the people they are trying to help. We want people who are reluctant to see health care providers at all to live healthy lives in spite of their disinclination to take on the role of patient. We want personalized medicine for whole people. Creating that is what this book is all about.

2 Why Else Do We Get Sick?

Without a doubt, genes and germs are major causes of disease. This chapter is about why *else* we get sick. We will argue that all the other causes account for more illness and disease than you may think,[1] and we will start to reveal the connections between more-or-less hidden environmental causes of disease and interpersonal relationships.

We have already pointed out that chronic diseases account for most deaths in developed countries. In fact, cancer and cardiovascular diseases alone account for more than half of deaths in the United States.[2] What is less well understood is how little of the burden of those diseases is attributable to genes. To sort this out, epidemiologists estimate the relative importance of genes versus environmental factors in causing disease by examining how often diseases are shared among family members. Sometimes twin studies are used to tease this apart in a more sophisticated way, by comparing the rate of a disease in identical twins (who share all their genes and some elements of their environment) with the rate in fraternal twins (who share only half of their genes and some elements of their environments). Stephen Rappaport, an epidemiologist at the School of Public Health at the University of California, estimates from these techniques that genes account for about 10% to 20% of breast and prostate cancer and only 1% to 3% of most other cancers. Furthermore, his data suggest that genes account for about 50% of deaths from vascular causes.[3] That leaves about half of vascular mortality and the vast majority of cancer mortality to be explained by environmental causes – which presents a problem because we don't really know what those environmental causes are. The usual suspects include smoking, alcohol, pollution, diet, obesity, and unsafe sex. If we look at cancer as an example, those factors in combination account for

34% of cancer mortality in developing countries and 37% in developed countries. That is a lot – and we will come back to some of those factors again because they are related to our thesis – but it still leaves about 65% of cancer unexplained.

We aren't doing much better than that in explaining other chronic diseases. We don't need to get lost in epidemiology; the point is that we still don't understand a great deal about the causes of chronic diseases, and the answers are not likely to be found in genetic analyses. We need some other ideas.

In this chapter we summarize four of those other ideas. Each is important to understanding the role of human relationships in disease. They range from the extremely familiar (the impact of stress on disease vulnerability) to the speculative (the role of inhibition of automatic processes). Let's start with the idea that we think is the coolest: the impact of the environment on genes.

Gene-environment interaction and epigenetics

Estimating the genetic influence on illness through twin and family studies may greatly underestimate the impact of genes if the disease depends on *interactions* between genes and the environment. Epidemiological estimates such as the ones that we reviewed in the previous section assume that since identical twins are born with identical DNA, they will also have an identical risk for diseases that are caused by genes. There was a time when that seemed like a safe assumption, but now we know that gene-environment interaction is the norm. Scientists who study this abbreviate these interactions as GxE ("G by E").

A straightforward (although imaginary) example of a GxE interaction would involve a disease that is the consequence of an infectious agent and a gene that increases the risk of infection for the person who is exposed to the bacteria or virus. The person would not be likely to get the disease unless he had *both* the vulnerability gene *and* exposure to the bacteria or virus. Since exposure is a necessary step in getting the disease, not everyone with the vulnerability gene is at the same risk of getting sick; it depends on each person's environment.

That interaction is simple enough, but it has recently become clear that GxE interactions often occur via something a little more complex and interesting: *epigenetic modification* of DNA. Epigenetics refers to a process by which genes are chemically turned on and turned off.

Genes are made out of long sequences of four simple molecules that make up DNA (guanine, adenosine, cytosine, and thymine, which as a group are called nucleotides). Their precise order in a strand of DNA (CCATAGCACGTT, etc.) is a code that is crucial to the gene's purpose.[4] A gene's code is used within a cell as the blueprint for making a protein. The purpose of a gene is exactly equal to the biological consequences of the protein that it codes for. If that protein is an enzyme, it will hurry a biochemical reaction along. If that protein is a receptor in a cell wall, it will allow a certain path of communication between other molecules to function. And so on.

It turns out that you can render a gene silent with a modest chemical change to the nucleotides in its DNA. If a chemical reaction results in a very simple bit of a molecule (a methyl group) being attached to the nucleotides in a gene's coding sequence, it stops the code from being read, which means that the protein that the gene codes for won't be made. This process of *methylation* is stable, whereas another simple change that attaches a different molecule at a different location (histone acetylation) makes a gene *more* available to be read and does so *reversibly*. Thus, methylation and histone acetylation are processes by which exposure to various events in people's environments can turn their genes on and off. You can't change the gene's code (i.e., if it codes for blue eyes, it can't be turned into a gene for green eyes), but you can render it silent.

Studies of the methylation of our DNA show that vast quantities of our genes are turned off at any given time and that patterns of methylation change over time. When the DNA of identical twins is studied, the patterns of methylation become more and more divergent as they age – their different exposures to various environmental events are changing which of their genes are working, in a very individual way.[5] Monozygotic twins start identical, but they don't stay identical – which is one reason that a disease that is caused by genes might show up in one identical twin and not the other. We are going to refer to epigenetic processes at various points in this book because they are important to understanding how interpersonal processes become translated into biological processes that are as fundamental as making proteins.

Stress and poorly regulated stress responses

Everybody knows that stress causes disease, right? Maybe not. As recently as 2007, experts in the field wrote a very cautious review of the evidence for this proposition in the *Journal of the American Medical*

Association in response to the impression that "despite widespread public belief that psychological stress leads to disease, the biomedical community remains sceptical."[6] The researchers found evidence that was strong enough to say the association was "established" for a few diseases: depression, HIV/AIDS, and cardiovascular disease. All by itself that is important because depression and cardiovascular disease are among the greatest contributors to the burden of chronic disease. For some respiratory diseases, infections, and autoimmune diseases, there was promising evidence that had not yet reached the same standard of rigour. For the rest of medicine, including the progression of some cancers that are widely reputed to be linked to stress, researchers found the studies were not robust enough for them to be sure of the conclusions. Finding that studies aren't strong enough to establish a link is different from finding that studies *disprove* the link; the former leads to uncertainty rather than refutation. But that finding does emphasize the need for caution and for specificity. When we talk about stress and disease, we need to specify *which* aspects of stress and *which* diseases.

It is helpful to start to discuss this subject from a position that is both precise and skeptical. By precise we mean that we need to specify exactly what we mean by *stress*; the word refers to many things and is understood differently by different people. By skeptical, we mean that we need to start by appreciating that stress is a ubiquitous part of life and usually doesn't make us sick. That is, understanding the link between stress and disease (and the even stronger relationship between stress and illness) means understanding the exceptions to our usual resilience.

In evolutionary terms, the link between stress and disease is quite new. Robert Sapolsky, in his book *Why Zebras Don't Get Ulcers*, described how diseases that are the result of stress had to wait, on the evolutionary timescale, until our species was living in a safe enough environment. We had to wait until we lived in a world in which we don't usually die in infancy, or by drinking tainted water, or as a tiger's dinner before stress had a chance to do us any harm.[7] That is because the adverse impact of stress on our health usually results from the very slow accumulation of damage over decades. Stress-related diseases are not diseases of childhood and are not usually diseases of young adulthood either. However, now that our expected longevity has doubled from around 40 years old to about 80 over the last century, stress has the opportunity to cause disease.

Now for some precision. *Stress* can be understood as referring to (1) an event or a circumstance (the stressor), followed by (2) an appraisal of how threatening that event is and whether or not we have the resources to deal with it effectively, followed by (3) biological, behavioural, and psychological consequences when our appraisal suggests that the event is likely to be more than we can handle routinely (the stress response).[8] A great deal of room exists for individual variations in the kinds of lives we lead (which affects the kinds of events we are exposed to) and in our appraisal of those events. People are quite different from one another in terms of how often they experience a stress response. We are going to talk a lot about interpersonal processes that affect exposure to stressors and appraisal later in the book. For now, let's leave those aside so that we can focus on the stress response.

The behavioural part of the stress response was famously described about a hundred years ago by Walter Cannon as "fight or flight."[9] Bearing this in mind, the biological aspects of the stress response are understood as the changes that are required to support running away or fighting. Cannon's phrase has been modified by Shelley Taylor and her colleagues at UCLA, who have argued that the idea of fight or flight in response to stress is a gendered concept.[10] While men tend towards fight or flight when they feel threatened, women may have additional responses to stressful circumstances, which Taylor's group call "tend and befriend." There does not seem to be much difference in the biology of stress between sexes, but Taylor suggests that women use these two behavioural strategies to reduce its impact. *Tending* refers to protecting themselves and their offspring, thus reducing distress. *Befriending* refers to maintaining social networks, which serve a similar purpose. Tend-and-befriend behaviours are very important to understanding how humans (regardless of gender) buffer the effects of environmental stress, and so we will return to them in the next chapter. For now we are homing in on the biology of stress, which is directly linked to fight or flight.

The biology of the stress response has been described as a complex and beautiful "neuro-symphony of stress."[11] The two systems at its core are linked: the autonomic nervous system (ANS) and the hypothalamic-pituitary-adrenal (HPA) axis. The neurosymphony is composed of a vast series of balanced, opposing forces – an exquisitely intricate counterpoint. We will not have to examine the physiological details of this symphony for most of our purposes, but the occasional dip below the surface will allow us to be admirably precise and is also worthwhile if only to foster awe of our amazing bodies.

The ANS includes two opposing arms. The first is the sympathetic nervous system (whose influence we will usually refer to simply as *sympathetic*), which is the accelerator of various processes needed for fight or flight, such as speeding up heart rate and constricting blood vessels to allow most of our blood to go to the organs we depend on while we are fighting or fleeing. Sympathetic nerves go to our adrenal glands, where they signal the release of adrenalin into the bloodstream, which has similar accelerator effects. The opposing arm is the parasympathetic nervous system, which generally acts as a brake on the same systems. Since the largest of the parasympathetic nerves travelling from the brain to the rest of the body is the vagus nerve, we usually refer to the braking influence of this half of the ANS as *vagal*.

The ANS has two particular characteristics that are relevant to our topic. First, although its nerves have their origins in the brain, they are not under direct voluntary control. As opposed to the voluntary portions of our brains that allow us to act as we choose (to speak what we intend to or to move an arm or a leg), the ANS mostly functions independently,[12] flying under the radar of consciousness. Second, it works very quickly. Compared with the slow work that is done by the hormones that are involved in stress responses, the ANS provides much more precise acceleration and braking of the body systems involved in responding to threats.

As for the hormones, the HPA is a system that works as a nervous and hormonal cascade: a series of signals start in the brain (in the hypothalamus, which also functions without conscious control), move down to the pituitary gland, which releases hormones into the bloodstream, and continue to the adrenal glands where pituitary hormones trigger the release of steroid hormones, especially cortisol, into the bloodstream. The HPA works much slower and for longer periods than the ANS; it does not kick in for a few hours after the onset of a stressor and then may continue to circulate for several hours or days. Cortisol influences cells throughout the body to change their function in a way that will support an extended period of responding to stress. Thus, cortisol promotes such functions as converting fats and proteins into sugar to replenish our energy stores when they are used up quickly in an extended period of fight or flight. Cortisol also acts on the brain to increase our appetite for food and to promote food-seeking behaviour.[13] As a result, cortisol is useful not only for extended periods of stress but also to help our bodies recover after stress.

Like the ANS, the HPA has an extensive system of built-in checks and balances, which in biological terms means that it is a negative feedback loop. Cortisol and related hormones circulating in the blood are one signal that dials HPA function down. It works to control itself.

We have evolved exquisitely controlled stress responses that play out across multiple systems for two good reasons. The first is that stressors come in many forms and so a one-size-fits-all stress response would not be very useful – far better that we can tailor our response to particular circumstances. The second reason is that several aspects of the stress response have harmful consequences if they are active for too long. Too much sympathetic drive leads to damage that is associated with many disease processes.[14] Chronically high levels of cortisol increase blood pressure, suppress immunity, kill certain nerve cells (especially those in the brain's hippocampus, which are important to learning and memory), and increase the risk of heart disease.[15]

If you graph the function of some aspect of the stress-response systems over time, as we have done in Figure 2.1, a pattern of optimal function is *spiky*. The response is robust when it is needed and is quickly dialled down again when it is not. This pattern holds true for both the ANS and the HPA, although the spike would occur over a different timescale for these systems. Health problems can result from three alternative patterns. The first of these is an exaggerated stress response in which the body responds out of proportion to what is required to deal with a stressor. The second suboptimal response we call *sluggish*, which refers to an inefficient return of the system to normal after the stress has passed. During this extended period of activity when the stress-response system is no longer needed, the stress response is doing more harm than good. An exaggerated stress response and a sluggish return to normal function can easily go hand in hand. The third pattern is one that can be called *blunted* because the response to stress isn't very robust in the first place. This lack of response may cause problems because the body doesn't get all the benefits of its stress-response system while it is facing a threat. Any of these patterns can have an effect on health over the long run but for different reasons.

How does this apply to you? Think of having a good aerobic workout, which will increase your heart rate substantially, and then monitoring your pulse afterward to see how much your heart rate has slowed

Figure 2.1 Variations on patterns of stress response

Normal stress response – nice and spiky

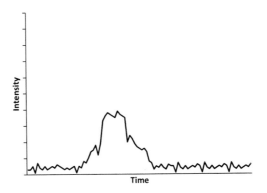

*Exaggerated stress response with sluggish return to baseline
(normal stress response for comparison in dotted grey line)*

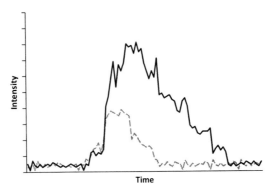

*Blunted stress response
(normal stress response for comparison in dotted grey line)*

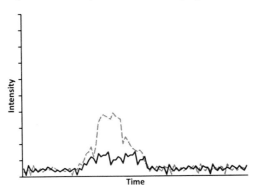

after resting for two minutes. The magnitude of this heart rate recovery is a good index of your cardiovascular fitness[16] and a reliable predictor of mortality over the next few years.[17] The increase in risk that comes from not being fit may not be huge for you as an individual,[18] but it is large enough to make a big difference to public health when that risk is multiplied by millions of unfit people. The point to emphasize for our purposes is that the prime force braking your heart rate after exercise is the vagal side of the ANS.[19] As a result you can readily observe your own ANS and see if it is spiky or sluggish, knowing that this pattern is directly related to your future health.

Now let's start to make the link between the biology of stress response and what happens *between* people. Our first example of the link between things that happen between individuals and the biology of the stress response results from elegant experiments designed by Michael Meaney of McGill University. These experiments show how interactions between individuals that are well within the range of "normal" behaviour can have lifelong effects on the physiology of stress. His experiments are with rats, not people, so we need to be cautious and not take them as directly demonstrating the power of "social" forces. Nonetheless, they demonstrate just how deeply we can investigate the biological consequences of interactions between individuals.

Meaney's model depends on observing how often a mother rat (a dam) licks and grooms her offspring (pups). Licking and grooming (LG) is a major source of tactile stimulation for rat pups. The behaviour also varies a fair amount from one dam to the next, so we can observe the consequences of pups being exposed to more or less LG. The basic observation, from which Meaney's research has followed, is that a pup that is exposed to more LG will grow up into an adult rat with a nice spiky cortisol response to stress, whereas a pup exposed to less LG will grow up into a rat with an exaggerated cortisol response.[20] By itself that observation would be an extraordinarily important piece of evidence that what happens between a mother and her infant has lifelong biological consequences. Those who want to take the leap from rats to humans do so by equating lots of LG interactions in rats to lots of high-quality mother-infant interaction in humans; and although we are resolutely cautious, it isn't a crazy leap. It leads you to wonder if many high-quality interactions between human mothers and infants would set up a child for a lifetime of nice and spiky stress responses.

In spite of how valuable Meaney's basic observation was, his group didn't stop with discovering the link between dam-pup interaction and adult stress response. They went on to do experiments that prove that the effects of LG are entirely derived from exposure to the dam-pup interactions, not from inheriting anything. Then, they examined the biology of the stress-response systems in rats that grew up with high or low LG to find out *how* early experience was changing biology.[21] Here detail matters; they found the difference in these rats' cortisol response to stress was caused by a difference in the numbers of specific receptors built by their cells to recognize and respond to cortisol (which are known as glucocorticoid receptors). These receptors are made out of a specific protein, which has to be built according to the code given by a specific length of DNA in the nuclei of the rats' cells. That brings us back to epigenetics. Meaney's group demonstrated that early LG interactions between a dam and her pup change the pattern of methylation of the pup's DNA – they turn up or turn down the genes that enable a rat to make the glucocorticoid receptors. The repeated tactile stimulation that a pup experiences during LG influences methylation of its DNA, which in turn determines whether its response to stress is nice and spiky or exaggerated. This is a textbook case of GxE interaction, where the E is all about what happens *between* individual members of a species.[22]

Our second example of a link between stress responses and interpersonal forces concerns the much more dramatic events that constitute psychological trauma. Trauma, in this sense, refers to a situation in which a person feels that he is in serious peril for reasons that are virtually completely beyond his control. Trauma does not have to be interpersonal, since a hurricane or a volcano may suffice to create that circumstance, but it usually is. The most common traumatic experiences are the result of war, physical or sexual abuse, car accidents, and assaults – all things that occur between people.[23]

Although it runs against our intuition, trauma of this sort does not always cause physical or emotional harm in the long run. In fact, a resilient response to trauma may be the norm. While most people experience at least one traumatic event of this kind in their lifetime, fewer than 10% develop post-traumatic stress disorder (PTSD), which is a particularly severe and dramatic form of the harm trauma can cause.[24] One of the differences between people who experience PTSD and those who do not after enduring similar exposures to trauma is a marked difference in their biological response to normal stressors.[25] Specifically, people who develop PTSD tend have *low* levels of stress hormones in their bloodstream and a blunted cortisol response to stress. If that difference in stress response runs in the opposite direction to your expectations, welcome to the club. Most chronic stress is associated with chronically *amplified* activity of our body's stress systems, much like what is observed in Meaney's low-LG rats. PTSD is associated with the opposite. Although it has not yet been fully worked out, this paradoxical suppression of cortisol is thought to be the result of an alteration in the equilibrium of opposing forces involved in controlling the HPA.

But here's the kicker: the low cortisol that is associated with PTSD appears to *precede* the trauma. This unusual pattern of stress physiology seems to be a marker of who will be vulnerable to developing PTSD if they are exposed to trauma and who will not rather than a consequence of the bad event. Furthermore, studies of the children of survivors of the Holocaust and of 9/11 suggest a sequence of events – first, children of parents with PTSD are more likely to get PTSD themselves; second, the link that passes on the risk does not seem to be a gene – it is GxE. In fact, two kinds of E have been identified that leave these children at risk of developing PTSD if exposed to trauma later in life. One is an exposure that occurs even before birth, when a mother's stress physiology may influence the programming of her child's developing stress-response system, leaving the baby with an HPA system that is blunted and under-responsive.[26] The second is that parents with PTSD are at some risk of abusing or neglecting their children in their early years, which affects the children's developing stress systems.[27] In either case, the most likely mechanism to explain the biological effects of these exposures is epigenetic. The sequence illustrates how vulnerability to interpersonal trauma (and trauma itself) can be passed down through generations and how this need not depend on a particular gene being transmitted from parent to child.

Our stress responses can be described as a symphony because they are both complex and beautiful. The complexity does not have to weigh us down as we argue for the importance of relationships to health because the take-home messages are quite simple. First, unhealthy patterns of stress response are usually only *relatively* unhealthy. They are only modest distortions of the complex interactions that we count on for survival, so their health consequences take many years to accumulate. Second, the biology of the stress response is a series of feedback loops;

we need to appreciate the overall equilibrium of its forces to understand how distortions in the stress response may affect health. Third, stress systems are strongly linked to interactions between individuals. We'll have much more to say about the third point as we proceed.

Hidden determinants of health behaviour

The third category of "hidden" determinants of health refers to those that are often unrecognized. We start with the true story of how a guy named Jerry made his first fortune. He went to the public library and collected some information that was freely available about various sources of scholarships to university (this was long before the Internet). Then Jerry advertised a scholarship-finding service; if you mailed him $25 he would send you information about how to get a scholarship. He offered a money-back guarantee. People sent him the $25 and he sent them the information, which was useless since it was not at all tailored to their particular situation. Hardly anyone asked for their money back. Jerry became rich with a business that was built on the premise that if you charge people $25 for useless information, they will usually not ask for their money back.

The point of this story, for our purposes, is that if we assume that people act in their own self-interest, this business model should fail, but instead it succeeded. What that assumption does not take into account are the real-world forces that Jerry readily intuited. These are forces like hope (which leads people who read an ad about getting a scholarship to imagine the key to a better life *for just $25!*), embarrassment about getting conned, laziness (why bother to request a refund when it is just $25?), and disillusionment (someone who sells this useless information for $25 probably wouldn't actually honour his money-back guarantee anyway).

We are telling the story of Jerry's first fortune because it provides an apt analogy to the story of the determinants of health behaviour. Some standard theories of health behaviour, as with classic economic theory, are quite powerful and very useful. However, also like classic economic theory, they leave out some other motivations for acting the way we do, primarily because the classic theories tend to assume that health behaviours are thoughtful choices.

For example, take the health belief model, which was devised in the 1950s to understand "the widespread failure of people to accept disease preventives or screening tests for early detection of asymptomatic disease."[28] To follow this model's logic, think about the specific example of choosing whether or not to get a vaccine to avoid getting the flu. The health belief model suggests that people make this choice based on a balance of variables:

- their perception of threat (how bad they think the flu is and how vulnerable they think they are to getting it)
- their perception of benefit (how likely they think it is that the vaccine will work)
- the barriers that they perceive to pursuing the strategy (such as how inconvenient or painful or expensive the vaccine is)
- cues to action (like being around people who are coughing or seeing ads for the vaccine)

The health belief model assumes that a person's perceptions of these things, rather than some objective truth, drive his or her choices, which is very sensible. If too many people are avoiding a useful intervention, like getting the flu shot, the health belief model directs us towards strategies that will change perceptions. We should help people to understand that having the flu is worse than they think or that the vaccine is more effective or safer than they think. Thinking about behaviour this way is valuable, and it has had successes. This is the kind of thinking, for example, that led to campaigns to increase the public perception of the harm caused by smoking, which have contributed to reductions in smoking over the last 50 years. On the other hand, this model locates all our decisional power in the thoughtful part of our brain. The health belief model is silent about how we arrive at our perceptions of threat and vulnerability and largely neglects the things we do automatically – which is most things.

Further explanatory models, the theory of reasoned action and its descendant, the theory of planned behaviour, are even more explicitly based on the premise that human behaviour is rational and voluntary.[29] The former theory suggests that people come to an intention about how they will act by balancing two evaluations: what they think the norm is among other people around them and their own attitude, based on their own beliefs about the health behaviour in question. The theory of reasoned action adds to this an evaluation of the resources that people believe they can bring to bear. These theories are broader, taking into account social norms and individual perceptions, but they are still rooted firmly in the most thoughtful parts of our brains.

Albert Bandura's social learning theory moves us closer to our destination. It describes how we model our behaviour on others' and then have that behaviour reinforced (or not) by external forces, like rewards, and by internal forces, like pride and satisfaction.[30]

Our intent is not to argue against these powerful theories. Rather, we want to talk about three elements that are underemphasized in the usual approaches to understanding why we act the way we do about our health. The first of these is an internal force that reinforces behaviour so it fits comfortably within Bandura's model but is a much stronger force than is usually acknowledged: the drive to *feel secure*. The second missing piece is how we act to regulate our emotions, with very little attention to our beliefs about the costs and benefits of our actions. Finally, classic theories of health behaviour neglect our extraordinary capacity to short-circuit our thinking brains with automatic brain processes that are unconscious.

To consider the last point first – the ways in which we short-circuit our intentions – let's return to the yo-yoing chart of Will's weight over the last five years that we introduced in the previous chapter (in Figure 1.1). According to the health belief model, Will should be in good shape. He believes that a BMI of 30 is bad for his long-term well-being and that losing weight would be healthy. He also believes there would be some other benefits to losing weight, such as looking more attractive and feeling more energetic. The barriers to losing weight are modest, primarily involving more careful purchasing of the food that aligns with a healthy diet. The cue to starting the process – a new diagnosis of hypertension – is salient and effective. So what went wrong?

Several things went wrong. One is that the cue and motivation that initiated the process got old. The consequences of hypertension are far in the future, if they occur at all,[31] and for day-to-day purposes, an essentially imaginary risk is hard to hold in mind. Another is that Will *likes* the food that makes him fat. While depriving himself of what he likes is easy when he is strongly motivated, he has many opportunities to give himself what he likes over time. Maintaining a healthier diet requires that when these opportunities arise, he *think* about what is best rather than automatically doing what he likes. Later in the book we will discuss the biology of *liking* – it is a powerful system of biochemical reinforcement of behaviour, not a trivial feeling of pleasure.

The contest between thinking and acting automatically is fundamental to being human. The tension describes a great deal of how our brains have evolved to function. The basic set-up is this. The older parts of our brains in evolutionary terms – the parts we share with humming-birds and crayfish – function automatically, completely out of aware-ness.[32] If we move a little higher[33] in the brain, we find functions, such as the apparatus that controls liking, that are not thoughtful but that do generate sensations and feelings. If we go higher still, into the cortex, a tension still exists between automatic thought and reflection. Nobel-Prize-winner Daniel Kahneman describes this tension in *Thinking, Fast and Slow*.[34] Most of the time we function very effectively as automaton-like beneficiaries of fast, relatively automatic thinking processes that are very efficient at dealing with familiar events. These processes are built to make choices with limited information, jump to standard con-clusions, and get on with things very quickly. When the traffic light turns red, we press on the brake without any thought about what it means. We ignore the green and red lights shining from the neon sign down the block. We may not even interrupt our conscious stream of thought (which is almost certainly not about driving) to do this. On the other hand, we have slower, reflective thought processes that are built for analysing complicated situations, spotting exceptions, revising the conclusions generated by fast thinking, and making hard decisions. Slow thought uses a great deal more energy than fast thought (liter-ally – it burns more glucose), and so we reserve it for tasks on which the effort will be well spent.[35]

At each level of the brain, the same pattern occurs: the lower sys-tem automatically does its thing, while a higher system occasionally intervenes by inhibiting that automatic action. Inhibition of automatic neural processes is effortful and slow. It has a high cost in terms of both energy consumption and efficiency. But it makes us reflective beings who can choose to lose weight to avoid an imaginary danger far in the future.

To link this bit of neurobiology back to Will's yo-yoing weight, let's consider one of Kahneman's main points: that slow, reflective thought processes depend on effort.[36] Will finds it quite easy to maintain a healthy pattern of eating for about 15 or 16 of his usual 17 waking hours. He is able to consider his intentions and his beliefs, and he is usually able to inhibit habits and preferences that would lead him to unhealthy choices. For most of the day, it is easy – and then, an hour or two before he goes to sleep, he gets tired. When he is tired, Will quite literally *changes his mind*. He doesn't care about his long-term goals. He tunes in to the appealing memory of how potato chips taste. And he returns to the mode of habitual patterns of consumption that he had been inhibiting for the rest of the day.

Although we will postpone talking about the powerful drive to feel secure until we can embed it in an understanding of how attachment relationships develop, we can foreshadow that discussion here by introducing the idea of affect regulation, which refers to all the things that we do to keep our emotions[37] in a tolerable range of intensity. Humans have a broad array of strategies for regulating emotions, ranging from private reflection (inhibiting an automatic thought that triggers distress with a more considered evaluation of the subject), to taking action to solve distressing problems, to seeking support and solace from others, to avoidance of thoughts and situations that make us feel bad. We can also manipulate our feelings directly or indirectly by consuming substances that change the way we feel or by engaging in activities, like sex or intense physical activity, that temporarily change our chemistry.

We can apply this perspective to the example of regulating weight, using the concept of emotional eating. Emotional eating refers to a pattern of eating in response to emotional cues rather than responding to hunger and satiety. It often occurs in an intense and problematic form in people who are at the extremes of the eating and weight continuum, for example, in people with anorexia nervosa, bulimia, or severe obesity. It also occurs in subtler forms, however. On an unusually stressful day or on a day that has gone exceptionally well, Will is prone to decide in the tired and fast-thinking later hours of the evening that he deserves a junk food reward. Or if he decides to have a glass of wine as a reward, that choice makes it just that much more appealing to give in to a further reward and that much harder to reflect on whether or not a bowl of chips aligns with his health beliefs.

To return to our polemic against the naive assumptions that guide popular responses to unhealthy behaviour, the point is that the forces that determine health behaviour are complex and often hidden. The reasons that we have trouble reducing the prevalence of smoking below 20%, or that we have an epidemic of obesity, or that it takes decades to convince people to wear seat belts, or that drunk driving continues to be a public health problem have very little to do with ignorance, sloth, or stubbornness.

Inhibition of automatic processes

The general neurological set-up that we described, in which lower brain processes are more automatic and critical higher processes that can inhibit them are effortful and used sparingly, extends even wider, and the implications for our well-being are profound. In the marshmallow test, which was first described in 1972, a child is offered a single marshmallow immediately but is told that if she is willing to wait for a time, she will be given two marshmallows.[38] How long she is willing to wait is a measure of her capacity to delay gratification, and delaying gratification requires active inhibition of an automatic drive.

What is astounding is how powerfully the capacity to delay gratification that is measured in the marshmallow test predicts the course of a person's life. Preschoolers who are able to wait for a second marshmallow grow into adolescents who do better at school, are more socially competent, and are described as verbally fluent, rational, planful, and capable of dealing effectively with frustration and stress.[39] Some argue that several or all of these good outcomes are a direct consequence of the advantages of being able to delay gratification. A broader perspective suggests that delaying gratification is just one example of a general phenomenon – the ability to inhibit and interrupt automatic processes – and that this ability is linked to a wide range of constructive social and psychological competencies.

Here we can return to the challenges that have been posed so far about understanding and promoting health: (1) much of the work of health care is caring for persons with no identifiable disease, (2) much of chronic disease is unexplained by known causes, and (3) most of the theoretically reversible behavioural causes of chronic disease are actually quite resistant to change.

In this book we argue that interpersonal processes, starting in our earliest interactions with those who parent us when we are infants, make a major contribution to our ability to think slowly and reflectively, and to inhibit automatic processes. From that perspective, the seemingly diverse collection of hidden determinants of disease that we have reviewed in this chapter are, in fact, all related.

Specifically, in analogy to what Michael Meaney has documented in rats, our earliest interactions change our biology, probably through epigenetic changes that modify the function of our DNA and definitely through modifications of the connections between different areas of our brains. The result of these developmental interactions is that a host of social, cognitive, and biological competencies tend to go hand in hand. People who find a certain kind of comfort and ease in close interpersonal relationships (which we will eventually come to call *secure attachment*), also tend to communicate clearly, to tolerate disappointment and stress effectively, to be able to reflect on things that go beyond whatever signal is most urgent in their immediate circumstance, and to be able to draw on others' support to get them through a rough patch. The same kids who are able to wait for a second marshmallow will grow into adults who have a nice, spiky biological stress response and who are able to make effective judgments about when to seek health care and when to wait out a physical discomfort that is not likely to be serious. They are also just a little more able to tolerate the discomfort that is required to quit smoking or to choose not to regulate distress with ice cream. The consequence is that, all other things being equal, they lead healthier, happier, longer, easier lives.

3 Health Happens between Us

At 76, Eric was a tough old bird. At least that is how the emergency department triage nurse described him after he drove himself to the hospital while his heart attack progressed. He recovered from that event as well as is possible; other than having to take a couple of extra pills, his life post–myocardial infarction was essentially the same as what came before – at least until his wife, Viola, got sick.

Viola's lung cancer spread quickly. Her last months were filled with pain from metastases in her bones and with morphine, hospitals, and home-care nurses. Eric was there for her in the same way as he had been for the previous 50 years: stoic, practical, silent, and strong. Nine months after Viola's cancer took her life, Eric died quietly in his sleep.

Eric's death occurring shortly after Viola's is an illustration of the *widowhood effect*, a tendency among couples for the death of one to precipitate the death of the other. The idea has been around for a long time, often expressed as dying of a broken heart, but it raises eyebrows among skeptics. "After all," the skeptic opines, "we all have to die sometime. Partners are usually similar in age and in lifestyle. Isn't it possible that couples sometimes die close in time by coincidence, and we just remember those deaths a little more vividly because they are more poignant?"

The argument is sensible, but we don't need to speculate because evidence exists that can settle the matter. A study of over half a million couples, published in the *New England Journal of Medicine* in 2006, showed that for people whose partners die or are hospitalized, the risk of death soon after increases, and the magnitude of the risk depends on the partners' type of illness. The riskiest diseases for remaining partners are the ones that create the most stress and disruption: dementia carried the highest risk, mental illness was next, then stroke, and then other causes of illness or death. The risk is a bit worse for husbands when their wives are sick, but the effect is found in both sexes.[1]

In this chapter we are interested in how health depends on what happens between people. The widowhood effect specifically is not important to us; the reasons for the effect, which also apply to other interpersonal determinants of health, are. We will discuss two important reasons that people affect each other's health: first, we cause each other stress; second, we calm and protect each other.

We cause each other stress

Because Eric loved Viola and spent his life with her, she almost certainly caused him a great deal of stress, as he did her. If you tried to sum up all the stress that Viola caused Eric, you would add increments of stress for all the days when he worried about her well-being, calmed her when she was frightened, cared for her when she was ill, and missed her when she was gone. This stress does not depend very much on Eric's personality or on Viola's; it is in the nature of a permanent, committed relationship. Eric's love and care was good for Viola's health, as hers was good for his health, but these benefits come with a price. Furthermore, unless Eric and Viola were unlike the rest of us, they also caused each other stress more directly, even if they tried to minimize the harm. Each would argue and injure, resent, neglect, and disappoint. In the words of a scholar of this subject, "support and strain are often found in the same relationships."[2]

While close relationships almost inevitably involve an element of mutual strain, in the special case in which one partner cares for another who is seriously ill, the strain is often pronounced. Caring for a partner who has dementia or mental illness, illnesses that often lead to dramatic and substantial changes in behaviour, has the clearest impact on the health of the caregiver. "Caregiver burden," which is the label given to this phenomenon, has been studied for more than two decades and is fairly well understood. The impact on caregivers' mental health is substantial: they are much more prone to depression than they would be without the strain of care. They feel less well, and their quality of life is diminished.[3] Caregivers' physical health also suffers, especially their cardiovascular health. The impact of the caregiving burden on mental health is greater than its impact on physical health, but the latter is still important. Even a weak force acting on a partner's physical health may be enough to tip the balance, as is demonstrated by the increased levels of mortality among caregiving partners.[4] More subtly, in women who care for a relative with Alzheimer's disease, a skin wound takes longer to heal than in women of the same age who don't have that caregiving burden, by about a week and a half.[5] Clearly, at least some of the things that happen between people who love each other can strain physical health.

Whatever the sources of stress that arise between people, the effects of stress tend to accumulate over time. Cumulative risks, by their nature, are difficult to detect at an individual level. Anecdotal evidence (i.e., familiar stories) will tend to lead us astray because most people know someone who is exposed to a risk factor and yet has not been affected by it – a centenarian smoker or a person who never wore a seat belt but survived a car accident. Furthermore, most people are quite inaccurate at trying to estimate the long-term cumulative risks of exposures that are not very harmful in the short term.[6] Good estimates of cumulative risk require scientific observation – studies that control for other sources of harm and carefully quantify exposure to potential risk factors. Studies of that sort have been able to identify the cumulative risks that arise from many different kinds of harmful exposures, such as drug side effects and symptoms of depression.[7] Some of the most convincing of these studies are ones that show a *dose-response gradient*, meaning that the more that someone is exposed to a potential risk factor, the higher the likelihood that she will experience harm in the long run.

One study that has been able to show a dose-effect gradient for harm following an interpersonal stress is the *Adverse Childhood Experiences (ACE) Study*, conducted by Vincent Felitti and his colleagues in San Diego. The ACE Study investigated childhood abuse and neglect, among other kinds of adversity. Unfortunately children are quite commonly exposed to very stressful experiences within their families.[8] Furthermore, recognition is growing that while experiencing one kind of adversity can be very challenging for a child, experiencing multiple kinds of adversity has a greater, cumulative effect.[9]

The ACE Study asked adults about their exposure in childhood to 10 kinds of adverse experiences: enduring physical, sexual, and emotional abuse and neglect; having parents die or separate; witnessing violence between family members; and growing up with family members who

Figure 3.1 Graded relationships between the number of types of adverse experiences a person had as a child (ACE Score) and various indicators of adult health

Risk of ischemic heart disease

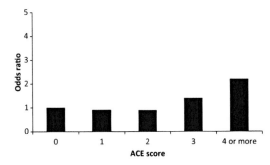

Risk of liver disease

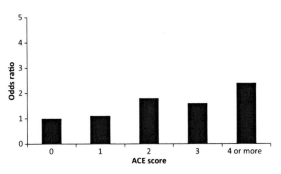

Risk of chronic respiratory disease

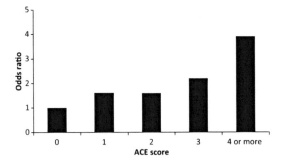

Each figure is based on data from the Adverse Childhood Experiences (ACE) Study by Vincent Felitti and colleagues. The ACE Score is the number of types of adverse experiences reported by each person. Risk of adult illness is reported with an odds ratio, with the risk for persons with ACE Score = 0 set at 1. Health behaviours (smoking and problem drinking) are reported as per cent prevalence.

Risk of needing many prescription drugs at ages 44 to 65

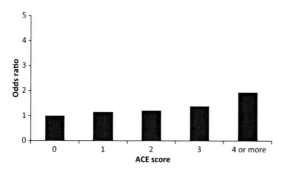

Percentage who smoke before age 14

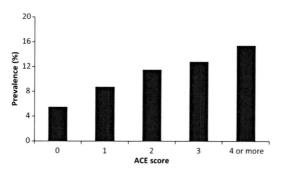

Percentage with problem drinking

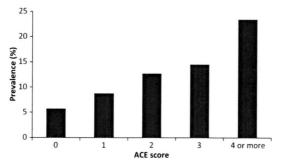

had problems with drugs or mental illness. The researchers then added up the number of kinds of exposure that each person reported and gave each of their research participants an *ACE Score* between 0 (no exposure to any of these adverse experiences) and 10 (exposure to all of them). Unfortunately, a score of 0 was not the most common; only about 40% of people reported being free of these kinds of experience. The importance of the study, however, is not in documenting how common it is to have difficult family experiences while growing up. Rather, the ACE Study has been able to study the cumulative effect on many aspects of adult health of experiencing *several* kinds of adversity. We have mapped out the results of a representative selection of the studies in Figure 3.1. What you see, in every example, is a dose-response gradient: the more exposure to adverse events, the higher the health risk. Whether we are talking about the likelihood of unhealthy behaviours, like smoking and drinking alcohol excessively, or the likelihood of developing the chronic diseases that are poised to place a $47 trillion burden on our economy in the next 20 years (see Chapter 1), a dose-response relationship exists between ACE scores and health.

We hope you are wondering how and why bad experiences in childhood could cause these outcomes and that you are creating some hypotheses of your own, because those questions bring us very close to the subjects we'll focus on in the rest of the book.

Of course, interpersonal stress does not always occur between loved ones or between family members. Forces that set large groups of people against one another, such as those that maintain social classes, also chip away at individual health. For example, the Whitehall Study, named because it was a very large study of the civil servants who worked at Whitehall in London, provided evidence that lower social class is associated with poorer health, a phenomenon that has been observed so consistently that it is completely beyond doubt.

Two aspects of the Whitehall Study are particularly important. The first is that it found a dose-response gradient of health across strata of social class. Indicators of the most common causes of mortality occurred most frequently among clerical and support staff (the lowest-status job category), somewhat less frequently among professionals and executives (the middle-status job category), and least frequently among administrators (the highest-status category). These results held true for ischemic heart disease, chronic respiratory diseases, smoking, and other important indicators of adult health.[10]

Second, note that the clerks and support staff who are at the bottom of the Whitehall gradient are still fairly well off compared with the general population. A clerical job in the British civil service is a decent job that provides a fair amount of security. So whatever it is about the differences in social class that are driving health outcomes among these civil servants, it isn't poverty, it isn't a lack of basic education, and it isn't a lack of access to healthy food or medical care. In most of the visible and obvious ways that distinctions are typically made within large groups of people, the civil servants of Whitehall are more similar to each other than different – and yet, their class differences are associated with gradations of health and health behaviour.[11]

What is going on here? Evidence from studies of non-human primates suggest that the stress that social hierarchies impose is not always rooted in an uneven distribution of resources; how the hierarchy is maintained also matters. Social hierarchies that are maintained through conflict and aggression (i.e., that are imposed on less powerful members of the group) are more stressful than similar hierarchies maintained through consensus.[12] Analogously, in humans, employees are healthier in workplaces with greater transparency and processes that support fair work practices than in workplaces that lack those indicators of justice.[13] So, although we cannot be sure, the differences in the lives of lower-class and higher-class civil servants that result in a health gradient over time may plausibly have something to do with interpersonal dynamics between the classes – stresses that result from conflict, aggression, injustice, and lack of control over their environment.

We have argued that stressors that occur between people are important determinants of health and that these effects occur on many levels – from the stressors that arise between individuals in committed relationships and families to the large-scale social forces that emerge from social hierarchies, inequality, and injustice. Of course, interpersonal stress is balanced (and ideally overbalanced) by interpersonal forces that act in the opposite direction: the social forces that bolster and support health.

We calm and protect each other

A groundbreaking study in Alameda County near San Francisco demonstrated the power of relationships on mortality.[14] In 1965 almost 7000 residents agreed to participate in a survey of social aspects of their lives, and when they were contacted again in 1974, those who had reported more support in 1965 were more likely to still be alive. It was a robust effect; it could not be explained by things that might differ between those who reported high or low levels of social support, such as health status in 1965, alcohol consumption, smoking, obesity, physical activity, or use of health services. Furthermore, when the study was repeated after another decade, the researchers found the same result.

Thanks to the Alameda County Study, and a huge amount of research that has followed, the effects of social support on health are now established. The way that social support influences heart disease has been especially well studied, and the results are impressive. Taken together, all the high-quality studies on this question appear to say that for people over 40, the risk of developing heart disease in the next 5 to 10 years is about doubled for persons who do not get much support from others. For people who already have heart disease, several studies have found that being socially isolated or unmarried increases mortality rates to three to four times the rates found in comparable heart patients with more support.[15]

Furthermore, different kinds of support and social connection may be linked to different kinds of health benefits. For example, compare the benefits of having a big social network with the benefits of subjectively feeling well supported. To investigate the former, Sheldon Cohen, a psychologist at Carnegie Mellon University in Pittsburgh, once found 276 healthy adults who were willing to spend five days in quarantine and to have a cold virus squirted up their nose (in exchange for $800). People received a *social network score* between 0 and 12, which summed up the number of kinds of social ties to people with whom they had frequent contact.[16] Using scrupulous methods to control for many of the variables that influence why one person gets a cold and another doesn't, Cohen and his colleagues found that the higher the social network score, the less likely a person was to get a cold after they were exposed to the virus. People with smaller social networks were almost twice as likely to get a cold as were people with six or more types of relationships.[17] Further studies confirmed that the diversity of a person's network is what protects against viral infection, not the perception of being well supported.

But the perception of being well supported, on the other hand, may serve to protect health in the face of major stressors. Once again, the evidence is strong. In one study that directly assessed the impact of confidante relationships on physical health, Elizabeth Maunsell and her colleagues at Laval University in Montreal followed women who

Figure 3.2 The relationship between major life events and mortality over seven years for men over 50 years old

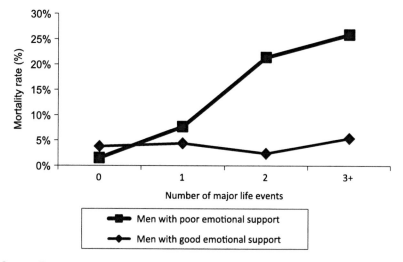

Source: Rosengren et al., *British Medical Journal*, 1993

had surgery for breast cancer for seven years after the surgery. Of the 224 women who participated in their study, 67 died over these years. When the survival rate was compared by number of confidantes (people whom the women had confided in or had discussed personal problems with in the three months after their surgery) each woman had, the results were striking: among the women with two or more confidantes, 76% survived; 1 confidante, 66%; no confidantes, 56%.[18]

As for men, in a Swedish study of men over 50, big events like retirement, or someone's death, or a financial crisis had a huge effect on mortality in men who perceived themselves as receiving little emotional support. This effect was so strong that during the study period, men who felt poorly supported experienced a mortality rate that rose steadily as more life events were experienced. No such link between life stress and mortality existed for the men who felt well supported. Viewing this in Figure 3.2 shows how strongly the perception of effective social support protects against the health impact of major stresses in these men's lives.

More recent investigations have extended the evidence to epigenetic processes. Socially isolated people tend to have higher than expected expression of genes that increase inflammation (and thus contribute to the many chronic diseases in which excessive inflammation plays a role) and to have lower than expected expression of genes that help to fight viruses.[19]

George Brown and Tirrill Harris conducted a landmark study in the 1970s that provides insights into the *kind* of relationships that buffer life stresses.[20] They interviewed young women who lived in the Camberwell district of London about the aspects of their lives that contributed to psychiatric illness, especially depression. Women who had recently experienced a major loss or life change were more than seven times as likely to be depressed as women who hadn't had that kind of change. However, among the women dealing with these stressors, having a confiding relationship with a husband or boyfriend was protective – the rate of depression was over three times as high in women who did not have such a relationship. Other kinds of supportive relationships, such as with a mother or sister whom the women had moved away from or with other friends, provided almost no protection at all against becoming depressed.[21] Two effects are at work here. The first is the one that we are driving home in this section: supportive relationships protect health.[22] The second foreshadows the larger topic of this book: some relationships have a more powerful effect on health than others, especially on aspects of health that are affected by stress. It isn't just a matter of whether relationships are perceived to be good or valuable; it is the functions that *certain people* serve in our lives. In Section Two of the book, we will make the case that *attachment relationships,* the close relationships in which we find feelings of security and safety, are the special ones that have most of the power to buffer stress.

Obviously we can't equate romantic partnerships and marriages with "good" support. We cause each other stress *and* we calm and protect each other but not in equal measure and in very different ways from one relationship to another. In the extreme, domestic violence (which is disproportionately directed towards women[23]) makes a relationship a very unsafe place. Short of that extreme, the balance point between stress and support is determined by complex and dynamically changing processes. Nonetheless, the kind of support that is available in some relationships is unique. A partner's death after a long marriage, as Eric experienced, leaves a hole in a person's life that cannot be filled with generic efforts at support by others, no matter how well intentioned and vigorous – a marriage simply cannot be replaced by casseroles from the neighbours.[24]

What are the special, supportive elements of these particular relationships? We can start by eliminating some candidates by using the following question as a test: "Could anyone provide this function under the right circumstances?" For example, committed partners do things for each other that support health in obvious ways – reminding each other to take pills, preparing food, driving to the doctor, and so forth. In the absence of a partner, any willing person could do the same things, so these will not help us to understand why very close relationships are particularly effective in promoting health. In contrast, in Section Two, we will focus on some emotional functions that are fulfilled *only* in our closest relationships: finding a place of emotional safety when we are troubled or having a reliable, secure base from which we can explore and express our most adventurous inclinations.

Summary of Section One

We have reviewed a perspective on the current state of affairs of health and health care that begs for a new way of understanding health and new approaches to practising health care. Here is what we have seen and argued, in brief.

Most of health care is concerned with attending to forms of suffering that are not caused by disease in the usual sense. Chronic diseases, nonetheless, are enormously costly and burdensome, a situation which is only going to get worse over time. The causes of chronic diseases are more poorly identified than is usually assumed; what *is* known favours the importance of environmental contributions to many diseases, especially those related to behaviours like smoking, overeating, being inactive, and drinking alcohol excessively. The other obvious candidate as a common environmental contributor to a wide range of ills is poorly regulated stress. For most of the suffering and burden that currently falls in the domain of health care, whether caused by conventional chronic diseases like coronary artery disease and diabetes or by the illness behaviours that cause so many symptoms, the logical place to intervene to provide the most direct benefit with the fewest adverse effects is at the level of behaviour – preventing disease, reducing the unintended harms that come from excessive medical investigation and treatment, and promoting resilient responses to diseases and to agents of disease. We have called this situation *vexing health care* because it runs counter to the very attractive idea that the one-two punch of a biomedical understanding of disease plus technological/pharmaceutical responses to this knowledge will be sufficient to find our way out of the extraordinary costs of our current dilemma. The situation is also vexing because the common sense solution is very difficult to implement.

As individuals and as a society, we aren't very good at modifying the behaviours that make us sick.

Of course, biology and molecular medicine in particular will be a major part of the solution. Furthermore, if we can understand how the environmental forces that are so important to illness and disease affect our molecular biology, it will help us to navigate a path to a less vexing version of health care. Social scientists talk about this link as the ways in which the environment gets under the skin. Interactions between the environment and our DNA, mediated through the epigenetic turning on and turning off of particular genes, is an example of how biomedical advances can help us to better understand *how* the environment matters to our health, which may lead us to more effective approaches for improving our health.

In this book we are arguing that some of the most important and least recognized environmental forces acting on our health, for better and for worse, are interpersonal – the things that happen between us. Having stated the premise and provided a sampling of evidence that interpersonal events that cause and that reduce stress are sometimes strong predictors of health outcomes, we are now poised to look at the science of close relationships more precisely.

Section Two is all about attachment relationships, which are a special category of human interactions. We will provide evidence that the biology and psychology of attachment bonds provide a bridge spanning the distance between the parts of the interpersonal environment that are most pertinent to health on one side and the biology and psychology of illness and disease on the other. In addition, we will explore how an attachment perspective provides a new and useful window into habitual behaviours, hidden motivations, and causes for acting in ways that on the surface we should simply change because they aren't good for us. Finally, we will discuss how understanding human attachment gives health care providers new tools for interacting with patients and otherwise unidentified opportunities to turn vexing health care into optimal health care by personalizing that care to meet each patient's strengths and needs.

SECTION TWO

Attachment and Health

4 What Is Attachment?

If it weren't for attachment relationships, our species would not exist. To understand what attachment is, and why our survival depends on it, we need to go back to the origins of human beings.

The evolutionary change that most distinguishes humans from our ancestors and peers is the dramatic development of our brain in size and complexity. One marker of just how valuable big brains have been to our species is how dearly we have been willing to pay for them. Although our brain constitutes only 2% of our body mass, it consumes 20% of the oxygen we breathe, 20% to 25% of our total energy, and 16 times the sugar required by muscle tissue – it is a metabolic hog.[1] Bigger and bigger brains must be of tremendous benefit because evolutionary forces have selected an extravagantly expensive upgrade.

The most important benefit that our big brains provide, in terms of our fitness as a species, is the capacity to flexibly adapt to constantly changing environments. We think about how to fix problems. We remember past accomplishments and use them as a guide to new challenges. We pass on our knowledge to the next generation. We plan. We modify harsh environments. We share tasks. We are a weed species, able to populate environments all over the world, from the desert to the Arctic. The value of our adaptability justifies the cost of our most expensive piece of equipment.

Our brain's size, however, led to a major evolutionary obstacle – the skull that houses a mature brain cannot fit through a pelvis. If a woman is going to have a strong enough pelvis to allow her to walk on two legs, then the birth canal can only be so large. And so at some point in our evolutionary ascent, two of our most important attributes came into conflict – bigger brains and bipedal locomotion had irreconcilable requirements for the size and shape of skulls and pelvic bones. How was the dilemma resolved? There was no choice but to get our most expensive and fragile organ out of the pelvis before the skull that houses it had grown too large to pass.

Enter a third evolutionary adaptation. The innovation that has allowed us to have both big brains and bipedal locomotion is that we are born premature, meaning long before we can survive independently. The consequence of this evolutionary solution is that children need care for many years, to keep them alive *and* to guide the development of their greatest biological advantage, their brain, so that it can grow and realize all its potential. While newborns of many species go through a period in which they depend on adults for care and protection, the *decade* or so in which human children grow their brains under the protection of their parents is extraordinary. Big brains, bipedal locomotion, and a long, dependent childhood allowed our species to make the huge leap from foraging primates to human beings.

You can probably see where this is going. If we are going to give birth to immature offspring and our survival as a species depends on caring for those youngsters for many years, during which they are completely dependent on adults for protection, nutrition, and learning, then our species needs a system that ensures that those first few years go according to plan. A vulnerable infant requires a reliable way of staying close to the adult who keeps him alive – and that is the attachment system. Attachment is essentially a behavioural system in which infants respond to signals and act in a way that promotes proximity to their parents or caregivers when it is needed. We will describe this system in more depth shortly – but we'll finish the evolutionary story first.

Newborn humans depend on adults for a longer time than any other primates, past or present. During this prolonged period of dependence, the mother and infant interact constantly.[2] Their dance occurs on many levels, from observable interactions like breastfeeding and play, to the mutual inter-regulation of brain neurochemistry, as we will see. Over time, this constant interaction helps the infant to develop a subtle skill, which is the capacity to imagine and appreciate what's up with Mom. This skill, called *mentalizing*, becomes more sophisticated over time, until it serves as the foundation of the intuition that allows individuals to be clued in to the subtle social back and forth of the groups in which we live.[3]

Mentalizing is the skill of being able to imagine what is going on in others' minds and how we appear from their perspective. Mentalizing, which depends on having a very large and complex brain, also arguably improves our species' reproductive fitness. The argument for this statement is that at a certain point in our evolutionary development, the point at which we could hunt and gather effectively, and hide from wolves and hurricanes – the point at which we had basic survival mastered – the biggest obstacle to an individual passing on genes more effectively than a peer became that peer, the tribe member who was competing for a partner. Those individuals who could intuit and understand others' motives and predict their behaviour had a big advantage. They gained in social power, and they often won the mating sweepstakes. By this argument, the selective advantage of social intelligence, the ever-so-gradual favouring of social intuition from one generation to the next, led humans to evolve into a deeply social species.[4]

Mentalizing has facilitated the development of cooperative social organization, sophisticated social constructs like justice, the ability to imagine and create narratives of the lives of others, and empathy. In other words, mentalizing has facilitated the development of much of civilization. Since highly nuanced mentalizing is a product of growing up within the near-constant interactions of an attachment relationship, mentalizing may be the primary evolutionary advantage conveyed by human attachment – the best reason that we have to care for and protect our infants' brains for so long.

Social organization, the evolution of big brains, and protected infant development exist in a self-reinforcing circle. Longer protected development allows for the development of larger brains, which in turn allows more sophisticated social communication, which enhances brain development and allows for more sophisticated ways for societies to protect and enhance the care of infants, and so on. The attachment system is intimately entwined with our emergence as the species that we are.

Minda is six months old. She reclines in a stroller in the shade in her backyard, happily batting at a colourful toy dangling from the overhanging canopy. Unexpectedly, a dog in the next yard starts barking from behind its fence. Minda wails and her father moves quickly to pick her up.

Minda and her father are demonstrating the attachment system at work.[5] During the years in which children require protected care, they can't always be near enough to touch their parents, so they need a way to rapidly get close to one of them when predators are lurking. The solution is the attachment system, which is made up of the child *and* the parenting adults who care for her. The attachment system is triggered by a sign of danger out in the world, such as the dog barking near Minda, or from an internal danger signal, such as when an unexpected pain causes a sudden alert. Once the system is triggered, infants and parents act to get the little one close to her protector. In this instance Minda cried, but under other circumstances she might have moved towards her father or started looking for him, or if he had been closer, might just have held on tightly. Her father responds in a way that is first protective and then soothing when the danger has passed. Finally, when everything is back to normal, the system is turned off again and they go back to other activities.

Minda settles down in her father's arms. They start making little faces at each other and she is amused. Soon she is wriggling, which is Minda's signal that she wants to be on her own again. Back in the stroller, she sticks part of the toy in her mouth and grins.

If the attachment system were always turned on, babies would never want to be apart from their parents, which would be a terrible impediment to growing into healthy and independent individuals. When it is turned off, however, another system kicks in – Minda's attention becomes directed at exploring her world, even if exploration extends no further than finding out what her toy feels like in her mouth. She follows her curiosity, which helps her to develop new skills and the confidence that will someday allow her to be comfortable with independence.

The attachment system does not reside within Minda, nor is it in her father; attachment occurs *between* Minda and her father. Minda cries and her father responds. Without her cry, nothing would happen. Without his response, Minda's cry would only make things worse (the dog would yap louder and louder). If we could transport Minda back in time to observe the evolutionary forces that selected the system, we would see that her crying would serve as a homing signal for predators only if it wasn't coupled with a parent's strong urge to care for her when she needs it. Attachment, with all its benefits, occurs in the *link* between Minda and her father. Donald Winnicott, a psychoanalyst of an earlier generation, provocatively summed up this irreducible union by saying, "There is no such thing as a baby, there is always a baby and someone."[6]

If the attachment system did nothing but keep infants physically close to their parents to protect the infants from predators, it would be of very little consequence to modern lives; avoiding predators is just not that high on our current list of priorities. However, one further achievement makes attachment bonds matter to us a great deal – the goal of the attachment system changes over time. When Minda's father picks her up and she feels safe and her fear diminishes, it feels good. Over time, children learn to use the attachment system to maximize the good feelings of security that have been associated with closeness rather than just seeking physical proximity itself. Children like Minda come to seek the welcome feeling of comfort and safety that arises from being near a loving protector, rather than the nearness itself. This simple shift in the goal of interactions between parents and infants allows children to develop far-reaching and flexible repertoires of skills and strategies that are directed towards feeling secure,[7] rather than being stuck with the single option of repeatedly clinging to a parent for protection.

For instance, as a child's experiences accumulate, she learns to use memories of soothing contact to calm herself when she is upset. This result only becomes possible because she has shifted her focus from wanting to *be near* her father or mother to wanting to recapture the good feeling that she has experienced when she is near them. Children also learn other strategies to achieve the goal of feeling secure. For example, they may rely on knowledge to avoid distress, such as knowing that help is not too far away if required. As the goal of the attachment system shifts in this small but crucial way, the system becomes much more than a survival trick; it develops into one of our most effective methods of regulating our emotions.

Jack and Diane are both arriving for their first day back at daycare after two weeks at home over the winter break. They are three years old. As their mothers leave them with Sapna, a favourite teacher, Diane runs over to the Lego table where her friends are already playing. Jack bursts into tears and grabs his mother's leg with both arms.

Now we are getting to the significant part – the ways in which our relationships to our parents grow into distinctly different ways of being in the world. In the beginning, we all draw from the same pool of attachment behaviours that we are born with: we cry, or cling, or follow to stay close to Mom or Dad. However, since in this book we are describing attachment to develop a model of *personalized* health care – a model that attends to individual differences in attachment behaviour that affect health – we need to understand how we end up taking very different paths from the same point of departure. Jack and Diane are acting differently because they are old enough to have developed different patterns of attachment.

One thing that leads us towards different patterns of attachment is that we learn from experience what to fear and how to find safety. Jack and Diane started with different genes and have lived different lives. Jack may be cautious about heading back into the hurly-burly of daycare, while Diane may feel reassured that she is in a good place to play and explore. Jack and Diane were each born, as we all are, with an exquisitely fine capacity to make links between fear and the most salient aspects of the situation that caused it. Our human ability to make those links has given us a powerful survival strategy during evolution. By remembering the context of frightening events, we learn to anticipate – to be wary of situations that may become dangerous, instead of just reacting to actual threats. Jack fears his mother's absence and does his best to make sure she stays. Just like Jack, we all react defensively to predictors of danger rather than waiting to actually be in danger; it's a smart thing to do. In a similar way, we also learn how to anticipate safety. We acquire a personal repertoire of signs that all is well and help is near. Learning about safety takes a little longer than learning about danger because our brains are hardwired to be excellent danger detectors; we can learn about dangers in a flash. The value of feeling safe is less than the value of being afraid at the right times (at least in evolutionary terms), so we have to work harder at acquiring knowledge about safety. But a sense of safety is still important; it allows Diane to play and explore. She develops the ability to do things for herself, and eventually she learns to deal with manageable threats on her own and to recover from manageable upsets.

Babies' brains make links between situations of danger or safety and their predictors. They also learn to predict whether or not someone will be there when they need them. How parents typically react to their babies' distress is one of the most important determinants of what those children come to expect from the world – after all, for most infants their relationship with their parents *is* their world. In the end, children develop complex mental models of what they can expect from themselves, from those who care for them, and from the world – and they develop these models when they are very young, certainly by 12 months and probably sooner.[8]

Some circumstances are virtually guaranteed to make any child feel frightened and uncertain. For children around their first birthday, being separated from Mom and Dad and left with a stranger will almost certainly do it. As distressing as this is for all children, it is remarkable how children in the same situation can behave so differently – because they are working from different mental models.

Psychologists who want to study and understand these differences may put a young child and one of her parents in what they call the *strange situation* (strange as in new to babies, not as in weird). The strange situation takes place in a playroom that is new to the toddler and is full of toys. A scripted series of events occurs involving the parent leaving the room and coming back, sometimes with a stranger present, sometimes not. The sequence of events, which is designed to be stressful enough to trigger attachment behaviour, occurs in the same way and in the same order every time, so we know that the differences we observe in children's behaviour come from the infant and parent who are participating, not from variations in the stressful circumstances.

Three common patterns are observed when children are stressed by the strange situation, and they can be seen most clearly when the child reunites with her parent after a brief but stressful separation. Consider how three children react to being reunited with their parent after about a minute alone in a playroom with a stranger.

Janice wants contact with her mother and runs to her with her arms open. She cries and her mother picks her up. Janice may or may not have been friendly with the stranger, it could go either way, but she is obviously much more interested in being with Mom. It only takes a short time, a minute or less, for Janice to settle down, and then she is ready to take her mother over to the toys to show her something interesting.

Janice is typical of kids with a secure pattern of attachment.[9] Her tears give us very little information about her attachment style because the strange situation is stressful for all kids.[10] We can tell that she is secure because of her wish to be reunited with her mother and because being back with her mother helps her to settle down quickly. Janice knows how to use this very important relationship to feel secure when she is threatened, and she knows how to use the security of that relationship as a base from which to go out on her own to explore.

When Theo's mother leaves the playroom, a casual observer might think that he was not distressed by being left alone. He keeps moving a toy car around and when the stranger comes in, he interacts with her in a way that is similar to his interaction with his mother – mostly ignoring her, occasionally looking over at what she is doing. When his mother comes back in the room, Theo looks like he might not have noticed. He ignores her at first and then offers a casual greeting, interrupted when he averts his eyes and then turns away. Theo masks his distress quite effectively, although the clues are there for a trained observer. If his mother were to pick Theo up, he wouldn't cling. In fact, he would be more likely to squirm, and he wouldn't resist being put back down.

Theo's attachment pattern is called *avoidant*.[11] The best clue to his style is in his apparent lack of concern when he is reunited with his mother. The essential feature of his interpersonal behaviour in the strange situation is that he conveys neither a sense of distress over the separation nor a desire for closeness on reunion. Importantly, Theo is not as nonchalant as he looks. The key to understanding Theo's lack of apparent distress is that his calm is a strategy to maintain a connection to his mother. Although thinking that *not* signalling an attachment need could be the best way to stay close to a parent is counter-intuitive, that is, in fact, how it works sometimes. The most effective way to stay close to a parent who is inclined to react hurtfully to neediness is to look like you are fine.

Astrid is easily distressed and hard to console. When her father leaves her alone, as he is instructed to do, she looks angry. When she is reunited with her father, she runs towards him crying, just like Janice ran to her mother. In fact, Astrid was crying most of the time that she was with the stranger. Her father scoops her up, but Astrid starts wriggling and looks away, all red in the face. She gets out of her father's arms and sits on the floor close by her father, not showing much interest in the toys around her, still sobbing.

Astrid's pattern of attachment is called *resistant*. Children with this pattern are more easily upset, are harder to console, and seem to express a mixture of emotions, especially the combination that Astrid shows: acting like she wants contact but getting mad and resisting when it is available, as if she were mad that it is too little, too late. A variation on this pattern would be a child who is upset but passive about doing anything about it.

Surprisingly, given how different their behaviour is, avoidant kids like Theo and resistant kids like Astrid have quite a bit in common during their first year of life. Both patterns represent forms of insecure attachment. Compared with secure children, both avoidant and resistant children cry more frequently, are more distressed by separations, express less positive and more negative emotions (especially anger), and are more likely to look away or walk away from a face-to-face interaction initiated by their parent. So even though avoidant kids don't look perturbed by events that cause stress to other infants and are more focused on exploration and play, they are not more resilient. Their muted expressiveness and lack of contact after a separation is based on insecurity rather than on confidence. The truth is easy to see by measuring the heart rates of children during the strange situation.[12] All children experience a faster heart rate during separation, and their hearts continue to beat quickly until they are reunited with their parent. But once they are reunited, secure infants return to their normal heart rate in less than a minute. On the other hand, both avoidant and resistant children experience a racing heart for much longer. Avoidant kids have a discrepancy between behaviour (which looks casual and unconcerned) and physiology (which reveals an amplified stress response). This fact lets us know that avoidant behaviour is a bluff, intended to mask underlying insecurity.

So, secure children find a balance between using contact for safety and comfort and enjoying exploration and play. Children with the other two patterns make different trade-offs between their needs for contact and for autonomy. One of these trade-offs emphasizes the strategies of seeking contact and signalling distress (*hyperactivating strategies*); the other emphasizes the value of distance and the appearance of self-sufficiency (*deactivating strategies*).[13] Children with either of these last two patterns have found the strategies that work best in their own particular situation, but the best that is available to them nonetheless leaves them prone to distress and unlikely to bounce back from it quickly, as revealed by their physiological agitation.

Most adults who have been around babies much can recognize the different attitudes towards separation and stressful events that we have just described. But what does this have to do with physical health? We can take a first step towards appreciating why close relationships affect health by recognizing that the attachment system is a biological system. In fact, it is somewhat of a meta-system because attachment regulates other biological systems. The ways that we interact with each other, at least in our closest relationships, control what is going on in our bodies.

The first insights into the biology of attachment came from observing monkeys who were raised without mothers. The little ones picked up the diaper material that was lining their cages and clung to it for comfort. In fact, they found diapers and towels far more attractive than things that are more obviously necessary – like a milk bottle. The monkeys also preferred a dummy wrapped in a soft towel over a hard wire dummy that had a feeding bottle attached; they were more attracted to the soft tactile feel of terrycloth than they were to food.[14] A photo that illustrates this preference can be found easily in an Internet image search (try typing "Harlow monkey reach milk" into the image finder in a search engine). In the photo a small monkey clings to a towel-wrapped dummy while stretching as far as it can to try to reach the milk bottle on a wire-mesh dummy sitting a few inches away. It clearly wants the milk, but it isn't willing to leave the soft dummy to get it. This reluctance gives us a clue about the powerful attraction of a certain kind of tactile experience for an infant: comfort is more attractive than food. In the real world babies don't need the feel of a towel but the soft and warm feel of skin. What is so striking about the orphaned monkeys' behaviour is that the need for this soft contact trumps more obvious biological drives. What is so important about that contact?

The answer to that question is not warm and fuzzy. It turns out that babies may need signals like the feel of skin to regulate very high-priority biological systems, such as temperature control and hunger. Most baby mammals, including humans, are born without the equipment they need to regulate their own temperature well, and yet bodies work only if they are at just the right temperature. So newborns need help. For example, the body temperature of rat pups, which has been studied particularly carefully, is controlled within the narrow optimal range by interactions between the pup and its mother. The pup doesn't control its own temperature; nor does its mother control it; rather, the pup's temperature is controlled by their interactions.[15] That point is worth repeating because this is an instance of our core theme: in early days of life, when temperature control is crucial to a pup's survival, it is controlled by *a relationship*.

One of the signals that allow that interaction to work depends on skin contact. A pup is warmed by skin-to-skin contact with its mother. Warmth is a signal that initiates activity in the pup. When it gets warmer, the pup starts running around and exploring its cage. That means no more skin contact and its temperature starts to drop. The mother rat may then initiate contact with her pup. It won't necessarily just sit still and sidle into her if left to its own devices, but she has another signal that makes the pup sit still – she licks and grooms it. As it settles down with her, its temperature starts to rise, until off it goes again. And so on.

The dam contributes two things to the system: a furnace and a signal to get the young pup to settle down with her. The pup also supplies two things: a drive to go off and explore when warm enough and a tendency to settle in to receive the grooming. Between the two of them, they can keep the pup's temperature just right, although neither one could manage it alone. This symbiosis is a very specific example of the "just right" or Goldilocks balance of physiology depending on interactions in an attachment relationship. Since the interactions involve the pup alternating between staying close and going off alone, it is also an example of how physiological regulation can be mirrored by the developmental balance between independence and dependent care.

The main point is that relationships regulate physiology, at least some of the time. This neat little example illustrates a couple of other principles as well. One of those principles is that the signals that keep attachment relationships working are quite specific and often pretty simple – by which we mean that they are not necessarily psychologically meaningful. Although we can use our poetic minds to construct an emotional connection between rat dams and pups, licking and grooming doesn't look a lot like love. But it doesn't matter whether or not little pups feel loved or whether their mothers feel loving; the system would work just fine without the feeling.

The second embedded principle concerns the *goals* of the system, which are ideal body temperature and an optimal balance between closeness and independent activity. The system's goals simply emerge, without any deliberate effort on the part of either pup or mother to recognize the goal at all. The loops of signals and responses that we described for rat pups and their dams end up controlling both the pup's temperature and the distance between pup and mother without the rats having to think about it. The system automatically figures out and regulates the optimal distance between pup and mother, even though no part of the system measures distances or even necessarily pays attention to them. It just emerges because of the way the system is constructed: temperature and distance go hand in hand. Even if rats had big brains and complicated desires, motivations, and feelings, they could find a balance of closeness and distance without using any of that equipment.

Approach and withdrawal between rat pups and mothers depends on signals that do not need to have any subjective feel, but in humans the *feeling of security* is a hallmark of attachment relationships. When we talk about attachment relationships in adults, we will use the feeling of security as a guide to which relationships serve attachment functions and which do not.

A man who had used opioid painkillers many times over the years, both as a prescription medication and as a street drug, described the feelings that opioids gave him as being "like someone you love has their arm around you."

This feeling provides another connection between our experience of attachment bonds and brain chemistry because evidence suggests that natural opioids (i.e., endorphins or endogenous opioids) may account for the good feeling that comes with being secure.[16]

We can divide human attachment relationships into phases. In the earliest periods of life, attachment may or may not feel like something, but it doesn't matter – we are like rat pups. It is sufficient that we have effective signals that keep infants and their caregivers at the appropriate physical distance. Later in development, physical proximity is no longer the most important goal. By this point, the feeling of security becomes more important and replaces physical closeness as the goal of our attachment system. Now, the biology of *feeling* secure becomes an important determinant of how we act. This feeling is the result, at least in part, of natural opioids that signal pleasure and reduce pain. In both cases our biology supports our closest relationships, and our relationships support our biology, even when it all works outside of conscious awareness.

While the brain processes that reduce pain and give pleasure are linked to security, the reverse is also true: social isolation is a form of pain. This connection is seen in some animals when preventing enjoyable contact between littermates triggers all the behaviours that the animals usually display when they are in physical pain. Remarkably, this response can be prevented by administering opioid painkillers before the animals are isolated.

Something similar occurs in humans. In 2003, Naomi Eisenberger and her colleagues found that human social exclusion is processed through some of the brain circuits that register physical pain.[17] Nerve signals that indicate pain are processed very quickly (like reflexes). Only afterward can more "thoughtful" brain processes work to understand what happened and stop the sensation of pain. In Eisenberger's study the experimenters used brain-imaging techniques to study the activity of their subjects' brains while the subjects played a computer game. The game involved a subject tossing a virtual ball back and forth with other players whom the subject believed to be real people playing from a remote location.[18] The game was set up so that after the other players threw the ball to the subject a few times, they would stop throwing the ball to the subject, about as mild a social exclusion as you could imagine. Participants reported that they felt ignored and excluded (so the game accomplished what it was intended to), and their brain scans showed that the areas that automatically detect pain responded to the social slight in the same way they do when physical pain occurs; the greater the subjective sense of distress, the greater the activation of this pain region. Furthermore, the more thoughtful, reflective brain areas that reduce physical pain kicked in as well to reduce distress and reduce the activity of the brain's pain areas. The conclusion from research like this is very striking, and it works in two directions. Social exclusion and isolation are forms of pain. Social interaction with parents, playmates, and partners is a form of pain relief. Of course, the science just confirms what anyone who has ever scraped a knee and had her mother kiss it better already knows.

So what is attachment? It is a behavioural system that solves the evolutionary problem of reconciling two otherwise incompatible achievements: bipedal locomotion and big brains. Furthermore, because of a self-reinforcing cycle of social attunement and brain development, infant-parent attachment lies at the root of the vast web of social competencies that are the hallmark of our species.

At an individual level, the attachment system is at its core a biological system, relying on simple signals that become psychologically meaningful only with experience. During childhood, feeling secure becomes a more important goal of the attachment system than actual protection from physical danger. Then – and importantly for personalized health care – individual experience[19] leads different people to emphasize different strategies to maximize their feelings of security. While these individual differences are easiest to recognize as patterns of behaviour, the attachment system remains closely tied to our biology. This connection can be seen in various ways, including the high degree of overlap between the biology of the social pain of isolation and responses to physical pain.

In the next chapter we will look more closely at the brain processes that regulate social interactions in attachment relations, and in turn, how experience in those early relationships changes our brains' early development.

5 Attachment Sculpts the Brain

In the previous chapter we described a virtuous cycle on an evolutionary timescale in which big brains fostered the development of nuanced social perceptions, which in turn fostered the evolution of even bigger brains. Something analogous happens on a briefer timescale during an individual's developmental years: a brain that is born with all the equipment required for nuanced social interactions is shaped by experience in those interactions. These in turn influence the way that an individual deals with other people for the rest of his or her life, such that well-attuned interactions during infancy and childhood guide brain development that will foster rich social interactions later. To understand how that works, we need to discuss the cognitive processes involved in these social interactions. These include expecting, reflecting on, and evaluating what is occurring socially, and retrieving representations of past social interactions from memory. We also need to clarify the brain processes that support these activities and how they come to differ between individuals.

Ahnaf was concerned about recent changes in his partner's behaviour. Simon was usually humorous, attentive to others' interests, and very social. Lately he seemed self-involved and unusually quiet. Ahnaf confided to a friend: "I am wondering if Simon is just stressed about his work or something or if he is reconsidering our relationship. I don't think he would tell me about that until he was certain that he had made up his mind."

Ahnaf provides an example of what cognitive psychologists refer to as theory of mind: the ability to think about what goes on in people's minds. He expresses a complicated idea. He has been thinking (a cognitive process) about what Simon is thinking and feeling (cognitive and emotional processes in another person) and reflecting on his awareness that others do not always express themselves fully or truthfully. We can speculate about what is going on in Simon's life, but we don't know. Separating out the elements of these ideas makes it clear that theory of mind is a very impressive social cognitive achievement. A different word for the process of thinking about what is going on in others' minds, which we introduced in the last chapter, is *mentalizing*.

Scientists have studied theory of mind by using tests that determine whether a person knows that someone else has a false belief. In the Sally-Anne test, a child is presented with a cartoon that tells the following story: Sally puts a ball in a basket and then goes away. Her friend, Anne, takes the ball out of the basket and puts it into a box while Sally is out of the room. When Sally comes back, where does she look for her ball?[1] Children who answer "in the box" demonstrate that they know the ball's true location. Children who answer "in the basket" demonstrate that they appreciate that Sally will have a misguided belief, which requires that they have developed a theory of mind, an achievement that is usually present by the age of six or seven.[2]

How do brains mentalize? It is useful to consider two networks in the cortex, each of which consists of several connected brain regions. Taken together with some lower brain systems that we will get to later, we can call these networks *the social brain*. Cognitive neuroscientist Matthew Lieberman has suggested that we name one of these cortical networks the X-system and the other the C-system.[3] The X-system (for the x in reflex) performs automatic functions that are processed very quickly. The X-system generates spontaneous, non-reflective responses to social events. Someone sticks out her hand to shake yours, and the X-system responds instantly ("Handshake coming in, activate the right elbow and hand!"). The X-system is fast and it works efficiently in states of high arousal, so it is good in urgent situations. On the other hand, the X-system does not contribute to wisdom because it is slow to learn when information from the environment changes. When Charlie Brown ran to kick the football that Lucy was going to pull out from underneath him, every single autumn throughout our childhood, his X-system was functioning flawlessly. Our experience of things that are processed in the X-system is that they are real observations of the world, rather than opinions or the results of calculations.

The C-system (for the c in reflective) is the slower system used for intentional, controlled processes. The C-system is not as good when quick decisions are needed to avoid harm because its function is impaired by cognitive load and by high arousal; the C-system gets easily flustered. The output of the C-system is not experienced as reality but as something self-generated. When Ahnaf makes an inference about the reasons for the changes in Simon's behaviour, his C-system is at work. In general, the X-system specializes in common situations, while the C-system is the home of exceptions and special cases.[4]

When a child reflects on Sally's false belief about her ball, the imaginative effort of mentalizing is done in the C-system.[5] Interestingly, thinking about external characteristics, like the colour of Sally's hair, can be processed in the automatic X-system, but the C-system is required to contemplate her inner world.[6] Similarly, reading a description of a person's behaviour (an external observation) activates the X-system, but making an inference from that description about the person's attitudes causes the C-system to kick in.[7] Your X-system notices that I am raising my arm, but your C-system is required to think about what I intend to accomplish with this movement. Mentalizing can also involve thinking about our own inner world. The critical distinction is that simply thinking is not mentalizing. Mentalizing occurs when we are thinking about thoughts, feelings, beliefs, and intentions.[8]

What is the C-system doing when we mentalize? The process of reflecting on someone else's inner world appears to require parts of the C-system to inhibit other brain activities. For example, the C-system inhibits attention to our own experience when we consider someone else's state of mind. This switch lets us appreciate that others have different points of view.[9] Here is another example of inhibition: controlled, effortful reflection on ourselves sometimes helps to diminish strong emotions. Thinking about feelings may dampen automatic emotional processes, an outcome that is exploited in some kinds of psychotherapy.[10] This technique is entirely analogous to the slow neurological signals that reduce automatic handling of pain stimuli, which we described in Chapter 4. The brain processes that allow us to mentalize are the same ones that allow us to put the brakes on strong emotions and on reflexive behavioural responses – so the ability of mental reflection to regulate the brain by slowing automatic functions is critical to many aspects of social effectiveness and health. Mentalizing is a very useful skill and a marker of a brain that is finely adapted to its social environment.

Health care professionals are familiar with the sort of difficulties that leave a person feeling stuck, perpetually repeating self-defeating patterns and having trouble adjusting to the reality that what used to work is no longer a useful strategy. In Chapter 2 we discussed Daniel Kahneman's insight that slow, high-energy-consumption systems of thought are required to overcome automatic cognitive processes. The X- and C-systems are a slightly different description of very similar neural processes. The difference is that they are focused on social cognition. What does social cognitive science add to our understanding?

The C-system has an important role in adapting behaviour to suit a changing environment. Its functions include evaluating the likelihood that an action will be associated with reward or punishment in the short term and in the long term.[11] In many species, including humans, an area of the C-system called the orbitofrontal cortex or OFC (orbitofrontal because it is located just above the eye sockets, or orbits, in the front of the brain) is necessary for changing a learned behavioural pattern when conditions change. If the OFC is damaged, a creature cannot adjust when something that used to be rewarding becomes aversive (which is called *reversal learning*). In addition to carrying out reversal learning, the OFC also enhances flexible behaviour by helping us to learn that the type of information required to assess a contingency has changed, which is called *strategy switching*.[12] A person may find, for instance that she needs to switch from evaluating the meaning of her partner's spoken words to interpreting his non-verbal body language to accurately interpret his frame of mind.[13] Not surprisingly, deficits in these skills lead to interpersonal problems. Difficulties with reversal learning and strategy switching in the social environment are core components of the sort of repetitive interpersonal problems that leave a person feeling stuck.

One reason that insecure patterns of attachment resist change over time is that insecure brains have difficulty with new social learning. This difficulty contributes to the trait-like stability of insecure patterns of attachment over time. It is part of the explanation for the common observation that an interpersonal pattern that has been shaped and reinforced during development tends to persist even when it is no longer rewarded in adolescence and adulthood.

Early experiences that facilitate the development of secure attachment are the same experiences that facilitate the growth and development of the OFC. A well-developed OFC enhances an individual's capacity to adapt to the changing social world throughout life. If early conditions are less favourable, the result is both insecure attachment and a less well-developed OFC. This outcome means that the person with childhood experiences that lead to insecurity has two problems to contend with – he or she responds to new social situations with old responses that are no longer adaptive and also finds it harder to change this response pattern.

Anwar and Lee are four years old. They are meeting with Willa, a psychology student working on her PhD. Willa offers them each the same simple choice: "I have chocolate chip cookies here, freshly baked. If you want, you can have one right now. But if you wait five minutes instead, I will give you two cookies. So you can choose one cookie right now but only one, or two cookies if you wait five minutes." Lee chooses to wait to get double the treat. Anwar has barely finished hearing about the choice when he grabs a cookie and munches it down, grinning at Lee who hasn't had a chance to taste them yet.

You may recognize that Willa is employing the marshmallow test that we described in Chapter 2. Add this scenario to our growing list of examples of the set of neurological activities in which automatic processes are inhibited by slower, reflective cortical circuits. We reintroduce the marshmallow test here because the ability to delay gratification, like other examples in this set, is influenced by the early parent-child interactions that determine patterns of attachment. Children with a secure pattern of attachment are more likely to wait for two cookies.[14] Our ability to inhibit automatic reflex processes is a core skill that underpins many aspects of our ability to get along with one another and function in our social world, including mentalizing.

Carol and her four-month-old son, Tyler, are playing. We are catching them at a particularly good moment and are privileged to witness a nearly ideal interaction. Not all interactions between Carol and Tyler go so well, but not all have to. What Carol is doing is easy and comes naturally; she is just having fun with her son. She is holding Tyler on her knee and tuning in to him. He starts to grin and Carol mirrors back a grin, a little bigger and more exaggerated than Tyler's. He likes this and grins wider and starts to giggle. He moves his little fist up and down. Carol does this too with her hand and then adds a gentle song, the pitch of her voice bouncing up and down between two tones in time with the hand play.

Although Carol isn't thinking about what she is doing, her communication with Tyler is very sophisticated. Her facial expression mirrors what she sees on his face, which gives Tyler the opportunity to see from the outside what he is experiencing on the inside. When he does something interesting, Carol emphasizes his expression by adding something beyond mirroring (like the little song that repeats the rhythm of his hand in its rhythm and tone). Through Carol's *marking* of his internal state, Tyler is given the opportunity to make a connection between two complementary modes of expression: kinaesthetic and auditory.[15] Carol's capacity to intuit Tyler's inner experience from his facial and bodily expressions and then to display expressions of this experience and elaborate on them contributes to his growing capacity to appreciate his own mental states. Almost effortlessly, she is teaching him to distinguish between various feelings and to fine-tune his interpretation of his feelings. He is learning about feelings, about faces, about interactions, and eventually about the difference between the self and the other. This process occurs because Carol gets him, and eventually he comes to appreciate that understanding. Carol's mentalizing helps Tyler to develop his own ability to mentalize.

Mentalizing isn't magic. Being able to intuit someone else's state of mind doesn't mean getting it right every time. It means being able to make a reasonable guess, to watch for more evidence, and to modify this guess as more information emerges. Mothers and fathers who are good at their parenting craft do not have a mystical ability to know what their children are experiencing, but they do hone their skills over time. If their opportunities to do that are limited by the competing demands that result from poverty or depression, for example, a child will have a very different experience growing up and is more likely to end up with an insecure attachment style.

Early interpersonal interactions almost certainly have a direct effect on the way that our C-system is wired.[16] The mechanism is simple in principle: frequently repeated, highly salient experiences result in a strengthening of the connections between the neurons that those experiences excite.[17] The process of neuronal connections being strengthened by experience is called *neural plasticity*. Although such plastic changes can occur throughout life, the brain is especially open to being shaped in this way during critical periods of development, which include the time when attachment bonds are most prominent in an infant's life. As a result, the structure and function of certain areas of the brain (and the connections between them) are shaped by consistently repeated experiences that exercise those areas. This shaping happens with visual experiences. Consistent exposure to certain kinds of visual stimuli alters the structure of the visual area of the cortex.[18] It also happens with exposure to languages, which alters the structure and function of areas of the brain that process language.[19] It would be extraordinarily surprising if the same thing did not happen in regions of the brain that are critical to social interactions, like the C-system.

When the repeated experiences that shape the brain are like the one between Carol and Tyler, the areas of the brain that support reflective thought and the inhibition of automatic reflex arousal are exercised. As they are exercised, the connections between these areas are reinforced. Parents with a well-developed capacity to keep their child in mind (i.e., to mentalize) are helping their child to develop a brain that is good at mentalizing too and helping their child to acquire the other benefits of cortical systems that inhibit reflex reactions and automatic thoughts: the ability to delay gratification, to pause and consider events rather than jumping to conclusions, and to calm and soothe themselves when they are in pain or overstimulated.[20] They are helping their child to develop a very well-regulated body, a body that is programmed to maintain health in the long run.

6 All Grown Up and Still Attached

The attachment system remains active and valuable throughout life, and the patterns that we develop as children adapt and mature in response to our changing circumstances as we grow.[1] One of the biggest adaptations is that the older we get, the less important parents are to our ability to feel secure. We become attached to others our own age. Peers start to fill the role our parents had and later romantic partners do the same. As a result, in adolescence and adulthood the nature of attachment bonds shift. But even as they mature and change, attachment relationships continue to influence our physical health.[2]

An example of the ways that interactions in attachment relationships foster good physical health emphasizes the point. This example concerns a small but powerful molecule in our bodies that has been dubbed "the bonding hormone" – oxytocin. Many of the good things that are much more likely to happen in attachment relationships than in other kinds of relationships cause oxytocin to be released into our systems: warm hugs, gentle stroking, welcome genital touches, and breastfeeding (which causes oxytocin release in the mother).[3] Once it is released, oxytocin makes us more receptive to intimate contact, more secure, and more trusting – a self-reinforcing virtuous circle.[4] Even more important to the story of attachment and health, oxytocin benefits several aspects of physical health by reducing inflammation, promoting wound healing, calming our responses to stress, and possibly even reducing our risk of heart disease.[5] At a fundamental biological level, we get something from our closest adult relationships that not only makes us feel better but also makes us healthier.

Oxytocin is just one small piece of the puzzle, but it demonstrates an important principle: not only do attachment relationships shape our health, but they also have an influence that is not available in other kinds of relationships. Attachment bonds are unique. But how can we tell exactly which relationships count? As we grow beyond receiving all our security from those who parent us, who is an attachment figure to us and who is not? To answer this question, we need to identify the things that happen in attachment relationships that distinguish them from friendships, business relationships, and other sorts of collaborations.

Here is a true story I (Bob) sometimes tell to students about a medical encounter. Although this story concerns the day that I had a vasectomy at the hospital where Jon and I work, I usually call this "a minor surgical procedure under a local anaesthetic" to avoid having students' faces scrunch up in horror.

On the day of the procedure my wife, Lynn, and I had planned that she would meet me at the hospital, but Lynn hadn't arrived when I was called into the room where the surgery would be performed. It took very little time before the operation was underway. The surgeon, whom I had met only once previously, went about his work like an efficient technician, essentially ignoring me. I was apprehensive about what he was doing but not able to see him from where I lay on the table. The nurse assisting him stood at the head of the table and, perhaps noticing that I looked nervous, put a hand on my shoulder. I didn't know her at all; I could barely see her behind me, yet her hand on my shoulder helped me to relax. Just then I heard steps coming down the tiled hallway and recognized them as Lynn's. I suddenly felt much more comfortable, although the only communication my wife and I had was through the familiar sound of her footsteps.

This is a simple story of the power of relationships in a health care setting, and I tell it to students because it illustrates how subtle those influences can be. The first point to emphasize is that I was frightened because the surgeon represented a threat. It doesn't matter that I had asked him to perform the procedure and that he was very professional about the whole thing, nor that I understood in an intellectual way that he was performing a service for me rather than threatening harm. Because of the way that human brains automatically detect threats of harm, a man standing over my genitals with a blade is still a threat even if he is a trained professional and he was invited. You can't turn off your harm-detecting device; you can only remind yourself to ignore its alarm.

The more important point to my story concerns the other relation-ships in this drama. Who is an attachment figure for me in the story of my surgery? The primary function of adult attachment relationships is to regulate distressing feelings.[6] The feeling of security that can come from being close to certain people identifies those people as having a privileged place in our attachment system.[7] That criterion is a helpful guide. The surgeon is clearly not an attachment figure. His primary role in this attachment drama is to serve as a source of danger. But the effect of Lynn's presence on my sense of security tells me that she is in a different category of people in my life. Physical proximity to her, as signalled by those familiar footfalls, makes me feel more secure even when we are separated by a wall. The nurse's role is less clear. Her mere presence is not enough to make me feel secure because I don't know her, but her hand on my shoulder does serve an attachment *function*. She is temporarily making me feel safer – presumably because her kind touch reminds me of the care and protection that I have received in my life from others who are closer to me.

Characteristics of an attachment bond

We can be a little more precise. The difference between attachment rela-tionships and every other kind of relationship is found in four defin-ing features: proximity seeking, separation distress, safe haven, and secure base.

Proximity seeking and separation distress

First, an attachment figure is someone to whom you like to be close. This function is most similar to the original proximity-seeking goal of the attachment system for infants: getting close to a protector at times of danger. When attachment researchers try to figure this out, they ask two questions. The first is, "Who is the person you most like to spend time with?"[8]

Jon: I like to spend time with the guys I play basketball with, but our relation-ships don't extend very much further than the court, the pub after the game, and the odd exchange of email jokes. They are great pals, but they are not attachment figures for me.

The first question doesn't sound very specific because there may be many people you like to spend time with who don't help you to regulate difficult emotions in any very substantial way. However, the word "most" in the question is getting at something more specific than basketball buddies. It is a kind of "desert island" question: If there were only one person you could spend time with, who would it be? Framed that way, the spending-time question is asking about someone who is special. In the example of Bob's medical procedure, Lynn fits this criterion but the nurse doesn't.[9]

The second question about closeness is, "Who is the person you don't like to be away from?"

Jon: When I travel out of town on my own, I don't sleep all that well. I miss having my wife, Nancy, in bed with me.

This is another way of figuring out who is helping to keep your feelings regulated. A two-person system doesn't function very well when one person is absent, so recognizing that things feel worse when someone is away is another way to identify that person as performing an attachment role. Kids *protest* separation from their parents; for adults, separation from an attachment figure is usually accompanied by an emotional experience of some kind of distress – hating to be away from or missing that person.

Safe haven

An attachment figure is someone you use as a sheltering harbour in stormy times. "Who is the person you want to be with when you are feeling upset or down?" is a question that very directly addresses the ability of an attachment figure to calm and soothe.

Jon: When I was a child, we went to a cottage by the ocean in the summer. We spent our time wandering across the tidal flats, climbing the cliffs, and running through the fields, often spinning a tale in our heads. Most of this time was unsupervised, and we understood that it was good and right to explore the terrain and try to figure out how things worked. Of course, sometimes it didn't work out well – once my brother and I had a jellyfish fight, thinking that if they were on sandbars they couldn't sting you anymore (wrong!), but at times like that we knew we could race back to our folks, who would fix the problem ... soothe the sting.

"Who is the person you would count on for advice?" is a more subtle indicator of someone in the safe haven role. It is not a question of who gives the best advice; any wise person might fill that role. The "you would count on" portion of the question will lead you to identify someone who serves your attachment needs.

Secure base

The fourth function of an attachment figure is to serve as a secure base. A person who fills this role for an adult may be proud and supportive of his partner's accomplishments ("Who is the person you would want to tell first if you achieved something good?") or is just reliable when it is his turn to provide strength and support ("Who is the person you can always count on?"). A parent who provides a secure base to a child fosters independent exploration and play. An adult attachment figure in the secure base role may foster his partner's creativity and accomplishment.

Bob: For a long while, I spent an hour or two on most nights writing this book. When Lynn went out of town on business for a couple of days, I had more time to write, but I didn't feel creative anymore.

If you think of whose name you would give in answer to each of those six questions, you will be identifying the person or people who serve attachment functions in your life. If you identify one person who serves all four of those functions, then you are thinking of someone with whom you share what Zeifman and Hazan call a "full-blown attachment bond."[10] The person who shares that bond with you, your attachment figure, is usually a romantic partner with whom you have been in a committed relationship for more than two years.[11] However, people in other roles (often parents and close friends) can serve *some* attachment functions.

When attachment functions are transferred from parents to peers during development, it follows a sequence. Proximity seeking to peers emerges first (and is observed between peers who are as young as three years old), whereas turning to peers for comfort when distressed emerges much later (sometime in late adolescence, at which point peers may be preferred to parents for this function). Using a peer as a secure base occurs only in late adolescence or early adulthood and usually corresponds to forming a full-blown attachment to a romantic partner.[12]

An attachment figure – a person in a relationship with *every* defining feature that we have just described – is in a very special category. Others may serve some of these functions in some circumstances, especially proximity seeking and safe haven. For health care providers, providing a safe haven can be a particularly important role at times. The nurse who put her hand on Bob's shoulder served this function for him (as indicated by the sense of security that her touch elicited) for a very short while, but during that time she was filling in for the full-blown attachment figures who were care providers when he was young and for Lynn (reminding Bob of them, actually). We will return to this idea in Chapter 11 when we discuss how attachment influences relationships between patients and health care providers.[13]

From childhood to old age, attachment processes continue to be activated by the same situations: danger, loss, and stress. Our patterns of attachment become visible at the times when we need to use close bonds to calm our distress and when we are in circumstances in which we need to trust others. Because we may only fully reveal our attachment style when we are threatened or afraid, it may happen that, as Warren Zevon once overstated, "you're a whole different person when you're scared."[14]

On the other hand, since situations of loss, danger, and extraordinary stress are special circumstances, attachment is often invisible. Your pattern of attachment is not apparent while you are engaged in routine, comfortable activities. Nonetheless, some situations are such reliable triggers of attachment phenomena that, within those circumstances, attachment phenomena are virtually always on display. Being seriously ill or coming to a hospital in distress are among those very reliable triggers, and so attachment, illness, and health care are natural partners. Although Bob might not want to admit it, as his surgery proceeded, a part of him felt just like a little kid in need of a calming hand again.

Patterns of adult attachment

Two couples sit in the reception area of a fertility clinic waiting to hear the results of the latest tests that will tell them if all their effort, discomfort, expense, and stress over four months of investigation and treatment have worked, or if it is time to start again or give up. In only a few moments in most people's lives do the stakes feel so high and the waiting so hard. Jamila and Greg have pulled two chairs up close to each other. They talk to each other quietly. Jamila looks worried and her hand is on Greg's knee. In the same clinic, Adam and Simone are sitting a few inches apart, facing forward, not talking at all. Adam's arms are crossed. He says something about where the car is parked, and Simone snaps back that they should have brought both their cars. Adam falls silent.

When a situation is threatening enough to trigger our attachment system, we display our own particular pattern of expectations, preferences, and action. Children separated from their parent and stuck briefly with a stranger in the strange situation test distinguish themselves by how they act when they are reunited with their parent. Similarly, as adults we distinguish ourselves during very stressful times by our preferences for closeness and support or for distance and self-reliance.

Secure attachment

The most fundamental distinction between patterns of attachment is between a secure pattern and all the other patterns. Secure attachment represents a balance that maximizes opportunities for feeling secure, while each of the other styles is designed to strive for security but tends to fall short of the goal, leaving people with those patterns feeling insecure. Secure attachment is the Goldilocks pattern, not too close and not too distant and, most importantly, not too rigidly stuck in one way of navigating interpersonal relationships. All the other patterns represent various types of insecure attachment.

When they first visited the fertility clinic, the nurse interviewed Jamila for almost an hour. In addition to her medical history, she told the nurse about the struggle that she and Greg had experienced with trying to have a child, their sorrow after her pregnancy three years earlier had ended in a miscarriage, and the discussions that had led them to decide to try fertility treatments.

How can we distinguish secure attachment from other patterns of attachment? Secure attachment has several markers. The first, surprisingly enough, has to do with storytelling; it is the ability to explain yourself clearly to someone else when you are under stress. Telling an accurate and engaging story about herself is a very complicated task that requires a combination of skills that set Jamila, and other people with a secure pattern, apart from the crowd. First, she is able to remember and express her story effectively. That means Jamila needs to select the most salient facts from all her thoughts and memories, to identify general trends from hundreds of detailed experiences, and to recall examples that back up her general conclusions. Then she needs to put the elements of her story in some sort of coherent order, according to time sequences or some other logical organizing principle.

Second, and just as important, Jamila is able to consider her audience. That means she can appreciate what the doctor and nurse need to know to feel engaged and to appreciate what she needs to tell them. Still other skills enhance effective storytelling: expressing emotions that are consistent with the story and enhance its impact, providing information that is mostly consistent, and reflecting on details that are inconsistent and either making appropriate revisions or at least acknowledging some uncertainty. All these storytelling skills are markers of a secure pattern of attachment.[15] Putting these qualities together, Jamila is able to tell a story that has *narrative coherence.*

Vince became a patient of mine (Jon) when he learned that he had an aggressive cancer. The first time we met, he made a point of discussing how his cancer was affecting Becka, his wife. Vince was concerned about Becka as well as himself and was able to appreciate what the impact of the disease might be for them both in the future. He described how she would worry about him if he were sidelined by the cancer treatment, how she would have to cope with the strain of his absence as her co-parent and manage their kids' schedules, and how she might be more afraid because she had recently had a friend die of cancer. He knew Becka's mind and wanted to make sure I did too.

Vince was displaying a second marker of secure attachment, which is mentalizing, the ability to "see others from the inside and ourselves from the outside."[16] Having an ability to step back from the immediacy of a difficult situation to intuit and imagine the perspectives of those around you can be profoundly helpful. For example, this skill allows a storyteller to appreciate what his audience needs to know for his story to have the greatest impact. For instance, Vince paused when he introduced his kids as part of the narrative and pointed them out to Jon in the picture he had beside his bed. His mentalizing is also apparent as a capacity for timely empathy, introspection, and reflection. We observed this same social skill in Carol's ability to tune in to her infant son's state of mind while they played and that four-year-olds demonstrate in the

Sally-Anne test. Vince shows how mentalizing can work in a medical conversation.

While mentalizing is a very useful skill, it is also a high standard to achieve. Consider the detective work that is required to make sensible inferences about another person's mind – something that is, after all, never directly observable. We observe the other person's behaviour, listen to what the person says, link these observations to the circumstances, bear in mind our past knowledge of this person, and compare and contrast what we know of her to our own mental states – all while under some pressure and mostly without explicitly thinking about any of these processes. We barely notice our interpretive efforts and might have trouble explaining how we "know" that someone else is hungry, or jealous, or probably not really agreeing but trying to be polite. It is a very sophisticated achievement to be able to understand how another person's beliefs, attitudes, intentions, and emotions motivate that person's behaviour.

When it was determined that Vince's cancer was untreatable, Becka was overwhelmed by the news. Vince was expecting that outcome and was able to listen while Becka cried and talked about how worried she was about how his dying would affect their kids. Later as he got sicker, Vince counted on Becka to do things for him that he no longer had the strength to do himself. She washed and fed him as he grew closer to dying.

A secure style is also apparent in the ways that people behave in relation to each other. Vince values connectedness to others, especially the give and take of the relationship that he and Becka have built. Reciprocity is an important clue. Vince does not always take the same role in his relationship with Becka; he is not always the helper or the chaser or the independent one. They each have the opportunity to trade roles as circumstances require. The back and forth in their relationship allows for mutual influence and support. Finally, reciprocity is connected to the idea of mutuality. Two secure people in a committed relationship are likely to genuinely share the burdens, responsibilities, and joys of their lives.

The oncology team did all they could to provide Vince with tests scheduled in a way that allowed him to get out of the hospital for his kids' hockey games.

Secure attachment tends to produce expectations of others that are realistic so that the demands that are placed on others are reasonable. In a health care setting, this makes a patient very easy to help, even if the care is complex or challenging. The ways in which the oncology team accommodated Vince are pretty clearly more than is required where we work. That kind of extra effort is likely to emerge only from relationships that are working very well. Here is another example of secure attachment in action:

Genevieve was in the emergency room with an unexplained chest pain. She had had a bad experience with an emergency room doctor in a previous hospital visit for a similar problem. He had been hurried, condescending, and in the end had discharged her without figuring out what was wrong or providing any relief. She was left to sort those things out with her family doctor the next day after a very uncomfortable night. When Genevieve briefly told the new doctor, on this second visit, about the previous ER experience so that he could understand why she was apprehensive, she was able to talk about her anger and her reasons for it without becoming frightened of the doctor in front of her or angry at him.

Although it sounds odd to put it this way, Genevieve demonstrated that at an emotional level she could tell two doctors apart; she didn't lump them both into one giant category of unpleasant, incompetent doctors (or men or people). Her capacity to step back mentally and reflect allowed her to understand these individuals in context and to describe the upsetting experience without re-enacting the conflict.

Genevieve has a small circle of very close confidantes, primarily her husband and her older sister, and a larger circle of close friends she spends time with and cares about but who would not be the first ones she would think to turn to in a tight spot. When she experienced chest pain at work, she asked a co-worker to help her with it – a friend but not a particularly close friend or confidante. Under those circumstances, she called on the most familiar and reliable person who was handy for support, but mostly to help her gather her thoughts and solve the problem of what steps to take next.
  It was different when her mother died. At that time she needed to talk to the two people who could listen and understand her best. She needed to cry and to laugh and remember her mother's idiosyncrasies and cry again, without anyone telling her that it was for the best, or that her mother was

in a better place, or that she would feel better soon. Her husband and sister were there for her.

Secure attachment makes it easier to draw on the supportive relationships in our lives for several reasons. First, a secure pattern of attachment fosters the kind of relationships that can provide effective support. The attitudes that accompany secure attachment – valuing close relationships and valuing reciprocity within those relationships – are the bedrock of healthy, emotionally intimate bonds. Second, the capacity to understand our confidantes by mentalizing and the flexibility to move between different positions within a close relationship (now providing support/now receiving it; now depending on a partner/now proceeding independently) are powerful tools for building and maintaining strong relationships. Finally, narrative coherence is a core aspect of secure attachment, and that ability to communicate clearly about our needs and emotions helps another person respond to us effectively. Secure attachment helps people to get effective support from others in many ways.

The way that a person behaves when she is angry is often another very useful indicator of her attachment style. The second ER doctor was able to understand Genevieve's expression of anger easily because it was obviously related to the emotional injury she had experienced in her previous visit and was more or less proportional to the event. Beyond being understandable, Genevieve's anger was constructive; it was directed towards remedying the problem. Often, people with a secure style are able to redirect anger into a declaration of healthy assertiveness – which affirms their right to an opinion without being hostile. Genevieve's ability to mentalize allowed her to alert someone new to the emotional territory that he was stepping into and to help prevent an inadvertently repeated injury.

Most people, no matter what their attachment style, use constructive problem solving as their first approach to dealing with stressful problems. A person with a secure style is often comfortable with using other coping skills as well – especially calling on others for practical and emotional support, and drawing on internal resources to soothe the distress by reflecting in solitude. A person with a secure style is adept at finding solace. Whether it is through engaging others in helpful ways or acting with purpose as an individual, a person with a secure pattern of attachment is marked by a force of self-agency that propels that person towards some sort of resolution of challenges (especially events that challenge personal relationships or an individual's safety and integrity) or at least a realistic understanding of the challenges that cannot be resolved.

Insecure attachment

Adults, as with children, can have various patterns of insecure attachment. One way of describing these patterns is to take the diagnostic approach of classifying people into different categories of attachment. These categories are descriptions of the prototypical ways in which adults manifest insecurity in close relationships – they answer the question, "In what way do you tend to express your insecurity?" Alternatively, a person's pattern of attachment can be described by placing that person at some point on a continuous measure of insecurity. This answers the question, "How severe does your insecurity tend to be?" If we were to use descriptions of body shapes as an analogy, the former description would be like sorting people into prototypical shapes (endomorph, mesomorph, ectomorph),[17] while the latter description would simply be a report of their height and weight.

For adult attachment, each approach has its virtues, but flipping back and forth between the two methods of description is confusing. We advocate a way of synthesizing these two approaches that is justified by its usefulness in health care.[18] It is based on the following basic premises.

- The two fundamental dimensions of attachment insecurity roughly correspond to the two primary interpersonal situations that make people feel insecure. Attachment *anxiety* corresponds to the degree to which being too isolated makes a person feel insecure. Attachment *avoidance* corresponds to the degree to which being too close makes a person feel insecure.[19]
- People with a secure pattern of attachment, which we have just described, tend to experience relatively small and tolerable amounts of each of these dimensions of insecurity.
- The *severity* of insecurity is often more important to its impact on health than the *type* of insecurity.
- For people who are prone to a moderate degree of insecurity, the type of insecurity they display can lead to quite different kinds of behaviour in health care interactions. For example, moderate attachment anxiety tends to lead to experiencing more symptoms

and using more health care resources, whereas moderate attachment avoidance tends to lead to underuse of health care resources and suppression of symptoms.

- When insecurity is extreme, a mixture of both dimensions of attachment insecurity is usually present, although it may not be an equal mixture.

In keeping with these principles, our plan is to describe three common situations in which insecure attachment is an issue: when attachment anxiety interferes with health (while attachment avoidance is low), when attachment avoidance interferes with health (while attachment anxiety is low), and when both attachment anxiety and attachment avoidance interfere with health. Since the last is a mouthful and the pattern of insecure attachment that combines attachment anxiety and attachment avoidance is more succinctly called *fearful attachment*, we will use that label to describe the situation where both types of insecurity are interfering with health care.[20]

When attachment anxiety interferes with health

Susan has never really had a sense that everything will be okay. She doesn't like being alone, and when she is worried or tense, she has trouble soothing herself. She relates this to her experience as a girl. Her father died when she was five, and after his death her mother fell apart. As Susan grew up, her mother was immersed in her own grief and anger at the loss of her husband and on top of that was worried about money. Susan's mother had a frantic way of coping with these problems – she was forever embarking on new money-making ventures and then abandoning these plans as quickly as they were hatched. Sometimes she blamed Susan for their plight. Other times she tried to tell Susan whom she should date or what career she should pursue, but the advice never really fit Susan's circumstances and didn't feel very helpful. Home never felt secure.

As an adult, Susan has had some helpful and caring people in her life, and she knows that being close to them feels good. The problem is that her first expectation, her default position, is that others are inconsistent and can't be counted on to appreciate her needs or to be there for her. She doesn't expect them to provide her with a safe haven. One of the things that her years with her mother taught her, however, was that she could maximize her chances of getting some care and attention if she sent out frequent and intense declarations of need. Susan was never rewarded for being subtle.

Today, Susan is at a walk-in clinic. She is trying to get some tests and some relief for a bloated sensation, nausea, and stomach pains that just don't seem to get better. She is in a similar situation to Genevieve's in the sense that she has previously had frustrating experiences with health care providers, but her response is different. When Dr Kinsman comes in, Susan motions her to come closer and tells Dr Kinsman about the specialists who have not been able to help. Susan starts to get upset all over again about how one said it is "in her head" but interrupts herself to describe the symptoms and to ask for a glass of water to take an antacid pill. She has had these symptoms – and others – on and off for quite a while, and she jumps back and forth in her description between different experiences that have alarmed her at different times. Quickly, both the time course of her experience and the pattern of her symptoms become muddied. Dr Kinsman asks how these problems have affected her life so far, and Susan grimaces and replies, "Oh, you can imagine."

As we have seen, secure attachment is characterized by the abilities to keep the other person in mind and to compose a coherent narrative. Susan's fear is too preoccupying to allow her to think about what a health professional needs to know to help her. Her frequent interruptions of herself, the multiple lines of narrative, vague words, lack of orienting context, and distress that seems out of proportion to the story that she is telling leave the doctor confused. Susan is presenting Dr Kinsman with the kind of incoherent narrative that is characteristic of high attachment anxiety when it is combined with low attachment avoidance.[21]

Health care providers are often confused by Susan because she conveys her distress so much more effectively than she conveys information. Even experienced health care providers sometimes feel overwhelmed because they are not very well trained to respond to interpersonal distress. At one point Dr Kinsman feels, in exasperation, as if she is expected to read Susan's mind. If Dr Kinsman were especially skilled in the intuition required to follow a story like Susan's, she might be rewarded with a comment indicating that "you understand me but others don't care." While this might be briefly gratifying, in the end Dr Kinsman wouldn't warm to it, because she wouldn't actually feel that she understands Susan very well at all. In the wrong hands or on a bad day, all this can easily be thrown back on Susan – her symptoms are "all in her head," she is "manipulative," she is "needy." Worse yet, she may get a new test, a new prescription, and another poorly defined diagnosis – anything to get her out of the office.

Dr Kinsman tries to communicate a plan for investigating Susan's symptoms, which needs to be done before she can suggest any treatment, and reassures Susan that her problems are not likely to be a sign of anything serious. Susan is not reassured. To the contrary: she thinks that Dr Kinsman is not taking her seriously and, sensing that the appointment is coming to an end, Susan starts to feel more distressed and hopeless about ever getting any relief.

What is happening here between Dr Kinsman and Susan illustrates a fundamental miscommunication. Dr Kinsman is, not unreasonably, focused on possible medical causes of the symptoms and their treatment. But Susan is preoccupied by fear. She experiences an unpleasant body sensation as a threat and fears what might come next. Although she is asking for a medical explanation for her suffering, she needs solace more than a diagnosis.

In her personal life, Susan wants close relationships but finds them troubling. One reason for this is that she feels too dependent, which isn't good for her self-esteem and leaves her feeling abandoned when she is alone. Unfortunately, she often ends up alone because her expressions of need can be daunting. Others often find her clingy, perhaps because even when she is close she doesn't feel fully secure, and it often leads to rejection.

Her years with her unpredictable mother have left her watchful and vigilant for others' states of mind. She has long antennae for detecting how others feel about her and when they might pull back or reject her. Her antennae are accurate (as when she correctly anticipates that Dr Kinsman is moving to end their meeting before she is satisfied), but they are too sensitive.[22] They set off alarms even for minor and transient potential rejections that would pass without causing problems if she could ignore them. They are also biased antennae because she is not as sensitive about detecting others' positive intentions. Susan's pattern of interpersonal vigilance is sometimes called a *hyperactivation* of the attachment system.[23]

To understand how Susan's pursuit of concern and care backfires, imagine a siren that is supposed to indicate fire. If the siren stays on when no fire is burning, or if it turns on every time the toaster burns a slice of bread, or if it cannot be turned off after the fire has been extinguished, it will soon be disregarded. If the siren is loud enough, people will either move away or dismantle it. The hair-trigger of the on switch and the lack of an off switch on Susan's alarm condemn her to constantly re-experience a kind of abandonment. So although the pattern was set in Susan's childhood, the memory of those experiences is not what influences her life; the here-and-now repetition of the pattern of abandonment keeps her fears distressingly current.

At the hospital, we often observe that people with intense attachment anxiety seems to benefit in the moment from a health care provider's attention but can't maintain the resulting feeling of security by themselves when the interaction ends. An inpatient may ring the call bell frequently and visibly relax once the nurse has responded and is providing some reassurance but then start to signal distress again as soon as the interaction is ending. This pattern sets up a bad ending. The nurse feels that the patient is acting as if he is entitled to more of her time than is reasonable; she is frustrated and feels compelled to interrupt and terminate the conversation unilaterally. Her turnaround, as she shifts from reassurance to managing his excessive expectations by asserting her power and distancing herself, reinforces her patient's expectation that the relationships he depends on will always end in rejection or loss.[24] When it is laid bare, it is an awful interaction; one person's anxiety and need prompts another person's hostility and rejection. Naturally, it is a vicious circle. The nurse's distancing serves only to amplify the patient's distress. Health care suffers when we get caught in these unhappy endings.

Susan is angry about a doctor's impatience with her in a previous interaction and describes it in a later conversation with Clay, a social worker. Clay wants to respond but feels he has no choices other than sympathetic collusion ("it's terrible that he treated you that way") or a re-enactment of Susan's victimization ("no wonder he treated you that way, you're so demanding"). He feels a little of both, but neither seems like the right thing to say.[25]

For a person with high attachment anxiety, the primary purpose of expressing any emotion is to maintain interpersonal contact. Anger is often expressed in a way that engages the other person, even if the engagement is not constructive. If Clay chooses to say one of the things that occur to him, he will participate in Susan's angry exchange rather than just hearing about it. Whichever he chooses, his participation will reinforce Susan's sense of injury. Because her narrative is organized this way, Susan maintains contact and engagement by sacrificing any movement towards a constructive resolution. She isn't able to step back from her feelings to being able to talk about them, and so the feelings persist. Her goal is not actually to solve the problem but to maintain her connection to the other person.

Susan has a large social network; she is frequently in touch with many people within her family and her community. Nonetheless, she does not get a lot of support from others. She makes little distinction between an inner circle and more peripheral contacts – from her perspective, everyone is a confidante. At the same time, she frequently feels let down by others and alone. To some extent this perception comes from within – she has a strong sense of need and little capacity to maintain the good feeling that comes from being with others. Truthfully, however, she is difficult to help. Her neediness puts some people off. When she feels that people are backing away, making offers that they can't follow through on, and letting her down, she is often right.

People like Susan with strong attachment anxiety may have many relationships, but their connection to others is full of conflict and tension. When Susan needs to count on people, her intense need to pull them in often leads them to pull back. As a result, she experiences the same self-fulfilling prophecy with friends that she did with her doctor – she expects them to abandon or reject her, and too often they do. Furthermore, a lack of reciprocity can be a problem for Susan. People with high attachment anxiety often find it difficult to provide support to others, and so they are less likely to benefit from the reciprocal nature of helping one another in long-term relationships.[26]

When attachment avoidance interferes with health

Cass has cancer. When he was first diagnosed, he was treated with chemotherapy to kill the cancer cells, which naturally made him feel tired and sick. In his case the chemotherapy killed so many cells that his kidneys were overwhelmed with cellular detritus and shut down, which greatly amplified his fatigue and malaise. Far from complaining about the burden of these symptoms, however, Cass just put up with it. He hadn't been expecting kidney failure as a possibility, and so he didn't question that he was urinating less and feeling worse and worse until he eventually got a fever that wouldn't go away. Even then, he was reluctant to go to the emergency department and "bother them," but his wife insisted, reminding him that they'd been told to look out for a fever, so it was his obligation to go to the hospital.

Cass apologized to the emergency department staff for needing help. He looked good for someone on chemotherapy, so it was surprising when routine tests showed that not only was Cass in kidney failure, but he also had early indications of pneumonia. After he was admitted into the hospital, his condition deteriorated rapidly, and he was soon in the intensive care unit (ICU) receiving dialysis to detoxify his blood and requiring a ventilator to breathe for him.

After the crisis, when Cass was recovering, a student was assigned to interview him to learn about his illness. She found Cass calm and cool. When she asked about how he had felt about his extraordinary time in hospital or about his cancer, he gave brief, polite, straight answers to her questions. It seemed there was very little to say. The conversation was pleasant; in fact, the student felt like she had a clear factual account of his illness by the time they'd finished. If she had been asked to describe Cass as a person, however, and give some sense of what made him tick, she'd have been at a loss.

When attachment avoidance is high and attachment anxiety is low, the attachment system is shut off or muted; proximity seeking is reduced, attachment figures may be considered unimportant, and signs of personal distress or vulnerability are suppressed. Because closeness and dependence cause distress, others may be approached with some level of mistrust, so situations that require dependence, intimacy, or vulnerability are avoided.

In terms of storytelling, when a person like Cass[27] recounts his personal history, it is usually notable for its lack of detail about his inner world and for his apparent lack of curiosity about the inner worlds of others. This is a different kind of incoherent narrative, in which the story makes sense from a distance but lacks the illustrative examples, the nuanced details, and the engaging emotion that would make it feel personal and real. Generalizations dominate over particulars ("I feel like anyone with cancer would") and expressions of emotion are muted. There seems to be little to say, and non-verbal cues ensure that Cass's listeners do not feel invited to enquire more deeply. Cass's narrative may even contradict itself since his words are often used to close off or control the dialogue rather than to accurately express his experience. His goal is not really to communicate but to guard against being perceived as needy or weak.

Cass talks about how his wife, Aileen, is dealing with his disease (actually he just calls her "the wife"). "She is doing pretty well. She's a Scot, you know, tough stock. She looks after the kids except for skating lessons, which I was doing before, so now her sister fills in there. My appointments are not interfering at all so far. I make sure I schedule them so they don't intrude on our routine. I'm sure it is hard on her but she is bearing up."

Although Cass loves his family, his descriptions of interpersonal interactions are not warm. They convey a sense of being scripted or following cultural rules that dictate how people should behave rather than giving the sense of real people interacting.[28]

Although this attachment pattern is based on the expectation that others will be rejecting, unresponsive, or hostile if we need their help, people with high attachment avoidance don't usually express that view. Complaining about how others treat you is like asking them to treat you better, and people like Cass have learned not to ask. Instead, a person with high attachment avoidance is likely to devalue the importance of relationships altogether. He is not usually socially isolated, but his connections to others tend to occur in casual relationships and the relationships that result from occupying a social role (such as co-worker, coach, or classmate). Those are not attachment relationships under most circumstances, which means that Cass tends to hang around with people that he does not need to count on for him to feel secure.

Cass has felt alone for as long as he can remember. His dad was a journeyman, and worked long hours, coming home to crash and recuperate before the next day's long physical labour. Unfortunately, Cass's mother believed his father was having an affair and would harangue him about it the minute he came through the door. Eventually Cass's father stopped protesting that she was wrong and simply refused to respond, at which point she would collapse into bed, sometimes for days at a time. Cass learned to do things for himself. For instance, in elementary school no one made him a lunch, so he located a bakery that would give him food if he swept out the shop.

Despite his impressive independence in those early years, Cass had one unsolvable dilemma: he was unable to tie his shoelaces in a bow because no one had shown him how. This caused problems for him every day because he had to get his shoes off and on again quickly for gym class or risk being teased by his peers. Although Cass had four older brothers, they didn't help; in his family each one looked out for himself.

As Cass saw it he had only two choices. Either he tied his laces in knots and endured the humiliation when he couldn't undo them, or he walked upstairs and awakened Mom to ask her for help. She would tie the laces into bows, but only after she hit him for waking her up. He decided the private injury was preferable to the public one, so he chose to start each day with a blow to his head from his mother.

Not surprisingly, Cass learned to avoid depending on others as much as possible. He rarely acknowledges the feelings of insecurity that lay beneath his seemingly confident public stance. Even when relating the frightening tale of his time in the intensive care unit, he speaks in the same calm, reserved tones.

A person with high attachment avoidance expects that others will be unavailable, unresponsive, ineffective, or rejecting. If that is what you expect, then it makes sense that you will rarely let others know when you are in distress or will rarely ask for their help and prefer to view yourself as competent and independent. As a result a person like Cass misses the health benefits of an integrated support network and strong emotional support.

Since attachment avoidance can be understood as a way that people defend themselves against feelings of insecurity, it makes sense that the more threatened highly avoidant people feel, the more they avoid intimacy. Highly avoidant individuals also tend to be less supportive of their partners as the partners express more intense anxiety – attachment avoidance leads them to shut down in the face of that distress.[29]

While expressions of emotions are often muted, if an exception exists, it is likely to be the expression of anger, which can, after all, be used to keep others at a distance. This expression of anger is very different from that seen in people who are high in attachment anxiety, where anger serves to pull people closer. A related, subtle way to create distance is through the deft use of logical debate, which has the effect of placing the person beyond criticism while limiting reciprocal or intimate communications. Alternatively, like Cass, a person may be simply aloof and inattentive.

As Cass's case illustrates, a person who is high in attachment avoidance may initially seem to present no problems in a health care setting. Independent patients are valuable in an under-resourced health system, and autonomy is a highly valued facet of personality, at least in Western culture. However, effective health care relies on collaboration, which can be undermined by mistrust or impatience with the expertise of professionals. Serious symptoms may be minimized or reported too late, as Cass came close to doing when he stayed at home while his kidneys failed. This determination to do things their way may lead to ignoring treatment suggestions. Whereas a person with high attachment anxiety (and low attachment avoidance) may have trouble ending an appointment, a person with high attachment avoidance (and low attachment anxiety) is more likely to have trouble making the appointment in the first place, may fail to arrive on schedule, or may leave prematurely because he is unwilling to tolerate a delay in the waiting room.

When fearful attachment interferes with health

Attachment insecurity is always a mixture of attachment anxiety and attachment avoidance, even when one of those dimensions predominates. Although Susan has a strong need to count on others and a lack of self-confidence that combine to keep her seeking closeness, all of which are characteristic of attachment anxiety, she is not optimistic about others' behaviour – her default position is that others will disappoint her – which is a stance that is more aligned with attachment avoidance. Similarly, while Cass emphasizes trust in his own abilities and a mistrust of counting on others that leads to distancing, as is characteristic of attachment avoidance, he is also aware of feeling lonely, frightened, and hopeless (especially when he tells the shoelace story), which reveals his underlying attachment anxiety. The reason that Susan and Cass come across so differently is a question of balance – where they ultimately found the best compromise between expressing the distress that they feel or clamming up and distancing themselves from both the feelings and the disappointing attachment figures.

Here is a more sophisticated version of that story of balance. A person has feelings of insecurity, such as fear of abandonment, the expectation of being rejected or punished when found inferior, or the inability to find solace from within (i.e., attachment anxiety). We all struggle with these feelings to some extent, but if they are too intense, we may need to push them away and silence them – which is accomplished by using the strategies that are typical of attachment avoidance, such as avoiding these feelings and the people who can cause them. If these defences prevail, what is visible is attachment avoidance. On the other hand, if the insecure feelings are strong and the avoidant defences are not, what is visible is attachment anxiety. When avoidant defences falter in the face of overwhelming stress, we can see a pattern in which expressions of insecurity or need for others and efforts at distancing or isolation are both evident. That pattern is called *fearful attachment*.[30]

When Joan had breast cancer she was referred to me (Jon) for advice because she felt unable to cope. Joan described how she resisted change in her life. For years she had held a clerical job archiving old files. She worked almost by herself, doing the same thing over and over again. She had mastered that task but was unwilling to try anything new because doing so made her anxious. Similarly, she still lived in the house in which she had grown up. She had nursed her parents through terminal illnesses and then she just stayed on even though it was too big for one person, and it cost more than she could afford to maintain. She had one social contact, a long-standing "friend" whom she actually experienced as a bully. But Joan was unable to assert herself, even over the choice of what movie they should see when they went out each week. She mentioned a boyfriend, but over time it became clear that he lived in another city. Indeed, he was living with another woman and his contact with Joan was limited to email. She was not able to assert her wish to see him in person.

When Joan was diagnosed with breast cancer, she suddenly needed to make many decisions. It was too much for her. Even though her distress was severe enough that her cancer doctor didn't believe that Joan would have the emotional strength to tolerate the necessary medical procedures, Joan had not asked for help. Without some mechanism for getting her support, Joan may simply have stayed at home, worrying about the growing lump in her breast but unable to risk the exposure that she would feel undergoing treatment. Luckily, a team comprising a psychiatrist, a social worker, nurses, and volunteers was able to prescribe support for her that she was able to accept, and she completed her treatments in time.

Like Cass, Joan employs a strategy of using interpersonal distance to reduce distress. However, when both dimensions of attachment insecurity are prominent, as they are for Joan, it leads to isolation. In her unhappy isolation, Joan does not appear confidently independent, as Cass can. Not surprisingly, because fearful attachment is characterized by a push and pull in different directions, different variants occur. One person may appear painfully shy – withdrawn and manifestly unhappy, or concerned but not asking for help, like Joan. Another person may appear perpetually angry, expressing distressing emotions much of the time but at the same time keeping those who might want to help at bay. A third may have a strong preference to *appear* self-reliant but simply be unable to contain her distress when a situation becomes too provocative.[31]

Because two kinds of insecurity are expressed, a person like Joan is likely to tell a story that lacks coherence, but many varieties of incoherence can occur. Lapses in coherence and mentalizing may take a form similar to that found with high attachment anxiety (intense emotion, excess words, multiple fragmented storylines, a lack of logical organization or effort to orient the listener) or like that found with high attachment avoidance (suppressed affect, minimal detail, a close, rigid, and sparse story) or a combination of the two – a mixture with an alternating emphasis that depends on circumstances.

A person with fearful attachment often experiences intense negative emotions and isn't able to regulate these feelings very effectively. Some, like Joan, may over-regulate and suppress difficult emotions or, if the circumstances allow, they may express their feelings in a way that appears exaggerated, such as when a very old grievance is finally aired with an intensity that catches the offending party completely by surprise.

Fearful attachment is particularly important in health care because it is uniquely associated with vulnerability to some health problems. This attachment pattern is associated with the highest rates of medically unexplained symptoms and with the lowest use of health care resources, which suggests an unhappy combination of distress and avoidance of medical help.[32] People with fearful attachment may also give health care providers the greatest interpersonal difficulty during their brief problem-solving interactions, which isn't good for health in the long run.[33]

Disorganized attachment

Disorganized attachment is a separate category that requires mention, even though it is not our primary focus. Each pattern we have described so far is an organized pattern; whether secure or insecure, people with any of these patterns have found the most adaptable balance available to them between expression versus suppression of emotion, and approach versus withdrawal in close relationships. Disorganized attachment finds no such point of balance. In children, disorganized attachment is the result of growing up in an environment of fear with no solution.[34] Imagine a child whose parent is frightening or even abusive. For that child, the person whom all her instincts tell her to turn to for protection and solace is also the person from whom she needs protection. No strategy exists that will allow her to adapt to her environment, and often she has no way to make sense of what she is experiencing. These circumstances lead to unpredictable and sometimes odd behaviour under conditions of stress; children become stuck or undone by fear and helplessness, and they may simply tune out and appear dazed rather than acting when they are afraid.[35] In adults with disorganized attachment, we see signs that they have never been able to resolve old traumas or losses. These may be subtle – as when a person who otherwise looks like they fit into one of the patterns of organized attachment becomes dissociated or overwhelmed by memories of trauma – or they may be dramatic, as occurs in the chaotic, unstable expressions of affect and interpersonal connection that are seen in some psychiatric conditions, such as borderline personality disorder. Karlen Lyons-Ruth defines adult disorganized attachment as including at least one of (1) inconsistent attitudes towards attachment figures, such as both devaluing and identifying with a hostile or helpless parent; (2) inconsistent use of both dismissing and preoccupied strategies; and (3) pervasive narrative incoherence.[36]

Unresolved trauma and disorganized attachment increase the risk of mental health problems substantially and have similarly potent effects on physical health and on the challenge of providing good health care. We de-emphasize this category in this book not because it is unimportant (it is very important), but because it is special. Our goal is to help health care professionals to provide personalized care for all patients; focusing our attention on those with the most extreme challenges would lead us towards a primer on mental health care, which is a narrower topic.[37]

Insecure attachment is not a disorder

Because we are paying close attention to the ways that insecure attachment can compromise and complicate health, it bears emphasizing that attachment is a theory of normal psychology – everybody has a pattern of attachment. Secure patterns are the statistical norm but not by much; about 60% of adults have a secure pattern of attachment.[38] Insecure patterns are not uniformly harmful – understood developmentally, they are the best relational style that is available to an individual under the circumstances of his or her upbringing. Insecure attachment is a compromise position, a trade-off between maintaining necessary relationships and minimizing problems that occur in those relationships. When we look across cultures, the consensus is that secure attachment is the most desirable position, but which variety of insecure pattern is favoured depends more on cultural values.[39] In Western cultures many aspects of attachment avoidance are valued and promoted – the archetype of the lone, tough, self-reliant drifter is a favourite movie character, and the idea that you can count on no one but yourself is often taken to be true.

Each of these perspectives, epidemiological, developmental, evolutionary, and cultural, supports the position that pathologizing attachment insecurity is unwise. Although insecurity increases health risks and the complexity of health care, it is not, in itself, a medical problem.

A quick approach to identifying patterns of attachment

The quickest way for an individual to identify his or her predominant pattern of attachment is to answer the questions in a standard survey. Several questionnaires have been found to produce accurate results.[40] We recommend that before you read further, you identify your own attachment style online here: http://www.web-research-design.net/cgi-bin/crq/crq.pl.[41]

The results of this survey will classify you into one of four types that correspond to the patterns of attachment discussed in this book: secure (low in both attachment anxiety and attachment avoidance), fearful (high in both attachment anxiety and attachment avoidance); preoccupied (high in attachment anxiety, low in attachment avoidance) or dismissing (low in attachment anxiety, high in attachment avoidance).

Feeling secure is good for you

In the remainder of Section Two, we are going to describe how understanding attachment illuminates the problems that we have called vexing health care and provides opportunities to personalize health care to reduce suffering and disease.

Susan has high attachment anxiety and low attachment avoidance. She is preoccupied with fear and a perpetual lack of comfort. Even when she has no disease, she experiences disturbing symptoms. She turns to over-the-counter drugs to calm herself, but they cause other symptoms, which creates more worry. She does not have many friends because people feel overwhelmed by the intensity of her need after a while and give up. She attempts to find closeness by entering into sexual relationships, but these are motivated by neediness and so are often impulsive, which has led to sexually transmitted infections, unsafe interactions with unpleasant men, loneliness, and self-blame.

Susan's over-exercised stress machinery increases her risk of certain illnesses. To complicate matters, her intense and usually unwarranted concern over her health has trained her doctors to under-react to her symptoms.

Taken together, these difficulties set Susan up to believe she is sick when she is not, to be vulnerable to stress-related diseases, and to have serious diseases treated poorly and late.

Susan's intense insecurity illuminates five paths by which insecure attachment interferes with good health.[42]

- Insecure attachment interferes with our bodies' ability to effectively regulate our stress-response systems.
- Insecure attachment promotes behaviours that increase the risk of getting sick, such as smoking and excessive use of non-prescription drugs.
- Insecure attachment promotes behaviour that interferes with effective health care, such as exaggerating symptoms or avoiding health care.
- Insecure attachment interferes with the health-promoting benefits of social support.
- Insecure attachment feeds into a vicious cycle of depression and disease risk.

Before discussing each of these paths, we need to take a short detour to address two questions that relate to basic assumptions of the model we are supporting.

Question 1: On average, how much worse is any particular risk factor for disease in a person with insecure attachment compared with a person with secure attachment?

Answer: Not much.

Question 2: So then, why should we care?

The power of a weak force

A dandelion, if its seed finds its way into just the right spot, can grow through concrete. A drip of water, if it persists, can carve a path through stone. All the evidence we have seen over our years studying attachment suggests that insecure attachment, like a dandelion or a drop of water, is a fairly weak force each time it acts to increase the risk of illness. Any model that attempts to link attachment to illness needs to explain how this weak force can have a large impact.

From an evolutionary perspective, it makes a great deal of sense that insecure attachment makes no more than a weak contribution to illness. Since about 40% of all human beings have insecure attachment, we would not survive as a species if this trait were a strong risk factor for serious illness. And yet our gene pool is full of variants that cause disease. Detrimental traits are preserved if they emerge at an age when they have no effect on reproductive success (e.g., genes that contribute to Alzheimer's disease), when they have been advantageous during most of our prehistory and have only recently become detrimental (e.g., genes for stress-related illnesses),[43] or when some balance exists between the gene's survival benefits and its costs (e.g., sickle-cell anemia).

In the case of insecure attachment, we should be clear that insecure patterns are generally advantageous. Insecure attachment is an adaptive response to a stressful developmental environment, which amounts to the best possible solution to some parent-child-environment mixes.[44] Humans are born with a highly developed capacity to adapt flexibly to a variety of environmental conditions, and insecure attachment is one consequence of that adaptive capacity. Having a variety of patterns of attachment present within our species increases our ability to adapt to diverse environments. Most of the serious health effects of insecure attachment also occur later in life, when they are unlikely to have much impact on reproductive success. A weak force needs time for its effects to accumulate, but given the increase in lifespan over history, we now have plenty of time in which to feel those effects.

How a weak force can have a big impact

Just because a force is weak does not mean its consequences are small. One way that its consequences grow is by working over a long time, like a constant drip of water that carves a path through stone over decades. Another is when the force's effects are multiplied because it affects many components of a system. Insecure attachment works in both of these ways.[45] This is one of the essential arguments that we are putting forth for the relevance of insecure attachment to public health. Insecure attachment is a weak force when it acts on any particular disease or any particular individual. But it exerts a powerful influence on society because it is very common, it acts over an entire lifetime, and its adverse effects are relevant to the most common causes of illness and death (including diabetes, cardiovascular diseases, and inflammatory diseases), the most common non-disease-related uses of the health care system (medically unexplained symptoms), and the most common

Figure 6.1 Paths by which a secure pattern of attachment reduces the risk and burden of illness and disease

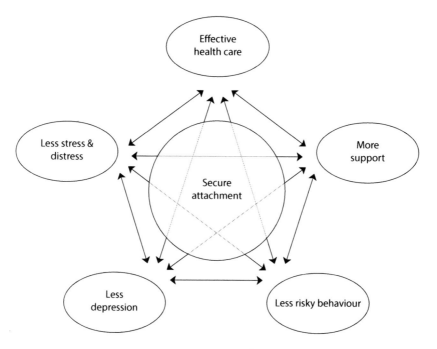

psychiatric illnesses (depression and anxiety disorders), which in turn contribute to reduced physical health.[46]

The other essential argument, which we are going to expand on in the remainder of this section, is that insecure attachment is an important force because it acts on so many of the determinants of health – if it doesn't get you one way, it will get you another. We provided a list of the main paths from insecure attachment to illness and disease as they relate to Susan. We finish with that list reframed more positively in Figure 6.1 as the five paths by which secure attachment contributes to health. The figure is designed to convey how tightly each of these paths is related to the others, but for the sake of clarity we will review them separately.

7 Depression

Our patients sometimes talk about *clinical depression*. Clinical depression isn't an official diagnostic term, but it serves a useful purpose. It distinguishes the disease, depression, from something more common – the mild, temporary, and normal low mood that often goes by the same name. Major depression, which is the official term, is a serious problem, leading many people to have a pervasive sense of emptiness, fatigue, lost purpose and motivation, diminished appetite, poor sleep, excessive guilt, and thoughts that the world would be a better place without them in it. Major depression is very common, affecting about 15% of people over their lives. Beyond its effects on attitudes and emotions, major depression makes a very substantial contribution to physical illness, suffering, and early death.

Three months after being hospitalized for a heart attack, Barbara attends cardiac rehab regularly. The section of heart muscle that died from lack of oxygen was small – but any such event is serious. She's dragging a bit now and reports that she finds it tough to get up and face the day. Her rehabilitation therapist is struck by the shift in her demeanour. Barbara's capacity to roll with the punches and adjust to challenges has been impressive, but now she looks like someone who is struggling rather than someone who is going to take this major health change in stride.

When the rehabilitation therapist asks how she is doing, Barbara acknowledges that she's disappointed in herself. Her parents both had heart disease at about her current age, and she had really believed she wouldn't follow the same path. Barbara has been thinking that she failed to prevent her own heart attack, that there must have been something else she could have done. She is oversleeping now, and sometimes wakes up tired, not seeing the point of trying to get up and follow her usual schedule. She really isn't sure that the future holds much hope for her having a rewarding life.

The rehabilitation therapist, concerned about this change, reassures Barbara that, in fact, she's done very well with her lifestyle and that her progress in rehab is great. In fact, she tells Barbara, this small heart attack may have served as an alarm, one that has allowed her to protect herself better in the future. Barbara smiles at her, appreciating the kind words, but her face quickly settles back into a forlorn expression.

Barbara has a secure attachment style, which gives her a leg up on dealing with depression quickly and effectively (although it does not make her immune to becoming depressed). Nonetheless, her rehabilitation therapist is right to be concerned. Barbara is experiencing the double challenge of the heart attack and then the depression, and she can't deal with them separately because they affect each other. Being depressed makes it harder to find the energy and the motivation for her rehab program and harder to remember to take her medication. When she is tired, she isn't sure why, since heart disease and depression both reduce her energy. To make matters worse, her depression tends to lead her to self-blaming explanations, such as that the real problem is that she is lazy. Not only does the combination of disease and depression interfere with her ability to function, but it also leads her to suffer more.[1] From a public health perspective, the combination of physical disease and depression is also very costly – it is a strong factor driving health care costs upward.[2]

Barbara's risk of major complications from coronary artery disease, including dying in the next few years, is almost doubled because of her depression. For those who are depressed in addition to having another serious disease, depression increases the severity of physical symptoms, makes treatment less effective, and increases mortality.[3] These consequences are true for many diseases, not just heart disease. The negative impact of depression on the costs of being sick is very significant.

Barbara is not alone in her situation by any means. Having a serious illness makes it much more likely that a person will become depressed. In fact, people who have a major physical illness are about twice as likely as those who are not ill to develop a new diagnosis of depression. The incentive is strong to recognize and cure the depression in people who have a combination of diagnoses.

Why does having major depression make such a large impact on disease, in terms of both suffering and medical outcomes? It is thought to work in many ways. Behaviourally, experiencing major depression may lead people to withdraw from life and to perceive things through a lens that filters out optimism, pleasure, and the ability to put things in perspective. This behaviour may make the experience of symptoms like pain and fatigue more intense. As well, the symptoms of depression include suppressed appetite, poor sleep, loss of sex drive, and fatigue, so depression can amplify symptoms that are already occurring because of physical disease. Being depressed also makes it harder for people to collaborate and participate in their treatment. It is harder to remember to take medications and to find the will and energy to attend appointments. Finally, the antidepressant medications that are used to treat the depression may cause problems with the other illness by adding to side effects.[4]

Since major depression can make having a disease worse in so many ways, it may not be surprising that being depressed also increases the risk that an otherwise healthy person will become physically ill. The evidence is particularly strong regarding disease of the heart and blood vessels. Among otherwise healthy people, being depressed increases the risk of developing coronary artery disease by somewhere between 50% and 100% and also doubles seven-year mortality.[5]

A little depression goes a long way

When the rehabilitation therapist sees Barbara again 10 days later, she finds her much as she was when she was at the start of rehab – a willing and capable narrator of her story. She details how her "blahs" have developed over the time since her MI, and although she is oversleeping, tired, and struggling with motivation, she tells the therapist that their last conversation was on a particularly bad day. Most days she is getting up, even though it's a struggle, and she is adamant about her faithful adherence to the rehabilitation program.

Barbara does find herself thrown off by various aches and pains – especially when she feels a twinge in her chest or arm, which feels like the first symptoms of the heart attack. At those times she has to work to regain a sense of being okay. She might call her family doctor, with whom she has a long-standing trusting relationship, to be reassured that she can let the symptom go without further investigation. She has some bad days, but feels like she's on the rebound now.

When we take a detailed look at how depression plays out in the lives of real people, we find that life does not fit neatly into compartmentalized pigeon-holes, such as the categories of depressed and not depressed. An important intermediate case exists in which a person experiences quite a few depressive symptoms but is not impaired enough to warrant a diagnosis of major depression. This situation goes by several names, but a useful one for our purposes is minor depression, which is a very common phenomenon, especially among older people. In one survey of people over the age of 60, 28% had major depression and 46% had minor depression, a shocking number,[6] especially because people with minor depression tend to have more health problems and to be more disabled than those who have no depression at all.[7]

Barbara appears to have minor depression. It will be valuable for her, both now and in the future course of her illness, that it has been recognized and she is getting the help she needs, because minor depression may have a major impact on the complications of heart disease. In fact, several studies have found that negative emotions in general are associated with increased cardiac mortality.[8] Even more commonly, minor depression reduces quality of life and increases health care costs because of more frequent symptoms and more medical visits and tests. Very often, after all the tests have been done, the cause of these physical symptoms remains unexplained.

Insecure attachment and depression

John Bowlby, the originator of attachment theory, predicted that attachment would be linked to depression. For example, when a parent dies when a child is still young, Bowlby expected the loss of a primary caregiver to be a fundamental challenge to the child's ability to maintain a sense of security. A child who has lost a parent has no control over the loss and may have little control over subsequent events. This lack of control can cause despair and lead the child to develop a belief that he is helpless to alter or respond effectively to traumatic events. An enduring belief in our helplessness to respond to adversity is a set-up for depression later in life.

The facts support this prediction. A study of girls whose mothers died before the girls were 11 years old found they were three times as likely to develop depression later in life as girls who did not experience that loss.[9] That is a huge difference in risk, and we have no reason to think it would be different in boys. The impact of a child being separated from a living parent may have an even greater effect than parental death.[10] Knowing that children in this circumstance can be helped is reassuring – the evidence also shows that a parent's death may have little or no damaging effects if the quality of the relationship with the surviving parent is good enough.[11]

Cass felt alone as a child. His dad was usually either away at work or asleep. His mother was often depressed, sometimes in bed for days at a time, and never up in the morning when he prepared for school. Although he became a self-reliant adult, he was prone to feeling depressed when illness interfered with his ability to look after himself.

Some of the parental behaviours and attitudes that contribute to insecure patterns of attachment also increase the risk for depression. For example, growing up with an emotionally unavailable parent increases the risk of depression. Similarly to the child whose parent dies, a child who repeatedly tries and fails to establish a secure attachment with a parent may develop a sense of himself as a failure. Cass was experiencing *learned helplessness*, in which repeated experiences of having no control over adverse events lead a person to stop trying, even when the situation changes such that more control is available. When animals used in experiments are trained to adopt a position of helplessness, it predictably leads to a state that looks very much like major depression (both with respect to their behaviour and to the changes in brain and bodily function that accompany major depression).[12] The reason that learned helplessness leads to depression is not the bad experience itself; the lack of control over it is the problem.

Early experiences of loss and dyscontrol can lead children to have low self-esteem, anxiety, negative moods, and discipline problems during adolescence. Each of these increases the risk of depression. A parent who consistently gives a child the message that she is incompetent or unlovable will impair his child's self-esteem and may cause her to have an exaggerated drive to be perfect to win her parent's love. Perfectionism is another path to depression. Not surprisingly, patterns of low self-esteem, a lack of confidence in the ability to effect change, and perfectionism, which are known to increase a person's lifetime risk of depression, are also core components of insecure patterns of attachment.[13] Overall, having an emotionally unavailable parent is as reliable a predictor of depression later in life as experiencing a parent's death early in life.

Insecurity also contributes to depression by increasing the amount of stress in our lives, but that topic deserves a full discussion all to itself, so we will leave it for the next chapter. Overall, little doubt remains that patterns of attachment are one of the more important factors that distinguish the 15% of us who will become depressed at some time in our lives from those who will not.[14]

The link between attachment and depression may be even more fundamental. In 1952, James Robertson, a social worker colleague of John Bowlby, brought a movie camera to work to record what was happening during routine hospitalizations of children at that time. *A Two-Year-Old Goes to Hospital* documented the distress of an independent and mature young girl named Laura who spent eight days in hospital for minor surgery.[15] Although Laura contains her feelings much more effectively than most children her age, most people cannot watch the film without feeling heartache and wanting to help as she protests for several days ("Don't like it. I want my Mommy") and then resigns herself to the situation, becoming unexpressive, self-contained, and cautious. One of Robertson's points was that Laura's settling after a few days in hospital was not a good adjustment but the result of despair and giving up.

Depression involves several processes that are triggered when an infant like Laura, who is separated from her parents, moves from "protest" to "despair."[16] The purpose of this shift is to shut down separation distress, which is unsustainable over long periods. In the environment in which these processes evolved, sustained separation distress would quickly lead to death either because the sustained crying would attract predators or because the intense physiological arousal that accompanies the protest phase would lead to exhaustion. So there needs to be a mechanism to shut it down after a time if reunion with the parent is not forthcoming. This process of shutting down is the despair that Robertson captured in his film of Laura. Of course, the shutdown process also needs to be self-correcting after a while. If this is right, then the questions we need to ask about depression are not why it occurs, but what circumstances trigger a process that was built into the system to regulate separation distress, and why this process sometimes fails to self-correct when it is no longer useful. Understanding attachment helps us to understand the former question. The answer to the latter question just isn't known yet.

Overall, insecure attachment and depression are closely linked. If we consider them separate entities, as an epidemiologist might, then we would say that insecure attachment is a risk factor for depression.

If we consider their antecedents, as a developmental psychologist would, we would say they are each, in part, consequences of similar challenges and deficits in developmental experience. If we observe the behaviour of vulnerable individuals whose attachment system is strongly challenged, as James Robertson did, we could go further and suggest that depression is, in part, a biological and behavioural variant of normal attachment behaviour – the consequence of an attachment system that finds itself helpless to obtain its intended goal of mobilizing the relationships that are required to feel secure. And the impact is clear: depressive symptoms are consistently linked to illness, each making the other worse.

A caveat and an intriguing question for the future

What we have discussed in this chapter tells a clear story of an infinite loop: serious illness increases the risk of depression; depression increases the risk of serious illness, disease, and death. It seems obvious that identifying and treating depression in people with medical illness is important not only to improve their quality of life but also to improve their long-term health prospects. This outcome should be especially true for people with cardiovascular disease where the evidence for these links is strongest.

So it is more than a little bit perplexing and frustrating that large-scale studies of the impact of identifying and treating depression in people with heart disease have found that treating depression has *not* improved cardiac outcomes. These studies have examined treating depression with either antidepressant drugs (sertraline or citalopram) or with short-term psychotherapy (cognitive-behavioural therapy or interpersonal psychotherapy), interventions that are well established to be effective treatments for depression. In these studies, the treatments for depression have succeeded in reducing depression as expected, but the reduction in depression hasn't had the expected impact on improving the prognosis of heart disease.[17]

Several possible explanations have been suggested, especially that it would take even larger studies to demonstrate a statistically significant finding. This explanation contains a discouraging implication: the effect of depression on cardiac outcome is strong, but the effect of treatment is weak. In our current research, we are pursuing a different explanation: maybe depression is not the *cause* of poor cardiac outcomes; it is just a marker of people who have poor cardiac outcomes for a different reason. Not surprisingly, we think that having depressive symptoms is a marker for insecure attachment. In this hypothesis, insecure attachment contributes to depression and, separately, insecure attachment contributes to cardiac risk. Some physical effects of insecure attachment that could have this effect – such as disturbances in the regulation of the autonomic nervous system (ANS) – are not necessarily a part of depression. At this point this is an unproven hypothesis – it is an intriguing question with big implications. If the hypothesis is true, then we need to do more than treat depression in people who have heart attacks. We need to do something that helps them with the broader impact of insecure attachment. That would be a major step towards fully personalized health care.

8 Attachment Is a Response to Stress

In Chapter 5 we talked about how Carol's focused, responsive attention to Tyler was helping him to identify and distinguish inner states and perceptions of himself and his mother. In the process, Carol was helping Tyler to learn to mentalize and to develop a secure pattern of attachment. Now, we want to expand on that idea to see how the very same interactions help Tyler to manage arousal and stress, both moment by moment and throughout his life. First, recall the type of interaction.

Four-month-old Tyler coos at his mother, Carol, and she coos back. He flashes a broad smile and she smiles back with an exaggerated happy face. He starts to giggle and makes a louder noise, and she makes a little raspberry sound back that startles him. He looks away and gets quiet. When he looks back, Carol is waiting for his gaze and gently smiles at him again.

If we monitored Tyler's heart rate, we could watch it rise and fall while he interacts with his mother. When Carol engages him in something interesting, his heart rate rises, as she did when mirroring and amplifying his expressions, which made him giggle and gesture. When she goes a bit too far for him (startling him with a raspberry), he experiences an even greater intensity of excitement, enough that he needs to look away and calm down. At various points in their play, Carol helps him to reduce his level of arousal either because it has become uncomfortably intense or just to help him to calmly enjoy quiet play. She does this in several ways. She holds him gently but securely on her lap, which is calming. Tyler is also calmed by the familiar rhythm in their communication, and by Carol gently rocking him and saying soft things. Very importantly, Carol respects Tyler's signal when he needs to interrupt their interaction by looking away. When he does this, it would be distressing to him if Carol were to try to override his need to disconnect by forcing her face into his averted field of vision or demanding his attention in some other way. Instead, Carol collaborates with Tyler in regulating his level of stimulation by respecting his signal that he needs to calm down and regroup on his own.

While Carol helps Tyler to regulate his level of excitement up and down within comfortable limits, Tyler's brain is making connections between the part of the cortex that is destined to become specialized for social functions (such as recognizing faces, intuiting others' mental states, and distinguishing between inner and outer phenomena) and the parts that are specialized for controlling arousal and distress. Over hundreds of interactions like this one, Carol is teaching Tyler to be an expert at using the social parts of his brain to calm his body down. The most important part of that equipment for Tyler during this interaction with his mother is his vagus nerve.

The vagus nerve is the powerful brake on physiological excitement that we discussed in Chapter 2. This brake allows for highly flexible fine-tuning of states of arousal because it works very fast – in thousandths of a second. In Tyler's heart, for example, the vagal brake slows his heart rate very efficiently. The function of the vagal brake is crucial for health. For example, our ability to slow our hearts efficiently after exercise, which is a mark of healthy vagal function, is a strong indicator of cardiovascular health and a predictor of longevity.

Carol's arousing and soothing behaviours maintain Tyler's level of attention within a comfortable range. Too little interaction and he will be distressed by boredom or isolation. Too much and he will be overwhelmed or frightened. Carol is acting as an external regulator of Tyler's nervous system. As she does this she is programming Tyler's vagal brake to finely tune the intensity of arousal he experiences. Under these conditions of optimal stimulation, Tyler is able to play, which means to explore and learn. On the other side of the interaction, while Tyler is enjoying the Goldilocks zone of neither too much excitement nor too little, Carol receives useful and subtle cues about what he is thinking and feeling, because his face is very expressive when he is in this zone (compared with when he is falling asleep or crying, when his facial expressions are not at all subtle and convey a much smaller amount of information about his inner state). In this way, Tyler's vagal brake is not only responding to social communication but also contributing to the quality of that interaction. This mutual influence between interpersonal interactions and vagal control of arousal continues to be important throughout our lives because we use our vagal brake to hone our alert attention to others (foot off the brake) and to pause and reflect on what is happening (foot on the brake).[1]

Jia is a young woman who had just heard from her family doctor that she had brain metastases from breast cancer, the outcome she feared more than any other. As she sat talking to the clinic's nurse-clinician, sharing her distress and wondering when she would hear from her oncologist about the next steps, her cell phone went off in her pocket. The ring and vibration together caused Jia to startle so much that she actually leaped to her feet. Before she became fully upright she had already started to recalibrate. Her frightened facial expression shifted into a self-mocking rolling of her eyes.

The area of Jia's brain that responds automatically to possible danger[2] was on high alert because she had so recently received news of a serious threat to her well-being, which caused her exaggerated startle. The areas of her brain that allow for reflection and re-evaluation[3] then worked as quickly as they could to allow her to right herself. Someone with insecure attachment will need a little longer to right herself in this situation; the fact that Jia recalibrated this quickly suggests that she had an upbringing with a parent like Carol.

The very same interactions between Carol and Tyler that foster the development of secure attachment also train his vagus nerve to be an efficient brake on overstimulation. These same interactions teach Tyler to mentalize and help him to develop the capacity to delay gratification.[4] We have illustrated this fantastic cluster of social skills, which all depend on early life interactions, in Figure 8.1.

How does insecure attachment increase the impact of stress?

When we first described hidden determinants of health in Chapter 2, we distinguished stressors, which are the environmental events that threaten us, from our appraisal of these events and from the biological and psychological ways in which we respond to a perceived threat. Insecure patterns of attachment influence each of these three components: increasing the number of stressors that are experienced, biasing appraisal towards interpreting events as threatening, and altering the body's response to stressors. This section is concerned with the way that this outcome occurs, the variations in these processes that relate to different attachment styles, and the impact of these processes on health.

Figure 8.1 Four related benefits of parenting that is reciprocal, responsive, consistent, attuned, and not too scary

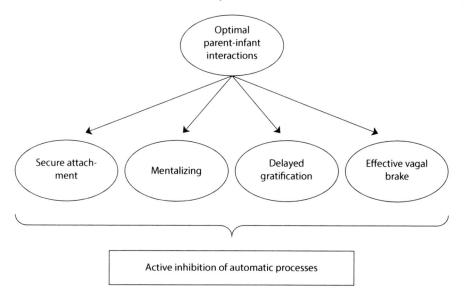

The reason that secure attachment, a well-developed capacity to mentalize and reflect, a well-developed capacity to use the vagal brake to calm down, and the capacity to put off immediate gratification of desires are related is that they are all developed and reinforced by the same experiences of reciprocal interactions in early life. These skills are not a random assortment of cognitive, physiological, and psychological capacities – they all rely on brain centres that actively work to inhibit automatic reactions: to pause, slow down, reconsider, and reflect.

Secure attachment reduces the impact of stress on our bodies in several ways. Figure 8.2 summarizes how processes associated with secure attachment – that is, mentalizing, the vagal brake on arousal and the ability to delay gratification – all contribute to a lesser impact of life stress.

One hallmark of our species is that we adapt very well to a wide range of conditions by having an efficient basic mechanism that can be easily programmed by local environments. So although the machinery of the body's systems that detect danger and respond to stress is essentially the same in all humans, important differences exist from one individual to the next in how the equipment ultimately works. Individual differences in stress reactivity therefore arise from genes, from the environment, and from the interaction between the two.

Figure 8.2 The corollaries of Figure 8.1: Capacities that tend to coexist with a secure pattern of attachment

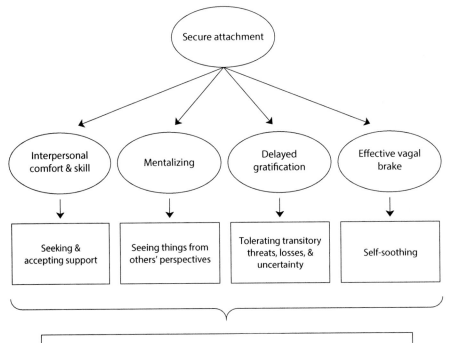

Because secure attachment results from the same processes that also lead to the other capacities detailed in Figure 8.1, it follows that when we identify a person with secure attachment, we are also usually identifying a person with a wide repertoire of characteristics and skills that reduce the occurrence and impact of stress in his or her life.

How we learn from early exposure to stress

The most obvious link between environmental conditions and the stress response is that persistently being exposed to stressful conditions during early childhood tends to result in greater reactivity to stress later in life.[5] This connection makes sense; someone who grows up in a high-stress environment is more likely to survive if she recognizes possible threats very quickly. Setting a low threshold to detect threats allows for quick detection, but it does so at a cost. The resulting danger detector is very sensitive and therefore overreacts (recurrent red alert) or never quite turns off (perpetual orange alert).

So we may imagine that exposure to early childhood stress amplifies subsequent stress reactivity, and its complement, optimal parental contact, reduces subsequent stress reactivity. Although that idea is appealing, the actual situation is quite a bit more complex. For one thing, a low-stress environment may also predispose a child to be highly reactive to stress. Since this is counter-intuitive, it requires some explanation.

Jesse is a creative child, always telling little stories, painting wild abstracts, and turning common objects into puppets and props in spontaneous mini-dramas. She is also fussy, sensitive to loud noises, feeling too cold or too hot, or itchy, or bothered to distraction by the feel of the tag of her shirt against her skin.

Syed is happy anywhere. He loves to play games with other kids, especially familiar ones. His paintings at daycare tend to be conventional – he looks at what the other kids are painting and makes something similar – but he enjoys making them. He likes his lunch, without being too concerned about what is served.

Thomas Boyce and Bruce Ellis argue that the survival of our species is best served if our numbers include people with a variety of patterns of stress response.[6] Since environmental conditions differ and change, a species is more likely to survive if it has a well-diversified portfolio of stress response patterns. In particular, two patterns that have been retained over evolution are found in the types of children who can be called *orchids* and *dandelions*. Orchids, like Jesse, are highly sensitive to their environment. They flourish and bloom in a supportive environment, but they are not robust in the face of adversity. Dandelions, like Syed, are more robust in an adverse environment but also less likely to bloom extravagantly in a highly nurturing environment.

Our species gains valuable diversity by retaining genes that produce both kinds of individuals: the orchids who are highly responsive to their environments and the dandelions who are more robust but less responsive. Here is an intriguing twist: Boyce and Ellis think that sensitivity to the environment is essentially the same thing as stress reactivity (i.e., creative sensitivity to a rich, pleasant environment and stressful sensitivity to an adverse environment hinge on the same low threshold

Figure 8.3 The U-shaped curve that links early environmental conditions to stress reactivity later in life

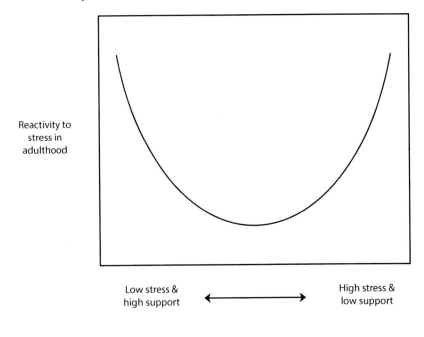

to stimulation). An invigorating attunement to the environment and sensitivity to its riches is the gift that an orchid experiences under conditions that are protective and supportive. Since that sensitivity is the same thing as being highly responsive to stress, Jesse may lack resilience in aversive conditions.

The orchids and dandelions argument is essentially about temperament – the genes that determine our personalities at birth. An analogous argument can be made about the effect of various environments on developing children. We already know that low-support/high-stress environments contribute to amplified stress reactivity. The odd fact that highly supportive/low-stress environments also promote high stress reactivity makes sense if we believe that high sensitivity to the environment and high stress reactivity are the same thing. In that case, a highly supportive, low-stress environment may tend to bring out the orchid in a child, so to speak. That means that under those circumstances, the sensitivity of the plasticity of our bodies' stress-response systems increases to optimize the benefits that can be obtained from the rich, supportive environment. If this sensitivity persists, the orchid nature that a low-stress/high-support early environment promotes will lead to high stress reactivity later in life.

If this idea is true, there should be a U-shaped relationship between a person's current stress reactivity and the stressfulness/stability of his or her early environment, with high reactivity at both extremes of early environment. Indeed, Boyce and Ellis measured how stress affects heart-rate variability in preschool kids and found the predicted curve.

Attachment and stress

Sian and Tracey are veteran paramedics. Dealing with medical emergencies and with scared people is their job, and they are usually not as stressed by these challenging experiences as others might imagine. It takes a certain kind of person to choose a career as a first responder to emergencies, a person who likes to help others but who does it with a thick skin (it is a career for a dandelion, not for an orchid). They act independently, think quickly on their feet, get the job done, and are not too concerned with the "touchy-feely" side of things. Like many paramedics, Sian and Tracey each have an interpersonal style that leans towards attachment avoidance. They are professionals who are well suited to their work.

One particular call for Sian and Tracey was more troublesome than usual. They arrived at a house to find an adult and a child both dead in the front hall. It wasn't clear what had happened but it was obvious that they had been dead for quite a few hours. Before they left the scene, the television cameras were already there.

Sian and Tracey call this a "critical incident," not because it was medically complicated (there was actually very little for them to do) but because it was emotionally troubling. Critical incidents tend to have certain characteristics that provoke strong emotional reactions, and this call had several of those red flags. That they could do nothing because it was too late to change the outcome was part of the trouble. True helplessness is very provocative for people who have chosen a career where quick, effective action can save lives. The fact that a child died is another red flag. Media scrutiny, a situation completely beyond their control, and a very bad outcome all combined to make this a call that Tracey and Sian would rather forget but wouldn't be likely to.

Sian and Tracey each had an uneasy evening and a bad night's sleep, and both were glad that the critical incident occurred on their last shift before a stretch of days off. Subsequently, however, things were different for them. Sian came back to work after a few days, more or less back to her usual self. The incident still troubled her but she was sleeping, interacting with her buddies and her family as usual, and focused on the job at hand. Tracey was still suffering. Her nights were still restless, she was irritable and snapping at her partner, and eating by herself at break instead of joining with her co-workers as was her usual habit. Why did the critical incident affect Sian and Tracey differently and what difference could that make for them in the long run?

Patterns of attachment provide part of the answer to the question of why some people are more prone to stress than others. Hans Selye, a pioneer of stress research, emphasized the importance of the response rather than the stimulus: "Stress is not so much what happens to you as how you take it."[7] Remember in Chapter 2 we described the intricate autonomic and hormonal *neurosymphony* that constitutes the human stress response.[8]

If Sian and Tracey had been wired to heart-rate monitors when they entered the grisly scene of their critical incident, the monitors would have shown that both paramedics experienced a surge in heart rate as they assessed the situation and tried to figure out what they could do. Sian's pounding heart returned to her usual 75 beats per minute as they were gathering up their equipment to leave the scene. Tracey would have looked about the same to anyone who was observing her, but her heart was still beating quickly even as they drove back to the ambulance station.

Resilient people are able to activate their stress response very quickly and shut it down quickly, in the pattern that we have called *spiky*. This ability to recover quickly is tied in with the ways that we relate to other people. Firefighters who report that they receive lots of support from others around them, for example, have a more intense cardiovascular response to stress and faster resolution of this stress response when the stressor has ceased – nice and spiky.[9] The link between secure attachment and vagal regulation of arousal explains why toddlers with secure attachment experience a spiky elevation in heart rate during the separation phase of the strange situation, with efficient recovery afterward, whereas toddlers with insecure attachment have a more sluggish recovery from tachycardia.[10] The same thing also occurs in adults: insecurity leads to a higher heart-rate response to stress[11] and less activity of the vagal brake on arousal.[12]

What is the connection between attachment insecurity and stress?

Attachment, as a system that organizes a dynamic connection between an infant and her care provider, is a defence system. Humans have several defence systems and they are all connected:

- Our skin and the lining of our digestive tract and respiratory system prevent unwanted foreign things from getting inside our bodies.
- Our immune system kills the foreign things that do manage to penetrate the barricades along our outer surfaces.
- Our stress systems (both the autonomic nervous system and the hypothalamic-pituitary-adrenal system) allow us to respond to environmental events with adaptive behaviours and a metabolism that suits the circumstances.

Since each of the defence systems communicates with and influences the others, it should not be a great surprise that the attachment system is also a part of this team and thus a highly connected member of our defence consortium.

One of the direct connections between the attachment system and the stress-response systems is that attachment events often signal danger and thus trigger a stress response. A second type of connection between attachment and stress systems is that attachment relationships may make an infant feel more secure and thus reduce the likelihood that an environmental event will be taken to signal danger.

Rhea and Les are twins. Rhea is playing by herself in the sandbox in their backyard. Les is on the side of the house digging in the garden with their mother. When a nearby car's horn blares unexpectedly, Rhea makes a startled little scream and cries, but Les is unperturbed. Les is just as susceptible to feel startled and afraid as Rhea is, but in this instance he is protected by being near his mom.

A third, less direct connection is that a secure attachment style makes it easier to have the kind of relationships with other people that are likely to provide a buffer against stress and help with coping. A fourth connection between attachment and stress response was illustrated by Carol and Tyler – interactions between parents, infants, and their larger environment during early development have a lasting influence on the connections between brain systems that regulate fear and our response to danger.

Since the attachment system is focused on detecting danger, people with insecure attachment unsurprisingly perceive threats more often – they have very long and sensitive antennae. Attachment anxiety, in particular, is all about not feeling secure on our own and responding to this challenge by amplifying the signs of distress that draw others near – feeling threatened and saying so is a core part of this style. A lot of evidence suggests that attachment anxiety is linked to high levels of perceived stress. For example, among Israelis living in areas targeted for missile attacks during the Gulf War, those with high attachment anxiety experienced more anxiety, more hostility, and more physical symptoms.[13] Under more controlled conditions, such as healthy people responding to standardized stresses in a laboratory, attachment anxiety is strongly linked to the intensity of distress that is perceived and reported.[14] As we see with Tracey, attachment avoidance also increases physiological vulnerability to stress, even in the absence of attachment anxiety.[15]

Although Sian and Tracey both tend to be avoidant of dependency and emotional vulnerability, Sian is closer to the secure end of the spectrum. She uses avoidant strategies to defend herself against emotional trouble, and they tend to work. She uses relationships on her own terms in a way that she finds comforting – although not a lot of emotional talk takes place between her life partner and her, she declares that on her first day off, they are going to be together and they are going to have a good time, so her partner takes the day off too. They go to an action movie and have a good dinner. In the evening she describes the bare bones of what happened at the critical incident to her partner and then truncates that conversation by declaring that "it's a piece of shit but there's nothing you can do about it." The rest of the evening is not bad, they have sex, and she settles to sleep thinking about other things. She is able to right herself after only a day or two of her social and emotional world feeling out of kilter.

Tracey, on the other hand, is a little more insecure. She finds that her avoidant attempts to defend herself against unpleasant thoughts and feelings after the critical incident don't succeed. She gets angry at herself for not being able to forget the image of walking in the front door of the house and seeing the dead child. She has two drinks before she goes to bed to try to drown out the image but it only leads to a more restless sleep. Her partner asks what is wrong, and she tells him to leave her alone and let her sort it out. All of this leads to worry, anger, and irritability that take a couple of weeks to settle down.

Janice Halpern is a psychiatrist who has a special interest in how first responders are affected by the stress of critical incidents. She did a large study of paramedics in Toronto and found that attachment insecurity affects how long it takes paramedics, like Sian and Tracey, to bounce back from a critical incident.[16] She found that reacting to critical incidents with insomnia and other signs of a persistent stress response is the norm, but insecure paramedics are even more likely to experience insomnia after a critical incident, and their insomnia resolves more slowly.[17]

This outcome makes sense. Since darkness and unconsciousness leave a person much more susceptible to night-time dangers, the secure ones who know that they can count on someone to watch over them sleep more soundly. In another study, our colleague Eileen Sloan tested this idea by studying the electrical brain patterns (EEG waves) of people with sleep problems. The idea was that people who are insecure remain vigilant for danger or separation and don't ever entirely relax. The idea is that hyper-vigilance during sleep might correspond to a pattern of disturbed sleep called *alpha intrusion* that had been recognized previously by sleep researchers. During most of normal deep sleep, EEG patterns consist of slow, rolling delta waves. In the alpha intrusion anomaly, bursts of faster (alpha) brain waves (that more typically occur in states of alertness) show up during delta sleep. People with alpha intrusion tend not to feel rested and have problems with pain and fatigue.[18] Sloan measured adult attachment in people who came to her for sleep studies and found, sure enough, that people who had a lot of alpha intrusion also had more attachment anxiety.[19]

If paramedics who are more insecure always remain vigilant, a critical incident is likely to throw their sleep further out of balance for a few days or weeks. Of course, we are using insomnia only to illustrate one aspect of a person's response to stress. The paramedic study showed that insecurity was also related to a slow recovery from irritability, social withdrawal, and signs of physical arousal (like a racing heart) after a critical incident.

The protective effects of proximity to an attachment figure

Being near to a responsive attachment figure is undoubtedly protective against the effects of stress for a securely attached infant or
adult – that is the nature of the safe haven function that an attachment figure serves.[20] The situation in other circumstances is more
complicated, however. For one thing, evidence shows that a sufficiently sensitive and responsive *stranger* can buffer the stress that
infants experience when separated from her mother.[21] Furthermore,
infants may respond to insensitive or intrusive attachment figures
with increased cortisol (i.e., a parent can be a source of stress rather
than a buffer).[22] So what an attachment figure *does* as well as who she
is makes the difference.[23]

It fits with these observations that adults with insecure attachment
have complicated responses to being close to their attachment figures.
In general, adults seek contact and closeness with their partner when
extended separation is imminent and in response to stress.[24] People
with high attachment anxiety are likely to seek proximity more persistently, without necessarily experiencing a secure feeling as a result,
and may be particularly sensitive to feeling unsupported by a weak
response.[25] Furthermore, being close to a partner may not buffer physiological responses to a stressor for people with high attachment anxiety.[26] Adults with high attachment avoidance, on the other hand, are
less likely to seek contact with a partner in response to stress. While
more avoidant people are prone to altered stress physiology in general,
this response is not improved by the presence of an attachment figure.
This lack of improvement is why it is so important to take an individual's pattern of attachment into account: it is simply not true that the
way that support from an attachment figure works for one person will
also apply to others.

More life, more stress

Finally, attachment insecurity may actually increase the number of
stressful events that occur in a person's life. That means not just an
increase in the number of events that are perceived to be stressful but
also an increase in the number of events that an objective observer
would say are likely to be stressful. This relationship is a bit counter-
intuitive, but it turns out to be true.

When we studied health care workers to test the relationship between attachment security and physical symptoms caused by stress, we decided to look at the number of major life events these hospital workers reported occurring over the previous six months – primarily because we thought that the burden of big events would add to the effects of work stress. What we found, surprisingly, was that the more insecure a person was, the more events they reported.[27] As we thought of why that might be, it started to seem obvious how one thing leads to another. Having some difficulty getting along with people leads to trouble at work and in relationships, which can lead to financial problems and relationship changes and so on.[28] Why, exactly, does attachment insecurity lead to a pattern in which people cause stressful events to occur in their lives? We think that the answer has to do with the skills that come with secure patterns of attachment, which allow people to tolerate minor problems without reacting in a way that triggers new events. Secure attachment is associated with a capacity to inhibit automatic reactions, to soothe oneself, and to reflect and mentalize in a way that allows a person to put things in context. Those skills allow a person to tolerate mild or transitory threats and injuries and to tolerate, at least for a little while, situations of uncertainty, loss, and rejection. Since some situations will pass without consequence if you leave them alone, that means those secure people need only to react to problems that are more severe and persistent – hence, fewer stressful life events.[29]

Attachment is linked to social support, to depression, and to stress because they are interwoven concepts. Our social nature as organisms and our big social brains are inextricably bound to each other in evolutionary codependence. The attachment behavioural system, which organizes the experience of stress (threat and response) into an interpersonal dance, both protects our big brains as they grow and shapes their growth by encoding our experiences of mutual regulation and dysregulation into biology. When all goes well, we learn to be expert at putting the brakes on automatic signals and systems, pausing to reflect, reading the cues from those whose presence matters most to us, and imagining their inner worlds. Those abilities facilitate both an easier life and adaptive responses to extraordinary challenges and threats when they occur.

Feeling insecure is a signal that this complex and beautiful neuro-symphony is not quite in tune. The signal triggers an urgent effort to set things right. If we can't find security, which feels like safety and solace, in someone else's gaze or arms or conversation, we turn to other means. The next chapter describes how our sometimes frantic need to use anything that works to feel secure is another way in which insecure attachment can lead to health problems.

9 Why Are So Many of Us Fat, Drunk, Stationary Smokers?

Let's unpack the title of this chapter a bit. It is, we admit, not true that most of us are obese *and* unhealthy drinkers *and* inactive *and* smokers. However, most North American adults *are* at least one of these. Consider some statistics that bring an empirical undeniability to what each of us already knows.

- In spite of a successful 50-year campaign of public education, policy development, and innovation in medical treatments, about one in five adults still smokes.[1]
- As of 2007–2009, almost a quarter of Canadian adults (and a third of Americans) were obese. More than half of us met the somewhat lower threshold of being overweight.[2]
- Over 25% of men and 10% of women drink alcohol heavily enough to contribute to social and health problems.[3]
- About 25% of Canadian teenagers do not include any form of physical activity in their leisure, and the sluggishness rises as we age to almost 40% of young adults and 50% of adults beyond the age of 35.[4]

Much of the prevalence of the leading causes of early death in Canada, the United States, and other Western countries can be attributed to individuals choosing to do things that cause injury and disease or failing to do things that are healthy, as we reviewed in Chapter 2. Furthermore, while behaviour has a huge impact on health and longevity, the list of risky behaviours that are known to make a big contribution to that influence is short: smoking, drinking alcohol in excess, eating unhealthily, and being inactive. We could expand the list a bit by including some behaviours that are either less common or increase the risk of a narrower range of unhealthy outcomes, like having unsafe sex, having an addiction to other substances, and being reckless in driving and recreation – but the list is still fairly short.

Gillian arrives at the restaurant for a business dinner. She always feels a little tense in these situations that seem in-between to her, partly like a social event with friends, partly like a business meeting. She acts differently in those two settings and isn't sure which set of rules applies to this one. She is pleased to see that she has arrived first because it will allow her to have a glass of wine while she waits for the others, exactly what she needs to calm her nerves.

Insecure attachment makes people more likely to behave in these unhealthy ways. At any point, the physiological and psychological consequences of insecurity provide a weak force that nudges these several causes of disease in the wrong direction. Working over many years, in many ways, on behaviours that affect many aspects of health, the influence of insecurity can be amplified into an important determinant of population health – the weak force begins a cascade.

Who cares what's good for us?

We have to start from an accurate but unfortunate premise. Almost everybody, secure or insecure, has trouble acting in ways that are in his or her long-term interest. Most of our lost years of life, as citizens of industrialized nations, are the consequence of unhealthy choices. The reasons for those choices are the topic of many other books and discussions, but for our purposes listing a few is enough.

- Fat, fructose, and salt taste good. Alcohol feels good. Smoking brings pleasure. Exercise is hard.
- Selling easily consumed forms of nicotine, alcohol, fat, salt, and passive entertainment is enormously profitable. The marketing of these products is extremely effective.
- Human psychology is much more focused on short-term appetites and goals than on long-term risks. In evolution, a strong attraction to high-calorie, high-fat foods has protected our species from starvation. Over that time it has also been advantageous for us to rest when we can.

- We are extraordinarily inaccurate calculators of true risks and benefits.[5]
- In our brains and bodies, nicotine and other addictive substances are agents that actively stimulate biological processes that evolved to serve useful purposes that have nothing to do with these drugs.

It's astounding that we ever make healthy choices when we have so much to overcome. People with insecure patterns of attachment have extra disadvantages. One difficulty is that most of the behaviours in question balance a short-term benefit against a long-term health risk. Insecure attachment makes the immediate benefit more valuable and so it tips the balance. A person who is high in attachment anxiety and who has little confidence in his capacity to cope with life's stresses on his own, coupled with insufficient support from others, may find that wine or cigarettes or chocolate cake provide a brief but welcome relief from constant tension. A person who is high in attachment avoidance, who does not want to express distress or ask others for assistance, may find that the time smoking a cigarette outside in solitude is a highly effective way to use an external device (a cigarette) to substitute for an internal process (emotional regulation) that isn't working optimally.

Direct biological links also exist between substance use and insecure attachment. To understand why patterns of attachment have anything at all to do with the biology of addictive molecules, we need to take a brief detour into the brain. Our brains have three parts. The brainstem is the stalk of the brain and is the oldest and most primitive part of the brain that we share with all other vertebrate species. The brainstem regulates the basic processes of animal life, such as breathing. The largest and most recently developed part of the brain is the cortex, which gives the brain its cauliflower-like shape and folded wavy surface. The cortex is the seat of language and consciousness, the part of the brain that controls all deliberate actions, perceives and interprets sensory information, and performs complex cognitive tasks like expecting, deliberating, understanding, interpreting, planning, and deciding.

At the top of the brainstem, but wedged beneath the cortex where it is hard to see from the outside, is the midbrain. The midbrain is less refined than the cortex but more refined than the brainstem. It includes a number of clusters of nerve cells that are important to attachment. Several brain areas that are important to our understanding of attachment and addiction lie in the region where the cortex and mid-brain are closely interconnected, which is sometimes loosely described as the mesolimbic region. "Mesolimbic" does not refer to a very specific location, but we are adopting it as a useful adjective because it saves us the trouble of overly fussy precision when we identify the locations of specific nerve centres in this region.

Wanting and liking: This is your brain on love

For many mammals the first hours and days of mother-infant inter-action after birth are directed towards the goal of optimal contact.[6] It doesn't take long, however, to move into the next, much longer devel-opmental period in which the infant can manage independently for a time but needs to be able to get close to his parent when circumstances demand, sometimes unexpectedly. The goal of the attachment system at this point is to optimize proximity rather than contact.

Two brain systems help keep an infant focused on the goal of main-taining optimal proximity to parents. The first system keeps us moti-vated to look for proximity (wanting) and the second one reinforces the good feeling that comes from having found the right degree of closeness (liking). Wanting is mediated by circuits of neurons in the mesolimbic area that communicate with each other by using the chemical dopamine. Liking is mediated by circuits of neurons that release different chemi-cals, known as endorphins or endogenous opioids. The powerful moti-vational and rewarding properties of these systems that evolved to keep us looking for and staying with things that are good for us also play an important role in addiction to drugs like cocaine and heroin.

It helps to distinguish the role of dopamine circuits in wanting things from the role of opioid circuits in liking the way those things feel. Thomas Insel, the director of the US National Institute of Men-tal Health, points out how this distinction helps us to understand the switch that occurs when a person who regularly uses an addictive sub-stance moves from simply liking the sensations that it causes to addic-tion. It is a substantial switch. Drinking a limited amount of alcohol, for example, brings feelings of pleasure – we like it. However, addiction comes with very little enjoyment; it is replaced by a strong sense of need. If we shift our attention from alcohol to a more powerfully addic-tive drug, the "jonesing" experienced by crack cocaine addicts in with-drawal is more powerful than virtually any other signal and may lead to personal ruin. For an addicts, where they once had pleasure, they now have preoccupation, intoxication, and compulsive drug seeking.[7] Insel points out a strikingly similar phenomenon that occurs in close relationships – the difference between the good feeling that comes from being secure in a romantic relationship and the compulsive, preoccupying drive towards proximity that is experienced by a person who has been jilted. A person with high attachment anxiety may experience a very similar feeling that is practically permanent rather than being a short-term reaction to lost love.

Gerry was a recovering addict who grew up in a neglectful and abusive family. He had succeeded in abstaining from alcohol and cocaine for several years and was now contemplating stopping smoking, which he considered a much greater challenge. While reflecting on his first cigarette at age 13 he said, "I have experienced cravings for drugs many times, I'm an expert at cravings. You know, I experienced cravings before I ever took a drug. I think my first cigarette was a response to craving. It felt great."

We need to wonder what Gerry's cravings were about before he'd experienced a drug. We can start by recognizing that these neurological systems for liking and wanting did not evolve to support drug addictions. Rather, they evolved to provide natural motivation and rewards for highly advantageous behaviours, including having sex, caring for our young, and seeking protection in attachment relationships. It was later in the evolution of our species that we discovered external substances that are potent triggers of these systems. Many drugs are addictive precisely because they directly stimulate wanting and liking while short-circuiting the desirable social interactions that these neural circuits are there to promote. Because of this shared circuitry, people whose experiences have literally left them wanting but not finding security (i.e., people with insecure attachment) may be more susceptible to addiction.

Thao Lan Le is a graduate student who decided to see just how common smoking, unhealthy drinking, and excessive weight are among patients of the family practice clinic at our hospital and if they are related to insecure attachment. She asked people coming to a routine appointment at the clinic to fill out a short survey. Almost all of them said yes (84%), so we can be sure that the 350 or so people who completed her survey were representative of the clinic's usual patients.[8]

Figure 9.1 The proportion of people with fearful attachment among people who meet a high threshold for health risk: current smoking, obesity (BMI > 30), or harmful patterns of alcohol consumption

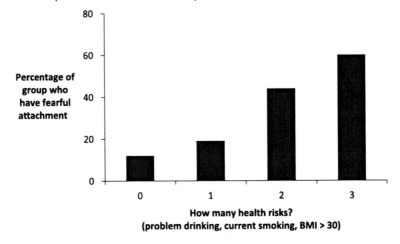

Not surprisingly, smoking and problems with drinking and over-weight were common. Even if we count behaviours only when they pass a high threshold, about 40% of family practice patients had at least one of them.[9] If we use a lower threshold, that problem rate rises to 80%. Meeting the low threshold is pretty clearly still a health problem. It means being overweight (BMI > 25) or drinking more than Cana-da's low-risk alcohol drinking guidelines suggest[10] or being a regular smoker at some time in your life. Worse, among these three health risks, people often report more than one. About 33% of the patients complet-ing the survey had just one health risk, but more than that (46%) had two or three of these health risks.[11]

When she looked at attachment insecurity, Thao Lan Le found a strong relationship between insecure attachment and these behaviourally based health risks. Not only are they related, but the relationship is also graded – the more severe the health risk (as indicated by high threshold risks or by multiple risks), the more insecurity is found. The relationship illustrated in Figure 9.1 is striking – among people with two or three high threshold risks, fearful attachment insecurity is the norm.

This pattern suggests that attachment insecurity might be related to these different behaviourally based health risks in a similar way. We think that this common link may derive from a one-two punch that insecure attachment directs towards the wanting and liking circuitry of our brains. Insecure attachment, especially when it includes both attachment anxiety and attachment avoidance, is experienced as *wanting*, which is literally a state of needing to find something that will allow us to feel better. This wanting is what explains Gerry's experience of feeling cravings that were ultimately satisfied by cigarettes but before he ever began to smoke. The second half of the one-two punch is that insecure attachment interferes with having that need satisfied by the solace of a close supportive relationship. If close relationships are fraught with fear of rejection, unmet needs, or mistrust, or are simply unavailable when they are needed, then feelings of insecurity and distress will persist. Something else, beyond support, is required, which is one way to understand Gerry's persistent addictions, drinking to overcome interpersonal discomfort – as Gillian did at the restaurant – emotional eating, and other emotional determinants of unhealthy and addictive behaviour.

Smoking

The forces that lead a person, usually a teenager,[12] to start smoking are different from the ones that make it hard to quit later. So if we want to reduce smoking, it makes sense to work on both sides – preventing teenagers from starting, and then helping those who do start smoking to quit, typically when they are adults. We need to look at those two situations separately to understand the role of attachment.

We can set the scene by referring back to the ACE Study, introduced in Chapter 3, which links adult health to childhood experiences with abuse, neglect, and other forms of adversity. That study found a strong graded relationship between ACE scores and smoking – the more adversity, the higher the proportion of smokers. Compared with those reporting no bad childhood experiences, persons with ACE scores of 5 or higher were more than three times as likely to be smokers at some point in their life, five times as likely to have started smoking by age 14, twice as likely to be smoking currently, and almost three times as likely to be smoking heavily.[13] Of course, not every teenager who starts to smoke comes to it from experiences of adversity, but the consequences of various forms of familial stress are an important and under-recognized risk factor, one that also substantially increases the risk of lifelong feelings of insecurity.

Both parents and peers can have strong influences on all sorts of choices that teenagers make, including the decision to start smoking or not. The choice to start smoking has been explained in two ways. One explanation emphasizes the reasons that individuals choose to smoke, such as their expectation that it will help them fit in with their social group or that it will help them lose weight or that they don't believe it will harm them.[14] The other approach is to view smoking as a deviant or delinquent behaviour and study the social forces that lead a teenager to deviate from social norms.[15] The quality of attachment of teenagers to parents has usually been studied by people who are interested in the second explanation. Their studies have consistently concluded that teenagers who have an insecure attachment to their parents are more likely to smoke.[16] For example, in a survey of over 28,000 14- and 15-year-olds in New Zealand, the rate of smoking was almost three times as high (28% versus 10%) in families where attachment to parents was the weakest.[17]

The link between attachment to parents and starting to smoke is more complicated than that, however, because another variable is involved: the influence of peers. Being influenced by peers as a teenager is not a sign of insecurity; it is inevitable and desirable as kids grow into adults. Adolescence is the period when attachment functions (such as whom we prefer to be close to and the use of a relationship as a safe haven) are gradually transferred from parents to peers.[18] The quality of a teen's attachment to her parents may affect the relative balance of the influences that she feels. Teens with a secure attachment to their parents experience a more balanced pull between the influence of their parents and the influence of their peers.[19]

Attachment security may have a stronger influence on the ability to quit smoking than it does on the choice to start. That idea makes sense because secure attachment comes with a cluster of abilities that would be very useful to a person who wants to quit smoking. Secure attachment may enhance a person's ability to tolerate the distress and craving of nicotine withdrawal in the service of a longer-term goal (a process that is not so different from the delayed gratification in the marshmallow test). Attachment also makes it easier to get support from a partner to help us quit, something that increases success.[20] If we think of how the biology of liking and wanting is linked to both addiction and insecurity, then people with secure attachment experience may possibly experience less intense cravings.[21]

The evidence supports the idea that smokers with secure attachment are more likely to quit successfully, both as teenagers[22] and later

in life. In Thao Lan Le's study, attachment anxiety was more important than attachment avoidance. Smokers with high attachment anxiety
were more likely to continue to smoke, and those with low attachment
anxiety were likely to have quit. For those patients of our family practice clinic, the previous smokers who had quit were the same, from an
attachment perspective, as those who had never smoked at all.[23] Most
smokers have tried to quit numerous times. Attachment insecurity is
one of the forces that make it hard to succeed – maybe because it makes
the cravings so difficult to resist.

Alcohol

As it did with smoking, the ACE Study also showed that childhood
adversity increases alcohol use, abuse, and dependence later in life. Each
category of experience measured in the ACE Study doubles or triples
the risk of starting to drink before age 15. Once again, a strong graded
relationship exists between the number of types of adverse exposure
and starting to drink alcohol before age 15.[24] Other research has confirmed that the relationship between childhood abuse and later alcohol
use is due, at least in part, to attachment style.[25] Studies of a direct link
between teenagers' attachment to parents and starting to drink support
the same general conclusions: parental bonds that leave children feeling
unsafe contribute to the choice to start drinking[26] and to drunkenness.[27]
As with smoking, peers are stronger forces than parents.[28] Furthermore,
a harmful loop can occur in that once teen substance use is initiated, it
can cause further impairment of attachment to parents.[29]

Drinking alcohol is different from smoking as a health risk because
it isn't always bad for you. Health care professionals divide people
in two ways: the first has to do with the amount that people drink;
the second has to do with the harm that drinking does. With respect
to quantity, it makes sense to consider three groups: those who never
or rarely drink, those who drink regularly at a rate that is generally
considered healthy, and those who drink an amount that often leads to
health problems. The distinctions can be made by using Canada's low-
risk alcohol drinking guidelines, which are based on an expert review
of the patterns of drinking that are linked to health risks; they are gender specific and defined by both total drinks per week and maximum
drinks per day.[30] The second important criterion is whether or not a
person has experienced the well-known social, occupational, and personal problems that suggest addiction. We are going to call this *harmful
drinking*.

Figure 9.2 The proportion of people with fearful attachment in people grouped by their pattern of drinking alcohol in the last month

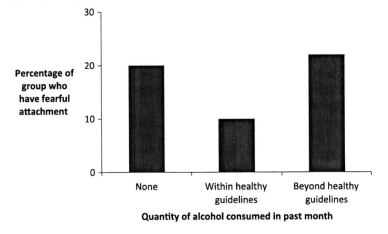

The clearest link between attachment and alcohol consumption in adults is that secure attachment is associated with lower rates of harmful drinking.[31] This association is likely to go both ways. On one hand, insecure attachment increases the risk of problem drinking for all the reasons that we are emphasizing in this chapter. For example, people with fearful attachment insecurity tend to drink as a way to cope with stress.[32] On the other hand, harmful drinking plays havoc with close relationships over time – exactly the kind of powerful interpersonal force that is likely to gradually change a person's attachment style towards greater insecurity.

If we look at how attachment is associated with the amount that people drink, we find some more subtle trends. Thao Lan Le is the first to do this, so we return to her study of family practice patients. The first thing to note is that drinking quite a bit was the norm: almost half (47%) drank enough to be beyond the low-risk alcohol drinking guidelines.[33] If we look at how this relates to attachment insecurity, we see something interesting. Figure 9.2 shows that attachment insecurity is associated with two patterns of drinking: drinking more than is healthy and not drinking at all. We can make sense of that by imagining the ways that a person who is feeling insecure might think about having a drink. While one person looks forward to the way that alcohol reduces the edge of the tension he feels, another doesn't like the sense of losing control that she experiences when she drinks and fears where drinking can lead (maybe because of the environment in which she grew up, with an alcoholic parent). The insecure person who prefers to reach for a drink may find it hard to restrain his consumption within a healthy limit.

These choices have an impact on health; the insecure person who chooses to abstain is making a healthier choice than the insecure person whose drinking leads to excess.[34] This is an example of a situation in which insecurity can lead to a healthier or a riskier choice. In our experience this example also illustrates a broader phenomenon – making healthier choices requires a person with insecure attachment to live a life that is a little more controlled, a little less varied than the secure person who can, for example, more easily drink alcohol in a healthy way. He may experience criticism for this rigidity at times ("relax, man, have a drink!") because his apparently excessive self-control is readily apparent, while his underlying sense of dysregulation is not. We see the same phenomena occur with choices made about diet or exercise (or for that matter dental hygiene and how often we should visit the doctor). A person with insecure attachment can find herself choosing between the lesser of evils: having a slightly obsessive adherence to healthy choices or opting to feel better in the moment without regard to long-term risks.

Eating and weight

Jo picks up the phone to call her mother and hangs it back up again. She knows that they need to talk because she won't be able to settle down and think of other things until they resolve the argument that started earlier today, but she can't bring herself to do it yet. It takes a while for Jo to work up her nerve. She rehearses the conversation that is yet to come and barely notices that as she does so she is eating the leftover pasta in the fridge until it is gone – "enough for two meals," she thinks, cursing herself.

Beyond sustenance, we eat for pleasure, for comfort, to reward ourselves, to explore, to bond with friends and loved ones, to pass the time, and out of sheer habit. Small wonder that the ways that we have found to manage our closest relationships and our emotions also influence what goes into our mouths. The health implications are obvious: unhealthy patterns of eating that lead to overweight are among the most widespread of the lifestyle factors that contribute to such serious chronic illnesses as heart disease and breast cancer.

The ACE Study found that verbal, physical, and sexual abuse in childhood increased the likelihood of obesity (BMI $\geq$ 30) as an adult. As it did with smoking and drinking, the ACE Study found a graded response between childhood exposure and adult health risk.[35] Once again, we see the incremental impact of a weak force on health that affects many people. The pattern is very similar to other examples of weak forces in this book: people become obese for other reasons (for, example, it occurs in 23% of people who have experienced no abuse), but exposure to childhood adversity is very common, and so the risk that it creates affects many people.[36]

Among teenagers and adults, fearful attachment is linked to both higher BMI and to higher waist-to-hip ratio.[37] In Thao Lan Le's study there was a graded, stepwise increase in the prevalence of fearful attachment, which depended on how high we draw the threshold for high BMI: 25% of people with BMI > 25, 37% of those with BMI > 30, 58% of those with BMI > 35.

Why do childhood adversity and attachment insecurity lead to excess weight? Much of this may relate to how insecurity leads people to feel about their bodies and to use food to manage emotions. Both youngsters and adults with insecure styles are more concerned about body shape, more dissatisfied with their own bodies, and more interested in cosmetic surgery.[38] The need for approval that is a component of attachment anxiety contributes to this body dissatisfaction.[39] Insecurity leads some people to feel that being loved and approved of depends on looking different from the way they do.

Attachment anxiety also leads to disinhibited eating,[40] presumably because insecurity leads people to use food to manage distressing feelings, as Jo does. Disinhibited eating means eating in response to negative emotions and injured self-esteem, periodic overeating, and difficulty resisting when others encourage one to eat. It is a strong predictor of future obesity. A person with high attachment anxiety can find herself in the conflicted position of being dissatisfied with how she looks, on one hand, and yet eating excessively in response to distressing feelings, on the other. A negative self-image leads to negative emotions, which lead to more eating and a worse self-image, and on it goes.

Sometimes the health effects of disturbed patterns of eating are even more immediate. For teenage girls with diabetes, eating thoughtfully with the goal of maintaining optimal levels of blood sugar is very important to health but often runs counter to the other forces that are part of being a teenager. Insecure attachment is one of the forces that tend to push girls with diabetes towards patterns of eating that have more to do with maintaining a sense of personal control and managing emotions than they do with controlling blood sugar.[41] Even something as common as night-time snacking, which tends to complicate control of diabetes, is more common among those with insecure attachment patterns.[42]

Our emphasis in this section is on obesity rather than being underweight, because we are focusing on the issues that affect the health of the most people. However, insecure attachment is also more common among those who restrict their food intake excessively (similar to the pattern we found with alcohol consumption). In the extreme, in disorders like anorexia nervosa, insecure attachment is the norm.[43] Anorexia nervosa is a very complex mental disorder, however, and beyond the scope of the kinds of issues that we are identifying as the sources of vexing health care.

Sex

The importance of safe sex practices has been in the public eye for three decades, emphasized by the rise of sexually transmitted infections that cannot be cured with antibiotics, including HIV/AIDS, hepatitis C, genital herpes, and cervical cancer caused by human papillomavirus. One of the most consistent observations over this time is that it is very hard to get human beings to behave in a way that is in their long-term interests – for example, to convince men to wear a condom – if it means denying or delaying the immediate gratification of a strong biological drive. Safe sex is not unique in this regard; it naturally calls to mind how frustrating it has been for public health professionals to convince well-informed and intelligent adults to quit smoking or to make healthy food choices. However, since sex is a fundamentally social interaction that often occurs in the context of an intimate pair relationship, it seems like a very likely forum for the enactment of attachment behaviour. Furthermore, since attachment security and the ability to delay gratification result from similar experiences during early development (as we discussed in Chapter 5), we expect that people with a secure attachment will have an advantage in pausing to reflect on the best interests of themselves and their partners.

Early in the history of the psychology of adult attachment, Phillip Shaver and Cynthia Hazan postulated that attachment security is directly linked to sexuality. They predicted that secure attachment would lead to sexual relationships that emphasize mutual intimacy and pleasure, whereas attachment avoidance would lead to emotional distance in sexual relationships, and attachment anxiety would lead people to use sex in the service of their needs for love and security.[44] In the light of the evidence that has accumulated since, these hypotheses were pretty close to the mark, although the situation is a little bit more complicated than first predicted.

Most of the research in this area concerns university and college students. Secure students have the most enduring relationships and are the most likely to be having sex; among those with steady partners, secure students are almost twice as likely to have relationships that include intercourse.[45] Secure students are also more likely to report that sex brings physical pleasure.[46] Attachment avoidance, on the other hand, seems to lead people in one of two directions. One is to abstain from sexual relationships.[47] Indeed, college students with high attachment avoidance report having been in love fewer times than secure students and are the least likely of any students surveyed to be having sex. The second way to avoid emotional intimacy is by engaging in uncommitted sex in casual relationships.[48] In line with this prediction, compared with secure students, students with high attachment avoidance purport to be more accepting of sex in the absence of commitment, love, or closeness.[49] This acceptance may suggest that young adults with high attachment avoidance choose between abstinence and non-intimate sex; or it may simply reveal an incongruity between attitudes (accepting of casual sex) and behaviours (having little sex in spite of the professed attitude). Attachment avoidance causing an incongruity between attitude and behaviour is a recurrent theme. In keeping with this tension, high attachment avoidance is associated with experiencing negative feelings, estrangement, and interfering thoughts during sex rather than experiencing pleasure.[50]

Attachment avoidance may also influence a person's motivations for having sex. Young people with high attachment avoidance are more likely than others to report that the object of having sex the first time was to lose their virginity, a goal that suggests they view sex as a personal accomplishment rather than as an intimate experience. These same individuals are unlikely to see sex as an expression of love or to have sex to achieve emotional closeness. They do, however, sometimes report using sex manipulatively to achieve some other goal.[51]

University students with high attachment anxiety report having been in love more frequently than other students but also report the shortest relationships, which suggests a desire for closeness but an emotional intensity that creates some difficulty in making it work.[52] When it comes to sex, since attachment anxiety is associated with a lack of assertiveness, low self-confidence, and a fear of abandonment, we expect these individuals to be vulnerable to going along with a partner's unwanted sexual advances.[53] Indeed, fear of losing her partner is a stronger motivation for sex among adolescent girls with high attachment anxiety than it is for others.

What about the aspects of sexual behaviour that put our health at risk, such as frequent unprotected sex with multiple partners? What about sexually transmitted infections? The ACE Study found a graded relationship between childhood adversity and sexually transmitted infections later in life. The prevalence of sexually transmitted infections in adulthood rose fivefold from those with no childhood exposures to those with six or seven exposures.[54]

The age at which you start having sex also has health implications because teenagers who start younger are likely to have more sexually transmitted infections over time. Teenagers who are high in anxious attachment start the earliest, and those with high attachment avoidance tend to start latest and to progress the slowest from kissing to petting to sex. Exceptions always exist – we can easily imagine a secure person with the maturity to establish a healthy intimate relationship at an earlier age than most, or a youth with attachment avoidance getting an early start, but not because he is looking for love.[55] Nonetheless, even with that degree of complexity, patterns of attachment are clearly closely related to the experiences of love and sex.

Summary

We have reviewed some of the evidence linking insecure patterns of attachment to risky choices concerning drinking alcohol, smoking, eating, and having sex. We would like to be able to talk about how attachment is related to poor physical fitness and other social behaviours that lead to health problems (such as talking on the cell phone while driving, a growing cause of accidental injury and death), but there simply is not enough evidence available yet to proceed beyond speculation on those topics.

Attachment security and insecurity clearly influence our choices about health in many ways. That is an important message in itself – one of the reasons that interpersonal dynamics are an important contributor to health is the diversity of their effects – they add up. Teenagers with insecure attachment tend to smoke and to drink at a younger age than those who are secure. The relative weakness of their bond to their parents appears to tip the balance towards greater influence by their peers at an age when they are vulnerable to developing lifelong patterns. Patterns of attachment are also linked to differences between individuals in the ways that their wanting and liking circuits function, which may cause a stronger desire or need for the feelings that substances bring. Furthermore, because people with insecure attachment often use strategies for coping that are not very effective, food, substances, and sex may provide some (short-term) relief that isn't available in other ways. Given the complexity of the interactions between types of insecurity and behaviour, the consistently with which research has corroborated the predictions of attachment theory is remarkable.

Acting in our own best interests is difficult for us all; insecure attachment just makes it harder.

10 I Don't Know What You Have, but I've Seen It Before and You Have It Bad

The title of this chapter is the punch line of an old and not very funny joke about disconcerting medical opinions. We resurrect the line here because it rings true in the experience of many health care providers when they are faced with a syndrome of difficult, unexplained physical symptoms, which is the topic of this chapter.

Bob's patient, Dustin Brandt

I felt that I already knew Dustin Brandt before he even walked into my office. The referral for the consultation, written by his family doctor in the typically terse form that such communications often take, said "chronic pain, irritable bowel, not working, won't take an antidepressant, please assess and treat." He had missed our first scheduled appointment because he felt too sick to drive. Today, he arrived 20 minutes early. When I greeted him in the waiting room he had a sheaf of papers in his hands – I recognized them as a stack of previous laboratory results and consultation reports. The thickness of the sheaf made my heart sink.

Dustin started telling me about how uncomfortable his trip to the hospital had been while we were still walking down the hall. I didn't interrupt, but I didn't respond either; it is a public space and lacks the privacy that I feel such a conversation requires. He was telling me that driving for a half hour is very tense because he never knows when he might suddenly need to find a bathroom. Once we got to my office, he sat down tentatively on the edge of the chair I offered, wincing as he changed position.

The next five minutes seemed to confirm my expectation. In a jumble of barely organized, half-finished sentences, Dustin told me that he had been suffering for over five years with a variety of health problems that had brought him to several medical specialists, as well as a naturopath and a chiropractor. None of the experts had given him a clear explanation of his symptoms, although he had settled on "irritable bowel" as a descriptor, in spite of the fact that he had more than just gastroenterological problems; headaches and back pain were also interfering with his life.

As I showed some interest in the symptoms he was describing and asked about others, Dustin at least partially endorsed most of the symptoms I asked him about but never with clarity.

Q: Is the pain in your gut worse after eating?

A: I had a reaction one time, and spicy ... you know, but they told me to not have gluten, and I like ... it's not the pain, it's the bloating. I get huge but of course it hurts.

Q: Have you had periods of dizziness?

A: Not so much dizzy as spinny, like when I had that pill ... whoa, that was bad ... not that I am against pills, but you know how sensitive it can be ... like that other time with Jacob, but it's bad, I know.

I suppressed the urge to ask a question I had first heard from a derisive teacher when I was in medical school: "Does it hurt behind your eyes when you pee?" The question is a cruel joke that I had found funny at the time.

We'll return to Dustin later, when we can be more thoughtful about him and not just react with the distancing hostility that Bob experienced at their first encounter.[1] Before that, let's review the ways in which his presentation is characteristic of people whose unexplained symptoms cause clinicians difficulty.

The first point to emphasize is that experiencing new physical symptoms that aren't explained by an injury or an identified disease is a normal part of life.[2] The threshold for symptoms causing problems, like interfering with activities or work, is much higher. Going to the doctor has a higher threshold yet; the average person experiences a new symptom every week or two but visits the doctor about three times a year.[3] These thresholds suggest a very broad pyramid. At the pyramid's base we find the exceedingly common experience of physical symptoms that have no specific explanation. In its higher tiers we find increasingly fewer experiences, those that correspond to symptoms that interfere with normal activities, and, a little higher in the pyramid, symptoms that require a professional opinion. Experiences at this level of the pyramid indicate a social transformation because by walking into a doctor's office a *person* becomes a *patient*.

Still higher tiers exist, each with fewer and fewer inhabitants. Once at the doctor's office, about half of the time symptoms will not be explained by any identifiable injury or disease, in spite of careful history, physical examination, and testing.[4] That means that crossing the threshold from person to patient often results in nothing more than the reassuring news that nothing serious seems to be wrong. To get to Dustin's situation, a person needs to climb even higher, beyond the usual effectiveness of reassurance, to the apex of the pyramid where we find the kinds of persistent, severe, and troublesome unexplained symptoms that lead to disability and seeing specialists.

What are the forces that drive a person like Dustin up the pyramid of difficult unexplained symptoms? Obviously, the intensity and persistence of the symptoms themselves and the degree to which they interfere with normal activities are crucial determinants. But other forces are at play as well, which are not as obvious and yet account for a great deal of the explanation of why one person rises up the pyramid while another sits nearer to its base.

Sensibly, Dustin's previous experience is likely to determine how seriously he takes a particular symptom, and how hopeful he feels that a medical setting will provide assistance or relief. Social and cultural attitudes and beliefs also often have a strong influence on the kinds of suffering that are deemed legitimate or worrisome. In this chapter we will be emphasizing the role of another determinant of medicalizing symptoms: the interpersonal forces that make unexplained symptoms into a difficult medical problem.

The role of attachment anxiety

No singular explanation exists of what causes new physical symptoms to arise. The boundary is often fuzzy between normal symptoms (e.g., shortness of breath from exertion) and indicators of concern (e.g., shortness of breath as a sign of asthma, heart failure, or panic). In addition, individuals vary quite widely in their tolerance of discomfort and even in their threshold for detecting a sensation. As a result, individuals have a lot of latitude to differ in their experience of physical symptoms even under similar circumstances.

One thing that influences our experience of physical symptoms is how much attention we pay to them, which depends what they mean to us. We are constantly receiving neural signals regarding myriad physical phenomena, most of which never penetrate conscious awareness.

Dr Sam Golden (from the Introduction), who recently suffered a heart attack, is much more attentive to chest symptoms than the next person because he knows that the stakes are high. A person who has been told that the hotel she slept in last night has a bed bug problem is likely to suddenly become quite interested in very subtle skin sensations. So individual differences in our sense of vulnerability to danger can affect how frequently we detect new symptoms. Vigilance for signs of danger is a central feature of attachment anxiety. The tendency to think of oneself as vulnerable raises the stakes; one person's transient discomfort becomes the insecure person's worrisome danger signal. Thus, the vigilance for signs of danger that is a core characteristic of attachment anxiety is one reason that people with this type of insecurity consistently report more symptoms of all types.[5]

Going to see a health professional for a new symptom is a big step, but a person with high attachment anxiety's bias towards seeking proximity and reassurance translates into a tendency to seek professional help more readily.[6] Very robust evidence shows that people with high attachment anxiety report symptoms of all kinds with greater frequency and intensity.[7] Once they are in the office, patients with high attachment anxiety, like Dustin, are also likely to receive more tests to reassure them that all is well.[8]

Even if he is initially reassured by normal test results, Dustin finds it hard to maintain this secure feeling. Doubts quickly creep in, and the solution to experiencing doubt and worry that is generated by attachment anxiety is seeking proximity to someone else. If a health care provider is able to temporarily meet the need for a safe haven, the stage is set for repeat visits from a patient like Dustin.[9] Unfortunately, he will benefit only briefly from that contact and then revert to ruminating anxiously about his symptoms when he is back on his own.

Next, three related characteristics of attachment anxiety tend to drive someone like Dustin up the pyramid of medicalization from primary care to specialists and consultations in hospital-based clinics. The first is that it is difficult for him to feel reassured by positive messages; he is always wondering, "What if you are wrong and there really is something serious going on?" Dustin's expectation that he will have a bad outcome can be almost unshakeable because certainty doesn't exist in health care.

A second characteristic, a cousin of vigilance, is the tendency to assume the worst possible outcome. Cognitive psychologists call this *catastrophization* because even a moderate chance of a bad outcome leads a person to expect catastrophe. It is very typical of people with high attachment anxiety to catastrophize, which in turn helps to perpetuate some physical symptoms, such as chronic pain.[10] For example, when neurologists decide that unexplained symptoms are benign, their accuracy is about 95%.[11] Someone like Dustin is prone to think, "What if I am in the 5%? I probably am because I'm not having any luck these days."

Thus a repeating sequence is set up in which symptoms lead to fear, which leads to a social interaction between a patient and provider that is frustrating for both. Reassurance fails, distress is amplified, help seeking is redoubled, and the symptoms (and more importantly the perceived threats implied by the symptoms) increase. Very often, the result of this process is to identify a new authority on whom to displace the dilemma, and a referral is made, where the most likely outcome is to have the entire frustrating cycle repeat itself.[12]

The role of attachment avoidance

In general, attachment avoidance biases the responses to physical symptoms in the opposite direction. An attitude of self-reliance and reluctance to depend on others or to appear vulnerable in their eyes biases a person with high attachment avoidance to tolerate symptoms without seeking help for them and to avoid taking on the role of a patient. People who are high in attachment avoidance tend to report symptoms less frequently[13] and to underuse medical resources relative to people with other attachment styles.[14] The added risk with attachment avoidance is that symptoms will be tolerated for too long and actual indicators of dangerous illness will be ignored. People in the community (who have not necessarily chosen to become patients) with high attachment avoidance are more likely to have chronic low back pain and headaches.[15]

Perhaps the greatest contribution of attachment avoidance to difficult, unexplained symptoms occurs when it presents in combination with attachment anxiety. Fearful attachment leads to very difficult interpersonal interactions, including interactions between patient and provider, which we will return to in the next chapter.

Fragmentation of the agents of care

An unintended consequence of the forces of fear and interpersonal need that drive difficult interactions for people with problematic, unexplained symptoms is that it is common for a great many care providers to become involved in a person's care.

In addition to his family doctor, Dustin has been referred to two gastroenterologists, a specialist in rheumatic diseases, and a neurologist. Although only one of the gastroenterologists offered to take on responsibility to treat his irritable bowel, Dustin has had intermittent contact with the other doctor "just in case." He has gone back to see the rheumatologist twice for an opinion about pain because she has a different approach than his other doctors, favouring more aggressive use of pain medication. The consultation with the neurologist didn't go well; Dustin felt that his concerns were being dismissed as imaginary. He left angry, wondering if he should find another neurologist. He sees a chiropractor who has provided some treatments that have reduced the pain he sometimes gets in his back when the rest of his symptoms are severe. Dustin also sees a naturopath intermittently, although he is not convinced of the benefit yet. Although it is difficult to get an appointment as quickly as he would like with his family doctor at times, Dustin has established a relationship with the receptionist and with the nurse in the clinic whom he finds reassuring. The circle of care expands farther when you look beyond the professionals. Dustin has a couple of friends he turns to regularly for advice, and he is highly engaged with an online support group that sometimes provides guidance about diet and raises concerns about medication. On the other hand, Dustin's wife, Lisa, has given him the message that she doesn't want to be a medical adviser, and she bows out of discussions about his symptoms quite quickly.

A wealth of experience and opinion can be an advantage in a complex situation. Dustin's circle of care, on the other hand, often generates uncertainty, contradiction, and more anxiety. A big part of the problem is that almost no organization or coordination exists among the many players. Very few of these professionals communicate with each other. Their advice comes with contradictions between experts that Dustin is left to resolve on his own. Most of them are not fully informed; it is confusing to interview Dustin about his symptoms and his treatment, and health care professionals can easily fall into the trap of providing advice prematurely without understanding the entire context.

Donald Winnicott dubbed this phenomenon "fragmentation of the agents of care."[16] Rather than being a well-designed and orchestrated care team that draws on the expertise of many, Dustin's care is a chaotic combination of ill-defined relationships, premature advice, incomplete understanding, and disorganized communication. Instead of a network, it is a pile of relationship shards.

Incoherent narratives

Dustin's relationships with those who provide care occur in a recurrent series of dyads. At the level of these individual conversations, the quality of the dialogue that occurs can be a strong determinate of the value of medical care that he receives. Just as his system of care is fragmented and disorganized, so goes Dustin's direct communication – his story is broken up and hard to follow. As we described in Chapter 6, attachment insecurity can interfere with clear communication, and an inability to convey a coherent story can turn an interaction that is merely complicated into a confusing and dissatisfying dead end.

Providers may contribute to difficulties by listening poorly, interrupting too quickly, interrogating instead of discussing, and lapsing into unnecessary technical jargon. One study found that physicians-in-training interrupted their patients' narratives an astonishing 12 seconds after they began.[17] Practising doctors typically only allow a few seconds longer.[18] Poor communication leaves the patient and provider at cross purposes, often feeling dissatisfied[19] and having widely different memories of what has taken place in their discussion.[20]

According to Paul Grice, four maxims define an ideal, logical, coherent, and collaborative contribution to dialogue: (1) be truthful and have evidence for what you say, (2) be succinct and yet complete, (3) be relevant to the topic, and (4) be clear and orderly.[21] Taken together these maxims compose a standard that none of us ever fully meets in conversation. When trying to explain ourselves to a health care professional, however, it is not a matter of meeting the standard but of how gravely our lapses interfere with getting treatment, relief, or reassurance. Attachment anxiety usually interferes substantially with all four of Grice's maxims.

With respect to the first maxim, we can safely assume that everyone who is in Dustin's situation is telling the truth. But attachment anxiety interferes with a person's ability to make helpful links between evidence and conclusions or between specific examples and general descriptions. This disconnect often takes the form of presenting a plethora of specific examples without being able to say what general phenomenon they are intended to illustrate, but sometimes it also takes the form of describing a general conclusion ("I'm allergic to everything!")

without being able to link the conclusion to examples that could serve as corroborating evidence. Either way, a patient whose high attachment anxiety has been mobilized by fear about the meaning of physical symptoms and by the pressure of trying to describe the situation to a health care provider often lacks the cognitive flexibility to move easily between the general and the particular, which can make it quite difficult for a provider to grasp the nature of the problem and to believe the story that she is hearing.

The second maxim is about the quantity of information presented – be succinct yet complete. In this case, attachment anxiety leads a person who is a patient to provide too much information. It is common for a medical assessment interview to take substantially longer for a person with this communication style, in part because he simply has so much to say. Fear drives over-inclusiveness – the obsessive need to say absolutely everything to be fully appreciated.

An over-inclusive barrage of anecdotes, concerns, beliefs, and caveats also contravenes the maxim of relevance. One of the reasons that a person like Dustin says too much is that he exercises little discretion over which pieces of information are relevant. Fear interferes with the mental reflection required to make that determination, and he is left with too many words and too few organizing ideas. It is well beyond him in those highly charged moments to be able to pause and reflect on his providers' point of view – to concentrate on what his care provider *needs to hear* to help Dustin.

Another factor that interferes with the apparent relevance of the elements of a narrative is that the purpose of the narrative may be misconstrued. An important idea behind our promotion of an attachment formulation to understand communication between a person with unexplained symptoms and a health care provider is that, for Dustin, the *primary* purpose of the meeting may be relational (using an interpersonal exchange with the provider to resolve a feeling of insecurity) rather than the medical problem-solving exercise that it appears to be and that the provider presumes it is. If this is the case, then a narrative that effectively conveys that a person is feeling great distress and keeps the provider engaged in a dialogue aimed at reducing that distress *is* relevant to the patient, even if much of it appears irrelevant to the task of making a diagnosis and providing a treatment recommendation.

Finally, it should be clear that a narrative characterized by an over-abundance of irrelevant content, weighted inflexibly towards too many facts and too few principles and generalizations, is also likely to be presented with a degree of disorganization that further interferes with effective collaboration. Indeed, rather than being a part of a collaboration, the health care provider in this interaction often feels as if she has been granted the full responsibility of discerning meaning, intuiting patterns, and even inferring the completion of thoughts, as the patient anxiously interrupts himself to move from one idea to the next. Temporal organization is often lacking, with confusion about the chronology of events that are being described and even between which are far in the past and which are more current. The characters in the patient's story may not be carefully identified or placed in content, such as when pronouns are used so extensively that people cannot be easily discerned (who does the patient mean by "she"?) or when proper names are used without first indicating a person's role in the narrative or relationship with the narrator (who is this "Jacob" that Dustin speaks of?).

Describing our health to a health care provider is a form of storytelling. Effective storytelling involves conveying emotion in a way that enriches the content of the story and keeps the listener engaged. Beyond Grice's maxims, which refer to the rhetorical content of speech, narrative coherence is further undermined by expressions of emotion that are disconcertingly intense relative to the content of the story (or, in the case of attachment avoidance, where a story has insufficient emotional expression to keep the listener engaged). In the end, the result is often that a health care provider feels confused and frustrated, and has great difficulty getting the information that she needs to exercise her expertise and offer optimal medical advice.

If you imagine that these same forces of incoherence are likely to be at work in each of the many professional and non-professional relationships involved in a system of fragmented care, it becomes clear that the fragmentation is not simply the result of inattention and expediency on the part of the health care providers or overindulgence in medicine on the part of the patient. Rather, *each conversation is fragmented* and each relationship is cobbled together out of shards of dialogue. Well-intentioned conclusions are drawn from incomplete information; premature guidance is patched together without certainty on the part of the provider or complete acceptance by the person looking for relief. Fragmentation of the system as a whole is in some ways simply a reflection of the much more fundamental pattern of individual emotional, cognitive, and interpersonal fragmentation.

Health care providers' contribution to the suboptimal care of unexplained symptoms

The patient's behaviour is not what makes the patient seem difficult; the experience it evokes in the health care provider, such as fear, hopelessness, helplessness, or hate, is what the provider cannot abide.[22] When a patient like Dustin, who is high in attachment anxiety, uses a confusing communication style with a health care provider, it tends to provoke such a troubling response. Distress that seems irresolvable, plus implicit or explicit requests for more time and more involvement than is convenient or available, plus suffering that yields no familiar diagnosis to suggest a course of treatment can trigger a strong emotional response in Dustin's health care provider. Which specific emotions are triggered varies among providers based on their own psychological characteristics (including their own attachment style), but all are likely to have feelings that are hard to tolerate, such as hostility, hopelessness, helplessness, or fear.

These feelings are not usually expressed directly. The provider doesn't want to have them, let alone acknowledge them to her patient. Neither the provider nor the patient would find any comfort in their expression. And yet disavowed strong feelings will inevitably affect the patient-provider interaction; health care professionals in this situation are prone to making poor decisions, guided by efforts to contain undesirable emotions rather than by what is best for the patient. Many outcomes are possible. Compared with a typical interaction, the medical interview may be truncated prematurely or may carry on interminably. Subtle signs of hostility may be expressed. A prescription or a referral may be presented summarily to end the interaction. The provider may show less certainty and confidence than usual. She may suggest that the problem is in the patient's head or that he just needs to calm down. The patient may then hear a disconcerting implied message: "I don't know what is going on but I know it is your fault." When we appreciate the troubles on both sides of the patient-provider interaction in a situation like Dustin's, no wonder it is hard to bring the matter to a satisfactory resolution.[23]

Dustin Brandt redux (the story in context)

Dustin's story turned out to be more complicated and much more interesting then it seemed at first. This is usually the case – it takes a lot of effort to appreciate a story that is fragmented and fraught – but the effort to understand can go hand in hand with building an alliance that is, in itself, a therapeutic intervention.

It was a big deal for Dustin to see a psychiatrist. Although he had seen several medical specialists over the five or six years that his health had come to dominate most of his daily life, seeing a psychiatrist felt like crossing a different kind of threshold. He worried that he was about to confirm what a few people had said and many more had seemed to silently imply – that his problems were all in his head, that he was complaining needlessly, and that there would be no relief from the symptoms that were virtually ruining his life.

He wanted to tell me that he hadn't always been like this. Seven years ago when he was graduating from university, he felt like his life was finally falling into place. Although he had always been shy, he had met a classmate, Lisa, in his third year of undergraduate economics. They started to date a year later, just before they graduated. Dustin felt good about the relationship and hoped that someday they would marry. He found an entry-level job at a big company in the financial industry and was enjoying the work and starting to make friends there. He wanted to tell me that before all these medical problems started, he was feeling like an adult with a solid future.

Even before relief of distress, many people with physical suffering yearn for an antidote to loneliness and the sense of not being understood or appreciated by another.

Although he wanted to tell his story, he couldn't get the words out. As soon as he started to talk about his health, he was overcome with worry. There were so many facts to convey; it was complicated, and he needed me to understand the nuances and the contradictions in his experience. He had one eye on the clock, expecting to be cut off or discharged, while also scanning for clues that might indicate what I thought of him. The more pressure he felt, the more inarticulate he became.

It is very helpful to recognize when a patient's narrative is becoming incoherent. If Bob isn't attuned to this, perhaps because he is caught up in the hostile feelings that were his first response, then this is a moment where he will become irritated and Dustin will perceive that his "inevitable" dismissal is imminent. Instead, Bob has a model in mind that explains Dustin's lapse in clarity as a response to threats to his sense of security. Seen from this angle, Dustin's incoherence becomes useful information instead of an irritant. Bob might offer at this point that they have the option of scheduling more time if needed to get the story straight – giving Dustin the flexibility he needs to relieve some of the pressure he feels. The underlying message that a health care professional needs to convey at this moment is, "I realize that it is hard to organize your story, and I will try to help you to construct it in a way that we can both understand."

In time, Dustin was able to convey a clearer narrative. He had always been a bit "high strung." He was a colicky baby and his mother had told him many times that he was "way more difficult than your sister." But he also was a smart kid and curious and happy enough when people would leave him alone with the solitary pastimes that he enjoyed.

Dustin started from a different place from his sister. His experience of his internal and external environment was more reactive, right from the start. It was a bad fit with his mother's preference for her easier child. Dustin was an orchid.

He was good at school but changes were hard for him. When kindergarten started, he refused to go, crying and grabbing on to his mother's leg. The teacher encouraged his mother to leave him in her charge, reassuring her that this was common and that he would settle down soon. His mother said that she would rather stay because "little Dusty" would feel better that way, but when he turned his back she slipped away immediately. ("It's a good trick," she told him years later, when he told her that he still remembered the shock of it and that he was inconsolable afterward.) For his first few years, he got stomach aches in the first weeks of September, often missing school because of it. In grade four, the stomach aches came back in December when his teacher left on maternity leave and a replacement took over.

Dustin's mother didn't understand what he needed – a more robust secure base than his sister – and this led to unhelpful behaviour. Her "good trick" amplified his attachment anxiety. Bob can help Dustin see that his needs for support are legitimate and, eventually, that his expectation that he will be too much for others no longer applies to all important relationships. Putting his story in context can begin to normalize Dustin's persistent anxiety and the sense of not being able to be understood that keeps him at a distance from others.

Dustin's descriptions of his parents were superficial. His father was not around very much because he travelled as part of his work and "was tired" when he was home. Dustin reported that his father "loved us and every-thing," but he wasn't able to provide any specific memories that demon-strated his father's feelings. His mother, on the other hand was ever-present. Dustin called her "pretty anxious," and the stories that he told of her sug-gested that she tended to do what was expedient rather than giving much thought to what Dustin needed.

Dustin's bland description of his father is also a mark of incoherence, because there really isn't anything in it that could help Bob to appre-ciate what the father was like or the quality of the relationship he had with Dustin, except that it seemed disengaged. Although much of Dustin's presentation is evidence of strong attachment anxiety, describing his father with an empty cliché is a mark of attachment avoidance.

Dustin's mother was doing her best, probably from an insecure base of her own and apparently without much support, and her style seems to have worked well enough with his sister. Nonetheless, her prefer-ence for expedience (as with her "good trick" at the kindergarten) privi-leged her own need over Dustin's. We can appreciate that as his needs for a consistent secure base and responsiveness to his reactivity were overruled time and time again, he learned to hide the vulnerability that he felt. Although Dustin comes across as having high attachment anxi-ety, it is mixed with some evidence of attachment avoidance.

Things changed for the better after puberty. Dustin found that even though he was socially awkward, he could gain his peers' acceptance by excelling in sports. It took Dustin a long time to warm up, but he valued the few close friends that he made in high school and stayed in touch afterward.

Operating from a place of competency, Dustin remains cautious of rela-tionships, but he *can* develop trust and has relationships that persist. This is a good sign – the lessons about aloneness and incompatibility with others from his early years are being overwritten.

University was surprisingly good. Dustin chose to go to a school out of town. Unlike his reactions to starting fresh at school in the early grades, Dustin thrived. He liked being away from his parents' home and loved being among smart and friendly peers who left him alone to find his own way. He surprised himself by joining a student club and played intramural sports. Although he had only a few good friends, he liked the community that surrounded him. In third year he met Lisa, and by the time he graduated he felt like he was finally finding his stride.

This successful phase is a positive sign about Dustin's capacity for resilience and is useful in his therapy because Bob can remind Dustin of his success and ask about what he did then that worked – a strategy to engage him in collaborating on current solutions.

Lisa and Dustin faced a major decision shortly after graduating. They found work in different cities – close enough to commute but not conveniently. It forced them to make choices about their relationship a little earlier than they would have otherwise wanted – would they live together, and if so where? They decided that they wanted to be together, and so they split the difference on the commuting inconvenience by living in a suburb midway between their jobs.

Rentals were hard to find, so the young professionals decided that they could buy a starter home if they each came up with half of a minimal down payment. For Dustin, that meant borrowing money from his parents, an entanglement that moved him in exactly the opposite direction of the independence in which he had been flourishing. His father seemed far from enthusiastic, pointing out that his retirement was not far off and that their resources were limited. His mother said that they would give Dustin whatever he needed before he even had a chance to explain his situation. But what followed were ambiguous statements that seemed to contradict that support – at least by inference. She muttered "harrumph" when he spoke of Lisa's excellent prospects with her employer. She spoke of how expensive it was to live these days but clammed up when he enquired further. Worse, she started to express opinions about the house they would buy – were they sure they wanted to live there? Dustin thought that his mother had some claim on those decisions, since she now had a financial stake. He started visiting his parents more, sometimes with Lisa and sometimes alone. Either way, he usually left with a headache.

Dustin found that life in the suburbs was less than what he had hoped for. He and Lisa had to leave early each morning, travelling in opposite directions, often returning late in the evening. They didn't have nearly as much time together as they had before graduating. They didn't have much contact with the neighbours. It was an isolating existence, and Dustin was losing his enthusiasm for this new stage of his life. He started to worry that Lisa wouldn't continue to want to be with him because they spent so little time together, and when they did his tension and unhappiness would interfere with their enjoyment.

Despite reasonable plans, Dustin finds his choices unwittingly precipitating isolation and an uneasy closeness to his parents. He has transferred many of his attachment needs, and in particular his secure base function, from his parents to Lisa, and having her less available reawakened old anxieties. Proximity to his parents doesn't help, and actually exacerbates his unease at this point.

Dustin started to worry that Lisa found other people more interesting than he was. He began to experience a feeling in the morning that hadn't been present for many years – he was afraid of starting the day, wishing that he didn't have to take the train to work. He now had diarrhea most mornings, which he recognized as a consequence of his anticipatory anxiety, and it sometimes made him late for work.

The most dramatic change came almost a year later. Dustin's mother discovered that she had advanced colon cancer. The next six months before she died were an agony of hope, disappointment, and suffering. A tumour in her spine caused intense pain, and she seemed to be a magnet for all the complications of treatment with radiation and chemotherapy. While she was in and out of hospital, Dustin had little choice but to be fully involved in her care. His father seemed to react to the worsening of his wife's health by becoming more withdrawn – working through the day and watching TV at night, often with headphones on "so I won't bother you, honey." Dustin's sister has her own family and had moved to a distant city. When something needed to be done, it fell to Dustin to do it. He started to miss work often enough that it was an issue for his employer.

We can't help but wonder if this was what it used to be like – if when Mom needed help raising the kids, Dad pulled away and left her to handle it on her own. No wonder expediency won out so often. Luckily for Mom, she had Dustin to fill the gap this time, and he did his best. But we can imagine that his emotions in this situation were a knot of hot wires. He may have felt sadness and grief about his mother's impending death, a reawakening of abandonment fears, resentment or rage at his father's abdication of responsibility, fear that Lisa or his workplace will find him to be much too difficult and reject or abandon him, and fear about his own bowel, to name a few.

Maintaining that pace became harder as Dustin's symptoms accumulated. He was not feeling like himself most of the time, although he had trouble saying exactly what was wrong. He felt "stupid," with lapses of attention and concentration that were becoming more common. He was constantly tired and sleeping poorly. Headaches and diarrhea became the norm.

These symptoms are best understood as the endpoint of chronic unresolved stress, sleep disruption, and overactivation of Dustin's sympathetic nervous system and hypothalamic-pituitary-adrenal axis. Chronic stress leaves most people feeling fatigued, cognitively impaired, physically sore, with perhaps an organ-specific symptom on top of it all, like Dustin's diarrhea.

The diarrhea was bad enough that Dustin saw his family doctor for the first time in years. He was told that he might have celiac disease and a referral to a gastroenterologist was made, although Dustin had to cancel it when another crisis in his mother's health arose. Just in case, Dustin started removing gluten from his diet.

Dustin's avoidance kept him away from the medical system until things were all but out of control. This was a problem in two ways: he had no ongoing relationship with a doctor he knew and trusted, and the doctor didn't know him either, so when he arrived with bad bowel symptoms, the doctor was obliged to rule out the worst case scenario. Dustin didn't have a calm reassuring first contact.

After a few months of this almost intolerable situation, Dustin had an episode that tilted the balance completely. He was leaving the house earlier and more quickly than he was comfortable doing to attend a medical appointment with his mother, feeling the pressure to carry on in spite of the uncomfortable feeling that his bowel "wasn't finished yet." Most unfortunately, his worst fear came true; he lost control of his bowels and had to return home to change his clothes. It was, he says, "completely humiliating." At that point Dustin stopped going to work.

In Dustin's story, we see a man who overcame his early insecurity by having a successful transition to his peer group and then to marriage, but circumstances pulled him back into his family. Then, his insecurities were reactivated, leaving him an amalgam of a scared kid and an adult who feels incompetent in spite of extraordinary efforts to support his dying mother. In this crisis, he lost his ability to regulate his emotions, his relationships, and his body.

When Dustin's mother died, his world seemed to fall completely apart. In spite of his worries, Lisa showed no sign of wanting out, but their relationship had changed. Dustin could find nothing to talk about except his health, and Lisa had made it clear that she didn't sign up to be his nurse or a one-person support group. Lisa was thriving in her new career and was focusing her energy on the positive part of her life. Dustin felt that they were strangers sharing a house. His symptoms persisted, and it became less and less common for him to leave the house at all, except for appointments. He saw one health care provider after another trying to find the explanation and the treatment that would put his life back on the rails.

Dustin's secure base, Lisa, had moved far enough away emotionally that she didn't effectively serve that function anymore. Dustin has all the old fears, plus a few new ones, and sees no way out.

On top of everything else Dustin was perplexed by his emotions. He expected to be relieved when his mother died, and he was to some extent. But the relief made him feel guilty. He was surprised at how much he missed his mother and how sad he felt. He was angry at his father for abdicating his responsibility when it mattered, and he dealt with this by cutting off all but the most perfunctory communication. What made all this worse was that it felt like he had to keep it to himself. Dustin's mother had been nothing but a negative force in his relationship with Lisa, and he felt it would be hard for her to listen with any sympathy or understanding to his grief and guilt. He couldn't really express his thoughts with any clarity anyway, so he just shut up.

If Lisa is unwilling to listen, it will further diminish her capacity to be a secure base for Dustin, but it's really an assumption on his part – Lisa might be more able to listen to him talk about his ambivalence towards his mother than he thinks. Seeing no other options, Dustin's oldest strategy, self-imposed isolation, wins out.

That's how things were for Dustin when he decided to accept his family doctor's advice that he should go and talk to a psychiatrist. He was simultaneously intensely looking forward to "someone who can finally hear me out and understand me" and horrified by the prospect that he was about to be found guilty of being weak and deficient, the author of all his own misfortune and, in his mother's words, "way more difficult" than all the more robust and normal people that he saw around him. Imagine what it would have been like for him if Bob had succumbed to the urge to reduce his suffering to a sick joke and a stereotype, to casually assume that Dustin could be known to him before his story was even heard. Imagine how little good it would have done Dustin to hear a reductive explanation of his suffering and receive a new diagnosis and a prescription for an antidepressant. That is the challenge a health care professional meets when trying to reverse the course of difficult, unexplained symptoms.

11 Trouble in the Patient-Provider Relationship

Jon: My dad was a physician in a different era. He came of age, so to speak, by serving as a navigator-bombardier in World War II, practised psychiatry in the 1950s and 1960s, and became the chair of the university's department of psychiatry. He was a thoughtful and highly respected clinician. Of course, I saw another side of him, the person behind the professional. When I was at university he drove me home some nights after finishing his practice for the day. One day, after a full schedule of difficult psychotherapeutic hours, I remember him getting into the car, lighting a cigarette, sucking so hard that he seemed to draw it down to a butt in one inhalation, and then finally speaking as he exhaled, "I've done nothing but take shit from borderlines all day!"

Health care professionals and patients have intense feelings about what happens between them more often than is acknowledged. These feelings are amplified in some situations, like psychotherapy, where clinicians are usually highly attuned to emotions, but they also emerge in other patient-provider interactions where a greater risk exists of unacknowledged or unrecognized feelings interfering with optimal care. This chapter is about what happens between health care providers and patients, especially when these interactions become challenging and unsatisfactory.

Trouble

It is not an indictment of health care providers, nor of patients, to notice that they sometimes exasperate each other. Patients are often frustrated by long waits, rudeness, and providers' intolerance of disagreement.[1] Providers tend to find patients difficult to get along with when they are angry, excessively needy, or unsatisfied with explanations and advice.[2] Such difficulty can't be solely attributed to either party but occurs *between* people.[3] Patterns of attachment provide a useful framework for understanding difficulty in provider-patient interactions for two reasons. First, health care almost inevitably provokes an attachment response in patients, especially when they are sick. A system designed to be switched on by the threat of personal peril is reliably activated by circumstances that include some combination of internal signals of danger (e.g., medical symptoms), external signs of danger (e.g., painful procedures, bad news, and uncertainty), exposure to strangers, and dependence on others for care. In encounters in which our attachment systems are activated, it makes sense that patterns of attachment will guide what happens in provider-patient interactions.

The second reason that attachment theory is a useful lens through which to view provider-patient difficulties is that when a patient is in the mode of activating strategies designed to help her feel more comfortable, she may use a health care provider to serve attachment functions, especially to act as a safe haven. Of course, not just any health care provider can fill that role (recall the surgeon in Bob's "minor surgery" story in Chapter 6); it needs to be someone who is trusted and in a position to offer comfort or protection.[4] We previously quoted Donald Winnicott saying, "There is no such thing as a baby, there is always a baby and someone,"[5] declaring the imperative that an infant always needs to be understood in the context of a crucially important relationship. After exploring adult attachment in Chapter 6 we might have extended that thought, less poetically, to say, "There is no such thing as an adult; there is always an adult and someone, even if it is only someone in mind." Although adults obviously function independently, we do not exercise our autonomy as solitary beings. We remain irreducibly social, bound to those around us to whom we are closest, to the memories of past relationships, and to the unremembered ways in which those relationships have shaped us. Now we can offer the medical version of that provocative paradox: "There is no such thing as a patient; there is always a patient and a health care provider."

None of us can enter the role of patient alone. The choice to become a patient is guided by attachment relationships, past and present, which influence whether or not we have symptoms, whether or not they bother us, whether or not we need them to be explained and treated, and whether or not we can trust another person to help us when we are in need. Furthermore, the role of patient is a social role. No patient exists without a provider of health care. A sick person is just a sick person until he enters the conversation in which he becomes a patient. And in that social role, the contribution of the other (doctor, nurse, chiropractor ...) cannot help but influence the medical outcome. We are never patients alone. As a result, difficulty in the patient-provider relationship can arise from attachment behaviour,[6] especially when attachment behaviour is not recognized for what it is – a patient is seeking feelings of security while the provider is focused only on the medical problem-solving task. These different goals put them at cross purposes and sets up frustrating miscommunications.

We found some evidence for the validity of an attachment formulation when we had the opportunity to work with a group of South African doctors who studied the impact of a patient's attachment style on emergency department visits, which are often highly charged, high-stakes physician-patient interactions. Patients are more distressed in the emergency department than in most other provider-patient interactions; many things compete for doctors' time and attention; the concern is greater about getting a diagnosis dangerously wrong. Furthermore, an emergency room patient and physician are very likely to be meeting each other for the first time. They have no interpersonal history that would allow each to give the other the benefit of the doubt.

Not surprisingly, among the patients who went to the emergency department of the Pretoria Academic Hospital, the physicians were far more likely to find the interaction difficult if the patient had an insecure attachment style. Physicians reported difficult interactions with almost none of the secure patients who attended the emergency department, with about 15% of those with high attachment avoidance or high attachment anxiety, and with 39% of those with fearful attachment.[7] These patients did not differ in the types of problems that brought them to the emergency department, many of which were quite complicated, but the nature of the conversation was very different with patients who had different patterns of attachment.[8] Of course, it is lopsided to measure the difficulty experienced by physicians without measuring the patients' dissatisfaction – we are guessing that the patients didn't find these interactions very satisfactory either.

On a patient's side, trouble in the provider-patient relationship may come in the form of finding a provider to be untrustworthy or unsupportive. A patient's ability to trust her physician may be a key component of a solid working alliance, especially when dealing with serious diseases, such as cancer, where trust facilitates effective communication and decision making, reduces fear, and improves treatment adherence. People with cancer feel more trusting of physicians whom they perceive to be technically competent, honest, and patient centred.[9] Although these are characteristics attributed to physicians, patient characteristics can be a strong determinant of their perceptions of doctors.[10] For cancer patients, for example, patterns of attachment are one determinant of patients' ability to trust doctors.[11] Let's look at how different patterns of insecure attachment challenge the provider-patient relationship.

High attachment anxiety

Susan experiences symptoms frequently and fears what they might mean. She often goes to the doctor in spite of the fact that she often doesn't find the interaction with her physician very helpful. She attends today because she is having dizzy spells. She has many worries. What if it happens when she is driving? What if it doesn't get better? What is causing it – a stroke? A tumour? Her doctor wants to know what she means by "dizzy." Susan replies, "You know, it's like that dizzy feeling, oh I hate that, you know ..."

When Susan walked into the clinic she entered a conversation, an interpersonal evaluation of her situation. Ideally this conversation would be a focused, collaborative, empathic problem-solving exercise. However, both Susan and her doctor are disadvantaged in obtaining that ideal. Susan is uncomfortable and anxious, a mental state that profoundly interferes with problem solving. Susan's incoherent narrative prevents her from conveying much information beyond a sense that she is distressed and needs help. Although she is badly in need of reassurance, the story Susan tells doesn't help her physician to develop a clear hypothesis; he tries to reassure her, but his efforts are premature because he doesn't fully understand what is going on.

Susan's doctor is in a hurry and is biased by previous similar encounters. He scans her story for patterns that suggest disease and makes diagnostic inferences very efficiently,[12] and so Susan has a short time to make her initial pitch. Her physician may quickly intuit that it will be difficult to end this interaction satisfactorily in the time available, which may lead him to shift his interactive style towards a pattern that is intended to contain Susan's emotion and impose closure rather than encouraging exploration. He uses narrow interrogative questions and leaps to reassurance and prescriptive advice instead of using open-ended questions, silent pauses, and empathic reflection, and clarifying when he is uncertain. Both parties are likely to end up feeling that they are working against each other. Each will find the other difficult and the interaction will be disappointing, if not aggravating.

If the interaction is poor enough, the doctor may default to trying to solve the medical question by doing more tests than usual. The results of the tests raise even more questions. Equivocal tests increase the intensity of Susan's apprehension. Even negative tests often do not actually reassure her.[13]

To make matters worse, when Susan doesn't feel satisfied after appointments like these, she often seeks help from other health care providers. The ones that she sticks with (her family doctor, a chiropractor, a naturopath, and her neighbour who is an anaesthetist) are distinguished more by their supportive and sympathetic manner than by their provision of useful explanations and solutions for her symptoms. Since these providers communicate with each other very little (or not at all), their support and advice is often inconsistent. Finally, to try to fix an ill-defined problem, her family doctor sometimes prescribes medication prematurely. It is well intentioned, but it tends to further muddy the water. One thing leads to another. Tests lead to more tests, and appointments lead to more appointments. Perhaps a consultation with a specialist is required. The cycle continues for as long as both the patient and the health care providers keep a narrow focus on the symptoms and do not attend sufficiently to Susan's underlying feelings of insecurity.

High attachment avoidance

Linda has been managing her diabetes since she was a young girl. She is now attending university, living in a different city from her family for the first time, and she is proud of what she has accomplished. It is a busy life and she loves the variety. She has never had problems with self-esteem, and she doesn't see why she should bother to worry about what others think of her. She manages her diet, does her blood tests to check on her glucose levels, and delivers her injections of insulin according to her own intuitions rather than strictly following the guidelines that she has been taught. It is not her style to feel self-conscious about finding a private place to give herself an injection or to make a special food request.

Like most of her classmates, Linda has a lifestyle that has become less predictable since coming to school. She goes to sleep later than she used to, except when she needs to crash and catch up. She has developed a student's pattern of drinking to excess on pub nights and weekends. In spite of running for exercise, for the first time in her life she is a few pounds above her ideal weight. When she got around to finding a doctor at the student health clinic to prescribe insulin rather than working with her old family doctor long distance, she was surprised that he was concerned about how she was managing her illness. She told him that she had it covered.

Her new doctor told her that, on the contrary, her lifestyle was unhealthy and she needed to get her diabetes under tighter control. He recommended that she increase the frequency of her glucose tests and that she see a diabetes educator to learn to adjust her insulin doses more effectively based on changes in her diet and exercise from day to day. Linda had seen a diabetes educator years ago, and she didn't think she had time now to repeat the process. The doctor wanted to see her again in two weeks. She left feeling criticized, and decided that rather than following his advice she would just go back to her family doctor when she was home for the next vacation.

Linda resents it when the doctor acts like he is the only one who understands her illness, and she resists authoritarian advice. She takes her medication and monitors her diet as she deems appropriate. Unfortunately her control of her diabetes is suffering. She found her childhood family doctor much easier to deal with. She always asked Linda what she thought was going on or what was important to her. Linda got the sense from that doctor's manner and how she treated patients that she was open to collaboration and "human" in a way that made her more approachable.

Adherence to professional advice is greater when patients are engaged in the problem-solving exercise and when the proposed solution is aligned with the patient's view of what the problem is. Even so, it is frequently hard for patients to fully adhere to a treatment plan. Many things may interfere, including the complexity of the medical regimen, the cost and side effects of treatment, and the often weak relationship between adherence and the perceived benefits of treatment (as in the case of continuing to take antibiotics when you are no longer feeling sick).

Attachment avoidance, as exemplified by Linda, can also interfere, especially when a patient with high attachment avoidance must interact with a health care provider who doesn't communicate effectively.[14]

Imagine what it feels like for someone like Linda to recognize and accept that she has a formidable disease that will require relinquishing any illusion of invulnerability at the same time that she is trying to establish a working relationship with a doctor who comes across as a control freak. The more she resists the patient role, the more prescriptive her doctor becomes, insisting on closer monitoring and tighter adherence to instructions. The doctor is simply advocating for the best practices of his profession. Nonetheless, it is a recipe for a stand-off and ineffective medical care.

Narrative coherence may also play a role. In contrast to Susan, who tends to say too much, a patient like Linda, whose feelings of insecurity are protected by avoidant strategies, may not give the physician enough information to work with. She may approach the doctor with apprehension about allowing him into her private world and may thus move to end the conversation prematurely, acting as if she has received what she needs without fully discussing the nature of the trouble. Her busy doctor may be grateful for a quick and apparently satisfactory appointment without pausing to enquire into her real concern. Worse yet for the quality of the conversation they are having, a patient with strong attachment avoidance like Linda may maintain interpersonal space through a critical or hostile attitude towards a health care provider. It takes a real professional on a good day to put up with much personal criticism for the sake of a full and empathic enquiry into a patient's condition when the patient herself doesn't seem inclined to figure it out.

The link between attachment avoidance and difficulties adhering to prescribed treatments introduces a dilemma for health care providers. How do we do something to help individuals with high attachment avoidance to improve their health without being intrusive and authoritarian, which makes them want to avoid medical care even more intently? Do we have to choose between driving away the very people that we would like to help and leaving them to their own devices? This dilemma demands creative solutions.

Fearful attachment

From an attachment perspective, we know that the same people who use health care resources the least experience the most unexplained symptoms. They make same-day crisis medical appointments more often than any other group and are also the most likely to cancel appointments.[15] These are clear examples of the tension that results when two conflicting attachment drives both come into play: anxious, hyper-vigilant amplification of signs of danger and need (which fuels symptoms) combines with mistrust and avoidance of seeking help. We can easily imagine that a person who is caught between the fear of danger and the fear of those who might be protective may elect to suffer in silence, frozen between isolation and interpersonal connection with no available position of comfort.

Su Mei finds that visits to her doctor cause tension, so she avoids them when she can. The wait is often long, which is inconvenient and sometimes stressful, but she sees her doctor as "having all the power," and so she doesn't complain. At the start of the appointment she feels that she needs to justify her visit by talking about all that she has tried before, implying that the doctor is her last resort, rather than simply saying she needs help. When he assures her that she is doing well, she understands this as meaning that he is used to seeing far sicker patients – he has more important things to do and he doesn't really appreciate her fear about her situation. As the appointment ends and the doctor recommends a course of action, Su Mei silently accepts it because she worries that he would be annoyed if she disagreed, but she isn't very likely to act on the plan because she hasn't fully participated in creating it – in fact, she hasn't even spoken about most of what concerns her.[16]

Understanding troublesome relationship moments from an attachment perspective opens up new opportunities to act more helpfully. Rather than seeing Su Mei as demanding and disorganized, the physician who is able to see her as frightened and in need of support is at a tremendous advantage, both in terms of getting her what she needs and in simply managing his or her own emotional responses to their interaction.

Now, what should we do about attachment insecurity as it affects disease and illness? That is the topic of Section Three, because we are now finally in a position to describe what relational health care might actually look like.

Summary of Section Two

Once you start to think about the impact of close relationships on health, you see the evidence just about everywhere. Here is what we have learned in Section Two.

Human social organization, the evolution of big brains, and protected infant development exist in a self-reinforcing cycle. During evolution, longer protected development has allowed for the development of larger brains, which in turn has facilitated more sophisticated social communication, which enhances brain development and allows for more sophisticated ways for societies to protect and enhance the care of infants. Our emergence as the species that we are has depended on attachment.

The first attachment is between infants and parents. From the start the system is regulated by simple biological signals and that in turn regulates an infant's biology, but it is not long before it is imbued with feeling and meaning. From that point on, attachment is about relating with others in whatever way we need to feel secure.

Crucial early interactions between infants and parents shape the development of connections between regions of the brain. Well-attuned early interactions foster the development of a social brain that is biased towards rich social interaction throughout life. Children whose genes and experience foster a state of affairs in which it is relatively easy to feel secure also develop subtle and sophisticated skills of social cognition – they become interested in what is going on in others' minds and in their own, are attentive to social cues, and desire reciprocity and intimate communication. At the same time, these budding social experts (whom we call secure) develop other valuable skills: the ability to soothe themselves when they are upset, to calm their bodies when they are overexcited, and to pause to consider what is best in the long run instead of acting immediately to gratify wants or react to threats. Each of these skills reinforces the others as elements of social competence and contributes to becoming a well-regulated individual.

Our early experiences shape the lens through which we perceive our social world and our responses to what we find there and lead to persistent and oftentimes permanent patterns of commerce between those we are closest to and ourselves. The permanence extends to our states of mind about those relationships and the ways in which we manage emotions and perceptions of threat. These patterns of attachment, whether secure or insecure, guide much of our experience in our most important adult relationships and have an enduring and important impact on our health.

Insecure attachment interferes with one of the most powerful protective forces for health and longevity available to humans: the emotional and practical support that we receive from others. Insecure attachment is intimately linked to the harmful effects of stress and promotes one of the most destructive forces for health, which is depression. Because we are hardwired to commit to whatever it takes to feel secure, insecure patterns of attachment drive us to behave in whatever ways will promote security or reduce insecurity in the short term, regardless of the long-term risk – all the more so because insecure attachment is usually accompanied by difficulty tolerating tension or distress long enough to let reflection on what is best in the long run modify our responses. The consequences of this drive to quickly ameliorate feelings of insecurity constitute some of the most important disease-promoting aspects of our lifestyles, especially obesity, alcoholism, and smoking.

Insecure patterns of attachment hide in plain sight wherever we see the core problems of vexing health care. They lead individuals to suffer excessively with symptoms that cannot be explained. They lead people to use relationships with health care providers to regulate feelings rather than to identify and treat diseases. Unrecognized, they play havoc with those relationships – causing dissatisfaction and difficulty for all involved.

In short, insecure patterns of attachment, although rarely recognized as such in the to and fro of relationships between health care providers and patients, are a major contributor to both disease and illness, and a source of many of the most vexing problems facing patients and providers alike. Furthermore, patterns of attachment provide one of the best and easiest ways in which to understand how to personalize health care – why *not* to provide exactly the same service for everyone who has the same health problem. That maybe equality, but it's clearly not smart. William Osler is widely quoted as having said that it is more important to know the patient than the disease, and attachment theory provides one of the most accessible and relevant ways for health care providers to do just that. *How* to do that is the focus of the final section of this book.

SECTION THREE

Relational Health Care

Introduction to Section Three:
Principles of Adaptation and Change

In retrospect, the fact that it was night-time, pelting rain, and I was sitting in a parked car with a dear friend who needed to share some bad news seems corny, like a movie scene overwrought with pathetic fallacy. In residency, Ken and I had gravitated to the same kind of work, pretty much running the psychiatric consultation-liaison service when he was the senior and I was the junior resident, and being the first residents in the system to join the Psychiatric Clinic for HIV Concerns. Although we worked with really ill people, illness hadn't touched either of us directly. We were young, active guys, raising families, playing baseball. He teased me about my propensity to cuss; I teased him about his hairline. That night he told me he had an inoperable and inevitably fatal brain tumour. "Jonnie," he said, "on Monday I was a doctor, and on Tuesday I became a patient."

At one time or another, we are all patients. Every time a health professional enters a clinic or a hospital in the role of patient, he has an opportunity to experience the many ways in which the culture of health care can fail to validate and respond to the human needs of people who are sick. He also has the opportunity to see how the system can make his challenge easier by being respectful, informative, interested, honest, accessible, reassuring, and responsive. When people who provide health care take an interpersonal perspective, the experience of patients improves.

This final section discusses how health care can adapt to better meet the diverse relational needs of patients. Since much of routine health care has been designed for the convenience of health care providers and institutions rather than for patients, it demands a degree of adaptability that can be difficult for people with insecure attachment to muster while they are feeling scared or unwell. Since about 40% of adults have insecure attachment (and it is even more common among people who have serious disease), a great many of our patients are trying to get the care they need in a system that is not designed to consider their interpersonal style.

The principles that guide our recommendations to clinicians, educators, and planners are simple.

1. Health care is better, and ultimately the health of patients is better, when it is provided in a way that is well matched to each patient's interpersonal style.
2. We emphasize how clinicians and patients can adapt their behaviour to suit individual differences in attachment style. We are much more interested in adaptation than we are in changing people's patterns of attachment.
3. Sometimes small changes have a big impact.
4. Prescriptions need to be practical – practising relational health care can't depend on becoming an expert in interpersonal psychology.

12 How Health Care Providers Can Adapt When Attachment Anxiety Interferes

Pain and fear trump everything else. A person who is in too much pain, or is too frightened, can't participate in a problem-solving exercise. Until she experiences some relief, she can't effectively collaborate with a health care provider to figure out what is wrong and what needs to be done. A patient with high attachment anxiety and low attachment avoidance is prone to fear and feels inadequate to meet health challenges alone.[1] In this chapter we will review the challenges that arise when a patient's attachment anxiety causes fear to interfere with health and health care, and we'll describe the 13 recommendations that are summarized below.

RECOMMENDATIONS FOR HEALTH CARE PROVIDERS ADAPTING TO A PATIENT WITH HIGH ATTACHMENT ANXIETY

1. Maintain unflappable calm.
2. Take a thoughtful history.
3. Take time.
4. Use specific techniques to reduce anxiety.
5. Allow your patient to use the resources that help him to feel more secure.
6. Break the contingency between expressing distress and getting care.
7. Be predictable, attentive, and supportive.
8. Use your observations about incoherence as useful information.
9. Use the skills of active listening.
10. Remember that anger starts with fear.

11. Teach healthy assertiveness.
12. Facilitate communication and coordination between agents of care.
13. Present the team as an integrated whole.

We have said that an interaction with a health care professional often triggers the attachment system because its circumstances involve an immediate or anticipated threat to our well-being. This is even more often the case for someone with high attachment anxiety because his threshold for detecting danger is low. He is wary and vigilant for signs of harm, and so the concerns that bring him into a medical setting frequently trigger his attachment system to respond in its characteristic ways.

Distress and symptoms

The most obvious aspect of anxious attachment that complicates health care is the distress that people with high attachment anxiety experience. Distress comes in many forms, including worry, fear, pessimism, and physical discomfort. People with high attachment anxiety report more unexplained symptoms and more intense symptoms in general.[2] They also worry more about what those symptoms mean. Worrying can take the form of *rumination* (turning the same bothersome ideas over and over in our minds), *catastrophizing* (assuming that the worst possible outcome), and *hypochondriasis* (a false belief that we have a serious illness).

Health care providers often find rumination, catastrophizing, hypochondriasis, and expressions of distress that are out of proportion to the apparent circumstances to be frustrating because they put the provider's understanding of the problem at odds with the patient's understanding; they can't agree about how to proceed. It can be helpful to realize that within the framework of attachment theory, it makes perfect sense for a person with high attachment anxiety to send out frequent signals of distress. We find that it often helps to bear in mind that a person with this style has learned through her hard-won experience that it is *adaptive* to make extra efforts to be sure that the ones on whom she depends for care are nearby and paying attention. We assume when we meet people with this style that sending out frequent distress signals is a behaviour that was reinforced, especially during our patient's developmental years, because it sometimes worked when other strategies did not. Seeing that a set of expectations or behaviours that don't seem effective in the current circumstances were learned when they were the most rational and effective response that was available helps to reduce the stigma and blame that can otherwise slip inadvertently into a difficult provider-patient interchange.

It also helps to realize that behaviour that has been repeatedly reinforced can operate as a *reflex*. When that happens, expressing frequent distress isn't a conscious choice – it happens automatically. These automatic expressions of distress or help seeking often occur even when a health care provider is being perfectly helpful and attentive. A person with high attachment anxiety simply does not have an effective off button for this type of communication.

It is difficult for a person with high attachment anxiety to control or regulate distress very effectively. He tends not to have access to the kind of support from others that is so effective in reducing distress and giving a person the opportunity to reflect. Lacking the opportunity to reflect, his ability to solve problems, or to be optimistic, or cope in similar ways may be limited. He may also have a limited capacity to tolerate minor distress long enough to see that it will pass. For all these reasons, it often falls to the health care provider to initiate the actions that will help a person with high attachment anxiety feel calmer and get the most out of his interaction with the health care system.

To help a patient who has high attachment anxiety, a health care professional should realize that she needs to help him feel more comfortable. A health care provider can do several things to accomplish this goal.

1. *Maintain unflappable calm.* A health care professional needs to demonstrate calm to help a patient to be calmer. An attitude of unflappable competence sets the stage for everything else that will happen. Having this composure is harder than it sounds. It requires a clinician to listen and respond empathically without accepting the catastrophic assumptions that may underlie a patient's worries *and* without appearing dismissive of the validity of his distress.

Maintaining a calm and competent manner also requires a professional to be able to tolerate whatever distress she may be feeling without immediately acting on it. A clinician in this situation needs to be able to reflect on her own feelings and imagine what might be going on in the patient's inner world – that is, to mentalize in the service of providing a calm and empathic presence.

2. Take a thoughtful history. It is easy to overlook the power of simple interventions, like taking a history. Taking a careful history of the concerns that are foremost in a patient's mind conveys the message that his distress is being taken seriously. If a clinician assumes that she already knows what is going on (as Bob was tempted to do when he first met Dustin Brandt), she will convey a lack of concern that trivializes the patient's most urgent concerns. This reaction has the undesirable effect of essentially *forcing* the patient to express his concern even more dramatically – how else is he going to be taken seriously? On the other hand, if a patient sees that the clinician is genuinely curious and competently pursuing hypotheses about his concerns, it allows him to relax the imperative to constantly express signals of distress to maintain his link to a source of safe haven.

A second benefit of a thoughtful history is that it can bolster a patient's capacity to cope. If a patient is feeling overwhelmed, asking about other situations in which he has faced major challenges and especially asking about what has worked well and what not so well can remind him that his personal resources are more robust than they may feel at the moment, and encourage him to draw again on the strategies and confidence that have previously been helpful.

Third, taking a careful history bolsters a health care professional's credibility to make suggestions. A professional who is attuned to the interpersonal dance that attachment anxiety demands is already anticipating that the end of the appointment is likely to be harder than the beginning. Anxiety will rise as separation looms. The result will be that at exactly the phase of the interview where the professional would like the patient to be able to absorb new information, collaborate on next steps, and be open to helpful suggestions, anxiety will once again be threatening to trump the practical tasks. Having taken a careful history and demonstrated some understanding of the situation *from the patient's perspective* gives a professional a strong advantage in being able to engage the patient in a collaborative end to their encounter when the time comes.

3. Take time. Rushing a patient who is feeling overwhelmed by attachment anxiety through an appointment is counterproductive. It has the effect of increasing his distress, which complicates all other aspects of assessment and of agreeing on investigation and treatment. The corollary is a paradox: taking your time will speed things up.

4. Use specific techniques to reduce anxiety. When a health care professional and a patient know each other somewhat (not usually at a first assessment), it can be beneficial to use specific techniques to help a patient to reduce anxiety. We say this usually needs to come later than a first visit because to be effective it depends on the patient understanding that he has *two* problems – the medical concern at hand plus the anxiety that is interfering with dealing with it effectively. Introducing specific anxiety-reduction techniques too soon tends to convey the inaccurate and unhelpful message that the professional thinks that the real problem is anxiety *and not* the medical concern for which the patient is seeking help.

Patients can learn and use many techniques to relax when distress is high. The professional's role is to teach these techniques; it is much more effective to teach a person how to relax than to do things that make him relax. That is why we favour teaching breathing exercises and imagery techniques or self-hypnosis rather than providing hypnosis or relaxing imagery or tranquilizing medications like benzodiazepines. To be sure, we use the latter as well as the former, but even then the intent is to build bridges towards a patient's ability to regulate her own distress.[3]

5. *Allow your patient to use the resources that help him to feel more comfortable.* We advise patients who are overwhelmed by anxiety in a medical context to write their concerns and questions out in advance and to bring a supportive person with them. Ideally this person can help the patient to feel more comfortable and therefore act more effectively in her own interests. Even if the person who serves this attachment need is not available, it helps to at least have a buddy – a person who can remember what was said and take care of practical things.

The corollary is that health care providers are wise to accommodate the presence of a buddy and to respect the questions and concerns that patients have written out. It sometimes happens that health care professionals adopt a dismissive or critical response to these manoeuvres. This may be a reflex reaction to the patient's underlying distress and neediness, or to a fear that it will endlessly lengthen the duration of the encounter – a response that is worth suppressing.

Neediness and dependence

Nobody wants to think that others find him clingy. For people with high attachment anxiety, this can be a very potent concern. Often, their experience has led them to observe that the need that they feel to be close to others drives people away. It can set up a loop in which a fear of being undesirable increases insecurity and triggers a self-fulfilling prophecy, as one person's urgent need to get closer provokes another person's need to enforce a comfortable distance.

In medical settings, this may translate into frequent appointments at an outpatient clinic[4] or overuse of emergency and drop-in services. For a hospitalized patient it can be measured by how often a patient presses the call bell to alert nurses to her needs. In these situations, a health care professional's first impulse is likely to be distancing. It is easy to invoke sensible ideas like limit setting, maintaining boundaries, and refusing to collude with helplessness to justify the distancing that is motivated by the simple reflex of "if you ask too much of me, I will push you away." This reflex is counterproductive.

At the level of public health, the need for reassuring contact that emerges from attachment anxiety is one of the sources of the overuse of health care services that the Institute of Medicine described as contributing to the "quality chasm" in current health care;[5] it is one of the driving forces behind what we have called vexing health care. At an individual level, the consequences are often even more pernicious – the cycle of help seeking and reflex distancing between patients and clinicians exacerbates the problems that each would like to resolve. It turns complicated interactions into frustrating and potentially harmful ones.

Attachment theory makes sense of this harmful cycle. Attachment anxiety is based on a set of cognitive filters that promote the views that "I am fragile and unworthy," and "You are inconsistent and unlikely to be there for me when I need you," which are linked to a strongly reinforced default strategy: "Be vigilant for signs that others are about to abandon me and send frequent distress signals to keep them engaged." When a professional realizes she is inadvertently re-enacting an attachment drama, opportunities to intervene more effectively open up. Here are a couple.

6. Break the contingency between expressing distress and getting care. One of the most important goals for a clinician trying to adapt her care for a patient with high attachment anxiety may be to interrupt the loop in which insecurity amplifies distress and help seeking, which leads health care professionals to set limits and distance themselves, which in turn amps up the patient's insecurity. In our experience the most effective way to do this is to *provide care before the patient asks for it.* That advice is so counter-intuitive that we will walk through this prescription step by step.

First, let's be clear about the rationale. When attachment anxiety interferes with a health care interaction, it is often because both patient and professional misconstrue the goals of the interaction. They can agree on the medical problem-solving goals: to identify and treat serious health problems if any are present. What they fail to recognize is that the medical problem-solving goal is secondary to the attachment goal: feeling secure. Since fear trumps everything, they can't get to the medical goal until they settle the fear down. They need to find a way to help the patient to stop scanning for signs that she is about to be misconstrued, abandoned, or rejected so that she can settle into the task.

To accomplish this we recommend predictable, frequent, reassuring contact that doesn't depend on the patient's asking for it. For a hospital inpatient, this may mean that the patient's nurse pops in every hour for a quick hello, a check of the intravenous line, and a question about pain. The result is that the patient is less inclined to anticipate catastrophes (such as no one being available with an analgesic when the current dose wears off). For a patient in primary care, it may mean a brief standing appointment. Although the prescription to meet so frequently *whether or not the patient has new complaints to consider* initially seems extravagant, the effects are paradoxically productive. As with the advice to take your time when speaking with a patient who has high attachment anxiety, having regularly scheduled appointments can decrease crisis appointments and decrease the use of emergency departments and walk-in clinics. Thus, in addition to the benefits that the patient experiences, a case can be made that regularly scheduled contact that is not contingent on distress makes health care more efficient and affordable.

7. Be predictable, attentive, and supportive. For regular, pre-emptive contact to work effectively to break the cycle of dependency and difficult interactions, the contact needs to be time limited and predictable – a 15-minute appointment needs to last 15 minutes. It is easy to err in either direction. On one hand, a patient's urgently expressed need pulls his clinician to demonstrate her concern and responsiveness by extending their time together. This need is often amplified when the time is ending because the anticipation of separation is an attachment trigger in its own right. On the other hand, the clinician's reflex desire to extricate herself from an overwhelming need may lead to a premature exit. So it takes discipline and diplomacy to maintain the time frame. Of course, it is very important that both parties have agreed to the plan in advance, including the length of the appointments. This arrangement doesn't have to be a kind of contract that feels threatening to the needy patient, but the parameters of the meetings should be clear and agreed on, otherwise each appointment's end will represent a new abandonment rather that what is intended: an opportunity for the health care professional to demonstrate that she is as good as her word, a highly predictable and reliable source of support.

A complementary message to health care professionals is that when you are there with your patient, you really need to *be* there. A clinician needs to be attentive, tuned in to her own thoughts and emotions, and straining to understand what her patient is experiencing. You don't need to have a solution or excellent advice about what to do, but you do need to be trying your hardest to appreciate your patient's situation and sometimes putting it into words with him or for him. In the same way that it is easy to want to truncate an interaction of this sort prematurely, tuning out a little bit is sometimes also attractive. This is not a time to look at the computer monitor.

A clinician who is trying to break ingrained cycles of distress and dependency is trying to be the consistent person her patient wasn't lucky enough to experience earlier in his life – she is trying to disconfirm his expectations of disappointment. She needs to be there with her patient, fully present, when she says that she will, be there reliably and often, and demonstrate that her reliability includes ending their time together according to plan to allow her patient to exercise his own capacity to manage for himself between visits. When a health care professional is able to pull this off, she provides an experience that is exactly the opposite of what her patient's schema has predicted, giving him a new positive experience that will help to extinguish the contingency between distress and support.

Fractured communication

In Chapter 6, we described narrative incoherence as a core feature of insecure patterns of attachment. When a patient with high attachment anxiety tries to tell his story, the narrative is hard to follow. Too many words are used to convey too little. Emotion and distress are conveyed emphatically, but the context that would make them understandable is often missing. Present and past are jumbled. The story's characters enter and exit without being introduced. Descriptors are vague. Thoughts are interrupted. At times, the listener is invited to substitute her own impressions for the narrator's experience. Overall, we summarize the flood of information that lacks organization or a clear communicative goal as "all evidence – no conclusion." It is the clinician's task to help her patient to express himself more clearly.

8. *Use your observations about incoherence as useful information.* The first step to helping a patient with high attachment anxiety to communicate more effectively is to recognize the attachment anxiety. The confusion that a health care professional feels in this circumstance, coupled with observations of the kind of dramatic, over-inclusive, fragmented, and vague expressions that we have just described is often the first best clue that attachment anxiety is interfering with the medical problem-solving exercise. In what is usually a stressful and frustrating interaction for a health care professional (and for her patient), recognizing the source of the incoherence can be a tremendous relief. Suddenly, an incoherent pattern of communication becomes a source of information and a therapeutic challenge – rather than just something that interferes with collecting information and providing care.

9. *Use the skills of active listening.* Active listening is a widely used set of techniques designed to maximize the clarity and accuracy of spoken communication. It employs skills that can make all the difference to appreciating a fragmented story. To listen actively involves a number of techniques, which include reflecting back your understanding of the story from time to time, usually in a paraphrased form, and inviting your patient to correct your impression. This allows the patient to see how well (or how poorly) his intended meaning is being conveyed and to take steps to improve your understanding. Your paraphrase can also have the effect of presenting a slightly more organized version of a patient's narrative, which both fortifies that narrative and models the reflective mental process that attachment anxiety undermines.

For a person with severe attachment anxiety and a very disorganized narrative, a health care professional may need to put a lot of emphasis on simple clarification. An example may help to show why. Here is a typical moment in a series of similar missteps and misunderstandings with a patient whose narrative is compromised by attachment anxiety:

As I listen to my new patient tell his distressing, confusing story, and I anticipate that my responses are going to be insufficient to provide the calm and direction that he needs, a new character enters the narrative without introduction. He says, "and naturally I'm worried what she will think," without providing me any clues as to who "she" refers to. If non-specific references such as this occur too frequently in a narrative it takes very little time before

I am hopelessly muddled. Worse, the narrative confusion occurs in concert with the interpersonal push and pull that tempts me to tune out from time to time, even briefly. As a result, when I hear of this unidentified "she," I experience a pang of guilty uncertainty – maybe "she" was introduced when I wasn't listening well. I think I should ask who she is, but I am concerned that I may be revealing my inattention and confirming my patient's expectation that he can't count on me to take him seriously.

In spite of my apprehension about the potential consequences of clarifying my patient's story, it is almost always the right thing to do. I need to understand my patient's story and I need to help my patient to become more easily understood. Frequent clarification of the elements that render a narrative confusing is a process that can be as valuable as it is painstaking.[6] If in the process I reveal that I cannot always listen attentively under these circumstances, that too will become an important part of the process of my patient understanding his impact on others – at least it will in time.

Anger

When attachment anxiety is high and attachment avoidance is low, the social purpose of anger is to keep the angry person and the other in proximity. It can be very difficult for a health care provider to respond without colluding or being inadvertently sucked into an undesirable argument.

10. Remember that anger starts with fear. Rather than choosing (or falling into) the role of sympathizer or aggressor, finding a third path is usually preferable, but it can be very challenging to see any alternative. One helpful point to keep in mind is that problems that stem from attachment anxiety almost always start with fear. In a situation like this a health care professional will need to use all her powers of mentalizing to *imagine* the fear that could be behind the anger, because it won't be apparent on the surface. In medical situations, anger about others who have been insufficiently attentive or supportive often result from a fear of rejection, isolation, or abandonment. Reframing anger as a consequence of fear may help a health care professional to feel more sympathetic and may open up possibilities for more effective responses.

Lack of agency

A person with high attachment anxiety can feel a desperate need to seek help from others. In fact, when attachment anxiety interferes with effective medical care, it is often because help seeking has overwhelmed other aspects of care. Paradoxically, in this circumstance the intense efforts applied to seeking help do not lead to more or better help. Help seeking is pronounced, but it is not effective.

Ineffective efforts to seek help are one aspect of a general lack of personal agency that is a core feature of attachment anxiety. A person with high attachment anxiety does not usually feel that he has much power. Often, he *knows* what the best next steps are in dealing with the matter at hand, but he doesn't take those steps.[7] He may rationalize his lack of initiative with pessimistic predictions of what the outcome would be if he tried or he may just fear the interpersonal consequences of assertiveness, preferring importuning (which conveys a lack of interpersonal power) to assertion (which connotes a level playing field).

Shoshonah is a senior nurse who has a heart valve problem for which she sees a very well-respected cardiologist for ongoing monitoring. Unhappily, she describes meeting him at a social event where "he didn't do anything wrong in an obvious way, but he was just sleazy if you know what I mean." Although it makes her uncomfortable to continue to see him as a patient, she doesn't make a change. She doesn't want to lose his expertise "just in case" and worries about how he would react if she switched doctors.

11. *Teach healthy assertiveness.* According to the *Oxford English Dictionary*, self-assertion is "insistence on recognition of one's own rights or claims." Assertiveness training can be a remedy to the lack of agency that a person with high attachment anxiety experiences. One of the advantages of identifying assertiveness as a specific treatment goal in this situation is that it leads to simple skills- and practice-based teaching, which may serve as a Trojan horse for a more powerful interpersonal change. As a communication skill, assertiveness is taught by distinguishing the simple statements of preferences, observations, and entitlements that characterize assertiveness ("Excuse me, I was in line first") from aggression ("Hey you, quit cutting in and get the hell to the back of the line") and passivity ("Mumble, mumble, never mind").

Another advantage of a focus on assertiveness is that life presents many relatively low-stakes opportunities to practise healthy assertiveness. Shoshonah doesn't have to start with the cardiologist; she can start with the line jumper at the grocery store. Practising in lower-stakes settings can lead to a more profound underlying transformation from a position in which she assumes powerlessness and vulnerability to the whims of others towards a position of relative balance. Many people experience this transformation as a very substantial change from passive resentment, resignation, or disempowerment to an active pursuit of their own goals and interests.

Fragmentation of the agents of care

One of the features of attachment anxiety that is most pernicious, at least when insecurity interferes with health care, is the diverse and disconnected patchwork of advisers and care providers who become engaged with a person who needs help, which is a recipe for ineffective health care.

12. Facilitate communication and coordination between agents of care. Very early on in the process of assessment and treatment of a patient with high attachment anxiety, we make a point of explicitly listing and discussing the people who are involved in her care. We find out who is providing more or less continuous care – the sort that allows the provider to reassess the value of previous steps and revise the treatment plan to suit – and who is involved in ways that are temporary or fractured. We ask about contradictions inherent in the advice from various sources and how the patient resolves these. If we have an opportunity to discuss how the lack of coordination undermines the patient's interests, without being too preachy about it, then we do that too. Finally, and most importantly, we suggest a plan to open the lines of communication and introduce some order to the chaos.

The steps involved in that plan depend on the circumstances, but some common elements usually apply. A useful starting point is to ask the patient's permission to include all the relevant players in communications by copying them on your letters and to ask them to do the same. We often ask for blanket consent to contact other important figures in the circle of care when we feel it would be helpful both to receive and to provide information. Asking for permission to use our discretion in this way demands a fair degree of trust – another reason that it is important for a health care professional to demonstrate active interest, empathy, and good faith throughout the process of assessment and treatment, to earn the trust that is required to provide good care.

Beyond open communication, a system such as this needs a coordinator. While this responsibility often falls to the patient herself, this is a case where the patient may not be the most effective coordinator of her care – at least not at first. A family doctor is often well placed to serve as coordinator, or another individual may be able to take on the role.

13. *Present the team as an integrated whole.*

Jon: When my daughter was hospitalized for 72 hours for an appendectomy, over three days she came in contact with 22 members of the health care team, the majority of whom did not introduce themselves by role – and some not even by name.

Health care can present a very confusing array of individuals to a person who is too preoccupied with her own suffering and worries to be making an effort to understand how the system works. For someone who is preoccupied by attachment anxiety, this barrage of individuals with their unknown agendas and affiliations can amplify anxiety or lead to unhelpful alliances (imagine disclosing all your greatest concerns and most urgent questions to a medical student and failing to mention them to your surgeon).

In this situation taking some extra steps to ensure that, as much as possible, the treatment team is functioning as a single coherent unit is helpful, as is presenting it as such to the patient. Communication, once again, is the foundation of an integrated system. In an inpatient setting, communication is fostered by good notes in the clinical record, inter-professional team rounds, an extra phone call when miscommunication or conflict arises, and special meetings of all concerned parties when care becomes complicated. Reducing the number of people from each service who are involved in a patient's care or appointing a point person who consistently communicates with the patient can also be useful, especially in teaching hospitals where each discipline may be represented by multiple professionals and trainees.

Depression and anxiety

We have emphasized that patterns of attachment are universal – everybody has one – and that even insecure patterns of attachment are adaptive in their contexts of origin. Attachment is a theory of normal psychology, and patterns of attachment are not diagnoses. At the same time, insecure patterns do increase the risk of illness and in particular the risk of experiencing major depression or an anxiety disorder. The magnitude of this risk relates to the severity or intensity of the insecurity.[8] Therefore, one aspect of adapting health care for a person with high attachment anxiety is to be vigilant for signs of mental illness and to arrange for effective treatment if required. Inpatient psychiatric consultation services and collaborative care strategies in primary care are effective strategies for accomplishing this.

Advice to patients

Health care providers are often well positioned to provide some guidance to patients about how they can act to minimize the adverse impact of their attachment patterns on health care. For a patient with high attachment anxiety, this advice is helpful in itself and has the added benefit of bolstering a patient's sense of having some control over interactions that often feel daunting.

We often coach patients to take the following steps.[9]

1. Maximize social support.
- Identify clear tasks when you are asking others for help. "I need help!" tends to feel overwhelming because it is vague, open-ended, and potentially all-encompassing. On the other hand, "Can you go with me to an appointment next Tuesday afternoon for two hours?" is a much more specific and limited request, which is much more likely to end satisfactorily for you both.
- Try not to set up supportive people to disappoint you. If you ask people for more than they can reasonably promise, well-meaning individuals will sometimes agree out of a reluctance to let you down or hurt your feelings. Try not to ask questions like, "Will you always be here for me?" The only sensible answer is "probably not," but forcing someone to say that (or worse, to make a promise that he or she can't keep) puts an unnecessary strain on your relationship.
- Bring a buddy to important medical interactions and ask if he or she can be present for at least part of the conversation. Anxiety plays havoc with being able to absorb information and ask good questions. A buddy can calm you down just by being there and, more importantly, can act as a second pair of ears. Choose your buddy carefully, however – it is *your* appointment, and you will benefit from a buddy who is good at discreet, attuned support, not someone who will impose her own agenda.

- Nurture your most important relationships with quality time that is *not* focused on your health or on supporting you.
- Demonstrate your ability to look after yourself. Providing support to someone who occasionally needs a hand in a challenging situation is fairly easy when you are confident that he can get back on his own feet when the crisis has passed.

2. Keep communication clear.
- Plan. Think about a scheduled interaction the day before it occurs. What do you hope to accomplish? Try to come up with an answer that identifies only one or two goals and identifies a goal that can realistically be achieved during the interaction. What is new? What is most important? Give priority to goals that are immediate and concrete ("I want to know what the physiotherapist thinks about the pain I get in my shin when I try to do the exercises she assigned").
- Make notes. Anxiety makes it hard to keep your focus, so having a reminder is helpful. After you have identified one or two questions or concerns that are your priority for the meeting, write them down. The notes are for you, little reminders to make sure you don't leave out something important. Don't bring in pages of notes or records for your health care professional to read unless you have been asked for them – she wants to talk with you, not read about you.
- Manage your anxiety. You may be aware of things that make your anxiety better or worse, which will allow you to manage the circumstance to your advantage. Maybe you need to know you have the rest of the day off, so you're not worried about the time spent waiting. Maybe the appointment will be easier for you to manage at a certain time of day. Maybe you need to ensure you get a good sleep the night before. Think about the circumstances that make interactions like these easier and what you can do to enact them.

3. Avoid having a large, fragmented treatment team.
- Open up communication between members of the team. Don't assume that clear communication will happen automatically. Provide a list of other health care providers who should be copied on all reports and letters to each of the main players in your network of professionals.

- Every circus needs a ringleader. A large collection of helpers is not actually a team unless at least one person knows who is doing what. Usually the best person for this role is your primary care physician, but many people don't have a consistent primary care physician and other possibilities can also work. Usually it is not ideal for *you* to be in the role of the team's manager, because if that were a strength of yours, the fragmentation would not occur in the first place. You should, however, be an active collaborator with your manager.
- Many health care relationships should end when the work is done. Whereas some health care relationships should be open-ended and potentially lifelong, such as your relationship with your primary health care provider or dentist, others, such as your relationship with a surgeon who fixes a knee injury, should last only as long as the problem requires the expert's attention.

4. Work on ways to reduce distress.

- You are probably better at managing anxiety about your health than you give yourself credit for. Think about the major challenges in your life and reflect on how you have coped with these events. The strategies that have worked for you in the past are often a good model for what will be useful again when you face crises in the future. Learning some specific techniques of relaxation and stress management, such as breathing and muscle-relaxation exercises, can also be helpful.

Attachment anxiety complicates many aspects of medical care. Worse, medical care complicates the lives of people who are high in attachment anxiety if it is practised without any effort to adapt to individual patients' needs. Fortunately, high attachment anxiety is not difficult to identify, and the adaptations that are required are often quite practical and effective.

13 How Health Care Providers Can Adapt When Attachment Avoidance Interferes

A person with high attachment avoidance and low attachment anxiety is in an invisible bind. On one hand, life has taught him that self-reliance is his best option to feel most secure most often. Emotional intimacy is uncomfortable, so expressing distress, even if he feels it, only makes him feel worse because it evokes a vulnerability that undermines the strength of character that he wants to project. On the other hand, he *does* feel insecure. And so the insecurity that he feels pushes him to appear even stronger. He sees no option but to dig in and distance himself further from those around him. Whatever he feels in private becomes hidden behind an impenetrable exterior. He becomes, as John Bowlby described it, *compulsively* self-reliant.[1]

The forces that reinforce avoidance extend further, however. Independence is highly valued in Western society, and fierce independence even more so. From cinematic heroes to the leaders of our governments and corporations, we admire those who have the strength to stand alone. In health care settings that are perpetually busy and understaffed, a patient who is adept at caring for herself is usually welcome. As a result, attachment avoidance is unlikely to be seen as a problem in itself. Only when this style interferes with collaboration, when reporting distress or accepting advice is crucial to health, is it likely to even appear on a health care professional's radar.

A person with high attachment avoidance prefers to manage his own health. The expectation that others will let him down when he needs them, or intrude into his comfort zone, or coerce him into taking actions that make him vulnerable or dependent, combined with the strong belief in following his own counsel, leads to a diminished capacity for collaboration. This bias towards independence can be an excellent strategy when it works, but it's a recipe for conflict when it doesn't. The problems that can emerge when attachment avoidance interferes with health, and the ways in which health care providers can adapt to reduce them, are largely the opposite of the problems and solutions discussed for people with high attachment anxiety. In this chapter we will review the common challenges and describe the value of 12 recommendations that are summarized in the table below.

RECOMMENDATIONS FOR HEALTH CARE PROVIDERS ADAPTING TO A PATIENT WITH HIGH ATTACHMENT AVOIDANCE

1. Offer scheduled follow-up instead of inviting the patient to call as needed.
2. Put more emphasis on objective measures of illness.
3. Respect your patient's need for independence.
4. Allow your patient to set the interpersonal distance.
5. When in a dialogue, follow.
6. Negotiate and reframe.
7. Use the principles and techniques of motivational interviewing.
8. Disconfirm negative expectations of you.
9. Mentalize your patient's needs and concerns.
10. Don't take anger personally.
11. Enquire with curiosity.
12. Facilitate the well-timed blurt.

Under-reporting of distress and symptoms

The primary consequence of attachment avoidance for interactions in the health care system is perhaps the most obvious: a person who does not like to acknowledge or express distress of any sort is unlikely to readily report symptoms.[2] The dilemma for health care providers is to try to identify health problems and assess health with insufficient information. A person with an avoidant style is much more likely to present too late than too early, and too infrequently rather than too often. She may appear to have no needs at all.

It is often not clear whether the lack of reporting symptoms is because a person with high attachment avoidance simply prefers not to express distress or because she is actually not aware of having the symptoms. Many symptoms, pain being the prime example, involve a substantial degree of subjective interpretation. Furthermore, large individual differences exist in the ability to detect and identify internal sensations, so attachment avoidance may sometimes be associated with experiencing fewer symptoms and not just with under-reporting.

1. *Offer scheduled follow-up instead of inviting the patient to call as needed.* When working with a patient who is high in attachment avoidance, health care professionals should make adaptations that reduce the potential for undetected illness and late identification of exacerbations of chronic disease. The practice of encouraging patients to call or make an appointment as needed based on how they are feeling, which is very sensible for a securely attached patient, may lead an avoidant person to show up too late. Instead, scheduling consistent appointments that allow for more continuity and for careful enquiry into problems that aren't immediately volunteered is helpful, even if they are scheduled at long intervals to accommodate the patient's reluctance to be dependent.

Even for people seen for a single consultation, we are in the habit of indicating that a second appointment is routine ("I usually see people twice, at least, so let's set up another time to meet in a few weeks"). Even if the intent of the interaction is only to provide an assessment and advice, a second conversation after establishing some degree of trust and alliance after the first meeting often allows for expression of more subtle aspects of a patient's experience.

2. *Put more emphasis on objective measures of illness.* Unfortunately, another recommendation for people who are high in avoidance and less likely to complain is that doing more testing is helpful. As with some of the other recommendations in this chapter, this is essentially the opposite advice that we give regarding patients who have high attachment anxiety. In that case excessive false alarms lead to excessive, low-yield investigations that can lead to unnecessary complications. With someone high in attachment avoidance, on the other hand, the balance of risk is less influenced by the harm that can be done by testing and more by the consequences of undetected disease. Needless to say, this does not mean extensive panels of blood tests for people who are apparently healthy, but it may mean, for example, following serum indicators of inflammation more frequently for patients with chronic

inflammatory diseases or putting more emphasis on the importance of sigmoidoscopies at regular intervals for a patient with colitis.[3]

Dislike of dependence and subordinate roles

We understand the avoidant person's habit of suppressing distress as a disinclination to be in the position of needing someone else's support. Whether or not it is strictly true for each individual, we generally make sense of this motivation by bringing to mind the prototypical developmental story of a person with high attachment avoidance, which is a narrative in which a child repeatedly and consistently finds that her parent is either unavailable during the times when she is injured or frightened, or is frankly punitive of expressions of distress at those times.

Twenty-five years ago, I (Jon) was at a picnic, standing and talking with the adults while the children played baseball. Jimmy, who was then about seven, came whimpering over to his father who was engaged in conversation with me. He had been hit in the head with a baseball and was fighting back tears while a big red welt formed on his cheek. "Well, Jim, if you play with the big boys, you're gonna get hurt," said his dad, turning his back on Jimmy and picking up with me where he had left off. The boy went back to the game and sorted it out on his own somehow.

Now in his early thirties, Jim is a police officer in a small town, a hockey player in his spare time, the father of two very independent young girls – and as self-reliant as they come. The point of the story, of course, is not about the power of the interaction that I happened to witness between Jimmy and his father; it is about the power of the thousand similar unwitnessed interactions that it represents.

For a health care provider, the value of keeping a story like Jim's in mind is that it allows you to mentalize a little more effectively. It can be helpful, for example, to bear in mind that a patient who doesn't mention the "detail" that she has noticed blood in her urine intermittently for the last three months is not being deceitful or unintelligent; she is simply following a rule that has been strongly reinforced in her life: "Look after yourself and act like everything is cool." Your effort at mentalizing may lead to the recognition (or at least the guess) that a patient like Jim may be frightened in spite of very little external evidence that he is feeling that way. It makes it clear that an important task of treatment is to provide the kind of relationship in which trust can be earned and defences temporarily relaxed enough to allow you into the patient's inner circle.

3. *Respect your patient's need for independence.* Recall Linda, the university student with diabetes introduced in Chapter 11, who decided to abandon follow-up at the student health clinic when a new doctor was too intrusive and controlling. Coming on like a bossy lecturer is a very ineffective strategy for a person with avoidant attachment. Linda doesn't lack information or guidance. If her control of her diabetes is slipping away, that may be something that she is able to identify as a problem and a goal for change, but it takes second place to feeling secure. A figure of authority who hasn't yet earned her trust acting as if he has status in her inner circle will never make it through the force field, never attain standing, and never have any valuable influence.

First things first. Until Linda develops some trust in you and believes that you have an appreciation of her and her situation, your advice won't affect in her behaviour. In other words, establishing a relationship that allows Linda to feel secure isn't a nicety or something that can be attended to after you deliver the medical recommendation; it is the necessary first step for the recommendation to have any impact. This is another circumstance in which a health care professional needs to realize that attending to feelings of insecurity trumps problem solving and providing expert advice. The physician must acknowledge Linda's need to manage her health independently before he will have a place in a problem-solving discussion. The first practical step to achieving this outcome is for the doctor to avoid assuming that he knows what is going on with Linda and instead ask her about it.

4. *Allow your patient to set the interpersonal distance.* Attending to social cues can help to set the scene constructively. Allow your patient to set the interpersonal distance in your interaction. This is especially important for a patient with high attachment avoidance because your intrusion into her comfort zone (physically or in terms of emotion and intimacy) may provoke a distancing response that prevents an effective collaboration. Ask before assuming it is okay to call her by her first name. If she is a hospitalized patient lying in bed, have a seat at the bedside to avoid hovering over her in a way that conveys dominance. Small signals can go a long way to establishing a good working relationship.

5. *When in a dialogue, follow.* In conversation, it is helpful to adopt a rhythm in which you *follow* an avoidant patient. Following means listening carefully and using your curiosity to ask questions that help to elaborate her narrative, which is often spare and to the point.

An avoidant person sometimes maintains interpersonal distance subtly by choosing phrases and words that have conventional, impersonal connotations. Remember Cass, in Chapter 6 describing his wife:

Cass talks about how his wife, Aileen, is dealing with his disease (actually he just calls her "the wife"). "She is doing pretty well. She's a Scot, you know, tough stock."

Certainly Cass loves his wife, but in conversation the choice of "the wife" rather than "my wife" or "Aileen" emphasizes her role over her individual identity and is slightly depersonalizing. His next sentence gives her credit for her personal strength but does so by assigning her to an ethnic stereotype, introducing an assumption that the listener knows and subscribes to the same stereotype. Making narrative choices that ask the listener to draw on a stock of conventional meanings and social norms is typical of a person with high attachment avoidance.

Following in this situation does not mean abdicating responsibility for the task; it refers to letting the patient speak first, listening intently, responding to what he has said, and looking for windows of opportunity to elaborate on his story and learn more about the things that are most relevant to the medical task. As opposed to a patient with high attachment anxiety, who may need a clinician to provide structure and organization to the dialogue to maintain a degree of coherence, overstructuring the dialogue with an avoidant person is likely to turn a conversation into an interrogation. A clinician who follows the narrative rather than leading it can do better.

"She looks after the kids except for skating lessons, which I was doing before, so now her sister fills in there. My appointments are not interfering at all so far. I make sure I schedule them so they don't intrude on our routine. I'm sure it is hard on her but she is bearing up."

A health care professional who hears this may find herself developing a curiosity about what she is *not* hearing: "Can you tell me more about how Aileen is coping with your illness? How do you think she feels about your absence?" or even a hypothesis to test: "I wonder if Aileen is more worried about your health than about your ability to do your part in the schedule?" Giving a patient like Cass the lead and then following up with genuine concern and attention to the aspects of his story that bear on his health serves to open a dialogue that left to its own momentum tends to move towards premature closure.

Non-adherence

High attachment avoidance is consistently linked to the tendency to not follow others' directions.[4] How can a health care professional overcome the reluctance to cooperate?

6. Negotiate and reframe. Although a self-reliant person usually doesn't like to be told what to do in an authoritative way, she may be quite comfortable in a negotiation between equals. By enquiring about the goals of a patient like Linda, a professional may be able to find some alignment between what the patient wants and what is good for the patient's health. Often, a useful part of the negotiation is the professional's recognition that being healthy is not as important to an avoidant person as being autonomous or self-reliant. This fact implies that being sick, in itself, may not be a strong motivator for change, even if the clinician thinks it should be. Rather, it may be more helpful to focus on how being sick interferes with autonomy. Health-related tasks, such as investigations and treatments, can often be reframed as steps that expedite a return to self-reliance or that maintain self-reliance. An avoidant person may be willing to temporarily accept an undesirable circumstance (such as attending multiple appointments for a course of treatment or being admitted to hospital) if it can genuinely be understood as a step towards re-establishing autonomy. Of course, the negotiation needs to be held in good faith – downplaying the costs or exaggerating the benefits of taking care of our health is pointless. In the end, misleading your patient in that way is likely to undermine her trust in you and harm the therapeutic alliance.

7. Use the principles and techniques of motivational interviewing. Motivational interviewing was developed as a method to help people with addictions make changes in their lives of their own accord by engaging them in a dialogue that helps them to move from contemplating change to taking action and then maintaining the gains that they make. Motivational interviewing has since been applied in many other situations in which the goal is to make difficult behavioural changes, including managing chronic disease.[5] This approach is particularly well suited to people with high attachment avoidance because respect for the patient's autonomy and decision-making authority is one of its central principles, and avoiding bossy confrontation ("rolling with the resistance") is a core technique.[6] Motivational interviewing emphasizes the need for a health care professional and patient to connect inter-personally and then for the professional to understand the patient's perceptions of what she needs, before proceeding together to address those needs. Techniques such as eliciting a patient's ambivalence about a behaviour by enquiring into the discrepancy between where she is and where she would like to be, for example, can be learned fairly eas-ily without expert training in motivational interviewing and can be incorporated into a medical interview.[7] This approach will helpfully remind a clinician to focus on the *patient's* goals and the costs and bene-fits of adhering to medical advice from the *patient's* point of view. After all, it is not adherence itself but what adherence is supposed to accom-plish that is relevant.

Rigid expectations that others will be inattentive or disappointing

A person with high attachment avoidance and low attachment anxi-ety expects others to be unavailable, inattentive, unresponsive, and unhelpful (including you, as the health care professional who presides over a circumstance that directly or indirectly exposes your patient to vulnerability). Worst of all, if it is present, is the expectation that others will exploit vulnerability – which is sometimes translated into the cyni-cal view that health care professionals have a stake in patients being sick because it's good for business.

Such negative expectations may be voiced explicitly, in which case a health care professional at least knows what he is up against. More often, however, the care provider has to intuit a patient's expectations based on the patient's behaviour or words. For example, the patient asking, "Have you ever had this operation?" in a certain tone of voice may be not actually be a question but rather an implied statement: "You could never understand what I am experiencing."

8. Disconfirm negative expectations of you. Identifying a patient's rela-tively fixed negative expectations of others provides an opportunity to promote change, especially for a health care professional who shares a continuous relationship with that person. By consistently acting in a way that is better than expected, a health care professional has the opportunity to negate the inflexibility of the negative expectation over time. The more exceptions a person finds to a rule, the less valuable the rule becomes.

This recommendation is more ambitious than most of the others in this chapter. Rather than being aimed at adapting medical practice to provide the best *response* to avoidance that is rooted in insecure attachment, we are now talking about making an effort to help a person who is high in attachment avoidance to *become more secure*. This kind of medical care borders on psychotherapy. Nonetheless, in a primary care relationship that has enough continuity to allow for the development of a robust therapeutic alliance (which includes trust, mutual respect, rapport, and a sense of mutual predictability) a constructive challenge of long-established patterns of attachment is sometimes possible.[8]

9. Mentalize your patient's needs and concerns. Being able to intuit what is going on in your patient's mind and then enquiring to confirm or disconfirm your hypothesis is very helpful. Such intuitions are often not exactly right, especially at the start, because an avoidant patient usually does not convey enough information to allow a health care provider to accurately appreciate what she is thinking and feeling. Shy reserve may look like arrogance; distancing anger may mask underlying fear.

Nonetheless, in the absence of other information, some basic assumptions are often a good starting point. Assuming that a highly avoidant patient feels more insecure that she lets on is fair, but acknowledging and discussing that fear is off limits until you are able to establish that you are an ally to be trusted. It is fair to assume that depending on others is undesirable to your patient and that she will not respond well when it is demanded (fight and flight being the two classic responses, since she perceives depending on others to be a threat). Assuming that she is proud of her independence and her personal effectiveness is also fair. When she is able to function in her preferred autonomous mode and when she is feeling healthy and strong, she probably feels quite good about herself. It would usually be correct to assume that your avoidant patient is able to participate quite effectively in a relationship that she believes is addressing her goals and is mutually respectful. Taken together, those assumptions form a schema, a set of plausible predictions about an avoidant patient, which can then be modified by your actual experience as your conversation progresses.

Anger

The interpersonal effects of expressed anger are a very useful clue to patterns of attachment. As opposed to the anger of a person with high attachment anxiety, which seems to enmesh others unwittingly in conflict, the anger of a person with high attachment avoidance creates interpersonal distance.

Many variations on this theme exist. A care provider may find herself on the receiving end of an adept, logical confrontation of the inconsistencies or deficits in a proposed course of investigation or treatment, feeling as if medical care has suddenly transformed into a debate against an opponent with superior debating skills. Or a patient might be indignant about a lack of responsibility or responsiveness shown by a health care professional and present herself not as a victim (as would be more typical with high attachment anxiety) but as a poorly served consumer who would take her business elsewhere if she had the option.[9] An avoidant patient's anger may or may not feel intimidating, but it always promotes distance. Anger is expressed in a manner that leaves her seemingly beyond entanglement, and leaves you, as a health care provider, uninvited to bridge the interpersonal gap.

10. Don't take anger personally. Several of the suggestions that have already been made can serve to calm or avoid angry confrontations. Mentalizing a patient's needs and wishes, engaging in a respectful negotiation, avoiding inadvertent indicators that you are exploiting the power differential that is inherent in a professional-patient relationship, and reframing the intrusions that health care makes into your patient's comfort zone as steps towards maintaining or regaining autonomy can all help to make the anger that a person with high attachment avoidance expresses into a more constructive force. To engage in these strategies, however, a clinician first needs to recognize anger as an interpersonal lever, rather than as a personal indictment. For example, a withering critique of your suggested plan need not signal a need to defend yourself. Rather, it signals that it is time, once again, to check in with your patient about her goals and concerns and to try to understand how the current circumstance looks and feels from her point of view.

Nothing more to say

The sense that everything has been said and nothing is left to discuss is close to being a *sine qua non* of high attachment avoidance. It is, at least, an extremely common response to the form of narrative incoherence that accompanies interpersonal avoidance.

The narrative style of this pattern of attachment serves to close enquiry and leave an avoidant person's inner world private. For one thing, expressions of emotion are usually quite muted. Rather than the inflections of vocal tone and prosody that often convey subtle clues about how a story feels to the storyteller and engage the listener in a complementary emotional experience, the narrative of a person with high attachment avoidance seems to present just the facts.

Worse than this, since the facts can rarely provide all the context needed to understand someone's intended meaning, the listener is left with ambiguous interpretations of a story that is spare enough to seem, on the surface, to be beyond such uncertainty. The ambiguity adds another layer of incoherence. Not only does the listener find himself with insufficient information to understand the speaker's world, but the story has also been presented so simply that to ask what it means may feel like a stupid question:

> Patient: ... and they locked the door to the clinic as I arrived, right in front of me.
> Clinician: How did that feel?
> Patient (irritated): How do you think it felt?

The story's lack of detail serves to close down communication. Often, descriptions are conventional (drawing on purportedly shared connotations rather than providing personal interpretations) and not elaborate. This is true whether the descriptions are evaluatively positive or negative. If a clinician asks a patient what her father was like when she was young, the answers "Good, normal, you know" and "Crappy, but that's behind me now" convey very different evaluations, but neither gives much information and neither conveys an invitation to ask more. The listener gets the impression that he is being provided with conclusions without having access to any of the evidence.

Similarly, such generalizations are not likely to be accompanied by illustrative examples. If a care provider asks for examples, a highly avoidant person may not remember any ("Nothing comes to mind, it was just always like that") or may provide examples that are contradictory or change the subject.

Contradiction between different aspects of the story does not, in itself, signal attachment avoidance. What's different about the contradictions of an avoidant person's narrative is her lack of reflection on the inconsistency and lack of apparent motivation to understand or resolve it. We can make sense of this by understanding the words of a person with high attachment avoidance as serving an interpersonal strategy more than a communicative goal. Her intent is not to help you to understand her experience; it is to prevent you from getting close enough to do any harm.

11. Enquire with curiosity. It is often helpful in this kind of conversation to choose your words and timing carefully. This prudence is made easier by the fact you often have very little pressure to speak up, which facilitates listening intently and looking for windows of opportunity. At an apt moment, it is helpful to enquire into your patient's experience with genuine curiosity. This query may require a brief justification when you have no social cues to indicate that questions are welcome, but a very few words will suffice. For example, in the case of the irritable response quoted above, a clinician might say, "I'm sure it didn't feel good. But I wonder more specifically exactly what it was like *for you.*"

12. Facilitate the well-timed blurt. Although it is not always a goal in this sort of interaction, a health care professional is sometimes able to establish a sufficient degree of understanding and acceptance that a patient with high attachment avoidance is willing to let down her guard briefly and express how she really feels. This is a delicate moment because if the patient feels, in the end, as if she has been tricked into revealing too much, or feels exploited or unsupported, the net effect will be harmful. However, if the patient's wish to express herself a little more directly and openly is genuine and if the clinician's response is accepting and non-judgmental, an exceptional moment of candour and emotional expression can feel very valuable to a patient and strongly reinforce the alliance between a clinician and patient. This moment can essentially be banked for the future, when a strong alliance will serve as a secure base from which to make changes in the service of health. We need to emphasize that the opportunity for a short period of exceptional self-expression is identified *by the patient.* Pressure from a clinician to say more than is comfortable almost always backfires.

Advice to patients

Advising a person who is high in attachment avoidance requires a fair degree of trust, but a health care professional who has established a good working relationship with an avoidant patient is sometimes in a position to help that person to have more effective interactions with other providers.

Here is how we coach patients when we have the opportunity.

1. Maximize effective self-management of health care.

- You can't manage a problem effectively if you don't acknowledge it exists. Minimize any tendency you might have to not think of health *at all*. We often see this, for example, when a person with a serious chronic disease decides that the most effective strategy is to try to live as if she is perfectly healthy, in the guise of not giving in. Pretending that things are fine when they are not only serves to reduce the number of options available to support a full and happy life.

- If tools are available to help you manage your health well with a minimum of interpersonal interaction, it is a good idea to take full advantage of these resources. For example, self-management is facilitated by a growing number of apps available to help people to monitor blood pressure, diet, exercise, and so forth, and self-management strategies and resources have been developed for a number of chronic illnesses.[10]

2. Negotiate and collaborate.

- As an adult who takes pride in the ability to look after your own interests autonomously, you may count effective negotiating skills among your strengths. Viewing health care as a negotiation and as an equal collaboration between partners with complementary goals may give you an approach that allows you to use health care professionals to your greatest advantage. It makes sense that you reject the patient role as it existed in antiquated models in which doctors gave orders and patients complied, but most providers of health care these days don't expect patients to be passively compliant. In fact, it would be quite reasonable for you to assess potential health care providers for their effectiveness as collaborators – to choose the team that best meets your needs to the extent that the parts of the health care system that are available to you works within those values.

3. Guard against minimizing symptoms and underusing health care.

- One of the simplest adjustments to make in the context of "routine maintenance and prevention" is to schedule regular appointments rather than calling in as necessary. If you make a point of not leaving the clinic or medical office without having made an appointment for the next meeting, you can make it easier for yourself to treat health care interactions as a routine aspect of life.
- A second adjustment is to accept that objective tests (blood tests and so forth) may be especially useful, because you tend to not be

a reliable witness to the state of your health. This acceptance is less the case in routine management of health (where objective tests have a minimal role) but can be more important in monitoring the waxing and waning of chronic diseases.[11]

4. Redefine what medical care means.

- One of the things that may keep you out of clinics, doctor's offices, and hospitals is that those are places for sick people – whereas you are *fine*. No problem. What if the purpose of the places is, instead, to keep you healthy and independent? Preventive health care reduces the need to depend on medical treatment and health care providers. If you have a temporary problem, medical care puts you back on the road to independence. Relinquishing your autonomy temporarily is simply expedient, a pit stop. *The purpose of excellent health care is to minimize the chances of needing more health care.*

The health care difficulties that arise for a person with high attachment avoidance are quite different from those that arise for a person with high attachment anxiety. The fact that the attachment-based perspective leads to different and opposite recommendations for patients with different patterns of insecure attachment is an indicator of how attending to relational aspects of health provides for a personalized medicine that can help to clarify and improve aspects of vexing health care that lead to overuse and underuse of the health care system.

14 How Health Care Providers Can Adapt When Fearful Attachment Interferes

A pattern of attachment that contains the influences of both attachment anxiety and attachment avoidance is the hardest pattern to tolerate for both the insecure person and the person who is trying to help. A person with fearful attachment has a great deal of difficulty feeling secure in *any* situation – let alone a medical setting in which her feelings of insecurity will almost certainly mobilize all her protective attachment strategies. The difficulty for a health care professional arises when these strategies are mutually contradictory, creating a complicated mixture of approach and withdrawal, or seeking help and then rejecting what is offered. Communication may be equally challenging. The situation demands patience, skill, and genuine concern to make the adaptations that can improve the situation. In this chapter we describe the value of 11 recommendations that are summarized in the table below.

RECOMMENDATIONS FOR HEALTH CARE PROVIDERS ADAPTING TO A PATIENT WITH FEARFUL ATTACHMENT

1. Let everything else wait while you put all your effort into establishing a trusting alliance.
2. Encourage clear and assertive expression of needs.
3. Help your patient to increase his or her agency.
4. Use the skills that work for attachment anxiety and the skills that work for attachment avoidance.
5. Focus on reducing attachment anxiety.

6. Break up tasks into manageable chunks.
7. Try to reduce the acute symptoms that interfere with focusing on other tasks.
8. Think of the patient as troubled rather than troubling.
9. Refer to your usual good standard of care.
10. Manage the treatment team.
11. Treat mental illness if it is present.

Tension between help seeking and help rejection, or anxious avoidance of health care professionals

Living with a high degree of both attachment anxiety and attachment avoidance means being pulled in two directions at once – towards those who could offer comfort or protection and also away from them, to the protection of isolation. In health care interactions, the most direct way in which this tension is expressed is through an inconsistent flip-flopping between seeking help and rejecting or avoiding it.[1] This inconsistency is probably why this form of insecure attachment so frequently causes difficulty for clinicians, who may respond very effectively to suffering and crisis but have few effective strategies to deal with the rejection of this treatment once it is offered.[2]

We bear in mind that a person with fearful attachment insecurity experiences a need for caring and human connection but finds that connection hard to achieve. Whether or not it is historically accurate for any particular person, it can be helpful for a health care professional to consider a prototypical developmental set-up that leads to mixed and severe insecurity. The prototype centres on the parent who is depended on for comfort and care behaving in a frightening way. In the most severe case, the parent is frightening because he or she is abusive or cruel, but lesser, sometimes quite subtle, sources of fear are also pertinent.[3] In a situation like this, a child becomes caught between the need to approach that parent for comfort and protection, because attachment is obligatory, and the repeated experience that approaching her parent makes things worse. People always learn from developmental experience. However, whereas developmental experience usually teaches a child how to manage relationships to feel as secure as possible, in this case experience teaches her that efforts to manage relationships are futile. No matter what she does, it will feel bad. The person she needs will be unavailable, or disappointing, or rejecting, or harmful, and very unlikely to be accepting, caring, and protective.

Using this template to understand a patient with fearful attachment insecurity helps a health care professional to appreciate her painful ambivalence about approaching and withdrawing from people who can provide care. In particular, a professional may be able to recognize when he has been cast in the role of a disappointing, frightening, exploitive, or negligent care provider in spite of his best intentions. Of course, *being cast* in such a role is a metaphor – the process we are describing is usually not conscious. A person who has had repeated experiences of a certain kind simply expects to experience more of the same.

It is quite sensible under circumstances such as these (even if they are as much *anticipated* as experienced) to avoid the whole problem by just not seeking health care whenever possible. Evidence bears this out – fearful attachment is characterized by the lowest health care use of any pattern of attachment.[4] Anxious avoidance of health care can lead to health problems and undermines opportunities for disease prevention. How can a health care provider best respond to this dilemma?

1. Let everything else wait while you put all your effort into establishing a trusting alliance. Once a health care professional appreciates the seemingly unresolvable interpersonal bind that a patient with fearful attachment perpetually experiences, she will realize that very little can be accomplished in a professional-patient relationship until an effective working alliance is established – and that requires thought and effort.[5] Unless the person has a medical emergency, solving health problems has to take a back seat to establishing trust.

Building an alliance is likely to call into play the strategies that are useful for patients with attachment anxiety or for patients with attachment avoidance. However, the balance between these may shift, and even when it is stable, it can be difficult to determine. These strategies include allowing the patient to set the interpersonal distance, taking time, following in dialogue, taking a careful history that focuses on personal strengths and coping, trying to genuinely understand what the patient's problems look like to the patient, not taking negative expectations personally, and providing effective techniques to reduce anxiety. In a sense, dealing with a patient with fearful attachment requires doing everything that is useful for other forms of insecurity – plus. That "plus" is the wisdom or intuition required to understand when to move in and when to hang back, when to support, and when to respect independence.

Certain attitudes that should be a part of *every* patient-professional encounter become critical to building trust with a new patient with fearful attachment insecurity. Although these attitudes are implicit in good health care, in this situation it is helpful to make them explicit:

- *Act in good faith.* Say what you mean and mean what you say. This is not an invitation to be thoughtlessly blunt – rather, it is a caution against, for example, promising more than you can deliver because it feels bad to admit your limits.
- *Be consistent and predictable.* A patient who finds it very challenging to approach a person in authority may need to choose his moments and prepare himself for the uncomfortable task of asking for help. You can make this much easier by acting in a way that is easy to predict.
- *Be patient.* Imagine how you would feel if you were trying to do something very uncomfortable (like jumping into a cold lake) or even terrifying (like skydiving). Reflect on what it feels like to be standing on the brink, reluctant to proceed. "Encouragement" to jump might just feel like an unwelcome push in the back and lead to a scramble away from the edge. Sometimes you just need to wait until your patient finds her moment.
- *Express compassion.* It will be very difficult and sometimes impossible to provide *solutions* for the problems that a patient in this circumstance is trying to express, especially if you are inclined to suggest solutions before establishing an alliance that she can trust. Instead, an acknowledgment of her suffering and genuine compassion for her situation are more likely to be welcome.[6]
- *Respect boundaries.* If you, as a health care provider, have the prototypical developmental set-up of fearful attachment in mind, then it is easy to understand how important it is to allow a patient with this attachment pattern to control access to her body and privacy – past breaches of personal space or integrity may be one of the sources of her insecurity. Whereas a person with a secure style is usually able to adapt fairly easily to the unusual social rules that are assumed in a patient-professional interaction even without formally addressing them (disrobing, allowing body parts to be touched or penetrated, providing embarrassing information, etc.), these actions may trigger stronger anxiety in a person with fearful attachment. Of course, medical interactions necessitate touch and impolite questions, but it is even more important than usual to ask first, to

not leave a patient exposed unnecessarily, to have a person of the patient's sex present during examinations, and so forth.

Extending this principle, a common error among health care trainees is asking a routine but intrusive question when it is not relevant to the current problem, out of a desire to be complete. It is especially important for someone with fearful attachment that intrusions into her comfort zone are justified.

- *Insist that boundaries be respected.* Similarly, patients with fearful attachment may have difficulty maintaining typical patient-professional boundaries. In the long run, consistent, firm, and friendly guidance about what behaviour works and what doesn't will support a trusting alliance. You don't need to overdo it (it is easy to make the error of responding to intense ambivalent need with excessive, inflexible power), but your usual standards of interaction with other patients should serve as a sensible guide. For example, if you don't usually engage in long telephone consultations with patients after hours, it is wise to maintain that boundary with patients with fearful attachment as well.

- *Listen, reflect, and enquire.* None of these guidelines should interfere with the main activities that support a trusting alliance within a patient-professional relationship: to listen well, collaborate in reflecting on the patient's situation, and use the information provided to guide further enquiry, led by compassion, curiosity, and the need to understand the patient's medical condition as fully as possible.

Powerlessness

People with fearful attachment experience more symptoms and distress than those with any other pattern of attachment and yet make the least use of the health care system, meaning that too often, they suffer in silence.[7] Underestimating what one is entitled to can play into this unhealthy bind. For example, patients with diabetes who had various patterns of attachment were interviewed about their medical care. Asked about how it feels to ask a physician for help, a person with fearful attachment said that he couldn't just say that he needed help, instead, "I feel like I have to justify it. I feel like I have to say, 'OK, I've done this, this, and this and you're my last resort.'"[8] Asking questions and seeking help can also be inhibited by a sense that health care professionals have all the power and see themselves as more important than patients. Patients may feel that it is risky to oppose the guidance they are offered or ask questions lest they alienate the powerful person they are counting on.

2. *Encourage clear and assertive expression of needs.* The most direct remedy for acting powerless is to learn assertiveness skills. In some cases where a lack of assertiveness poses a recurrent and crucial problem for a patient (as, for example, for someone with diabetes who requires ongoing and regular collaboration with his health care providers), it can be worth the effort to enrol in formal assertiveness training, where methods of communication and behaviour that enable individuals to speak up for what they are entitled to from others are learned and practised. More accessibly, patients who are reluctant to voice their concerns may benefit from simply being encouraged to speak up. The information that health care professionals view asking for help as a desirable behaviour can sometimes shift the balance to a more open and expressive relationship.

In Chapter 6, Cass's avoidance of the emergency department led him to suppress his complaints about the burden of his symptoms:

Cass just put up with it. He hadn't been expecting kidney failure as a possibility, and so he didn't question that he was urinating less and feeling worse and worse until he eventually got a fever that wouldn't go away. Even then, he was reluctant to go to the emergency department and "bother them," but his wife insisted, reminding him that they'd been told to look out for fever, so it was his obligation to go to the hospital ... Cass apologized to the emergency department staff for needing help."

Cass primarily experienced attachment insecurity in the form of attachment avoidance (and so his insecure attachment was not fearful) but the example still applies. What was useful in overcoming his reluctance to complain was the information that his health care team *wanted* him to report a fever, combined with some supportive pressure from his wife.

3. *Help your patient to increase his or her agency.* Beyond facilitating a patient's expressions of distress or concern, it is valuable to actively look for opportunities to encourage a patient to *act* in his own interests. It is remarkable how often, with certain patterns of insecure attachment, a person *knows* what someone in his situation would have to do to feel more secure, and yet he doesn't do it. For a health care provider, looking for such situations provides windows of opportunity to discuss, in much practical detail, exactly what the best plan of action would be and

to explore the pros and cons of this action and some of the anticipated obstacles. Such a discussion often uses the principles of motivational interviewing, as discussed in the previous chapter, and can facilitate a patient choosing to take action, where before he felt stuck.

Incoherent narrative

Fearful attachment can severely disrupt the coherence of an individual's communication, at least in the moments when she is feeling most insecure, although the form that this takes may be quite idiosyncratic. Since attachment anxiety pushes for more words and more intense emotion while attachment avoidance pushes for the opposite, the patterns of expression that result from the equal pressure of opposites can be complex (e.g., a pained expression while an individual tries to find words but says very little). Alternatively, communication may be inconsistent, as occurs when pressured expressions of intense distress alternate with excessive self-containment. It is difficult for a health care professional to read and respond to these mixed messages.[9]

4. *Use the skills that work for attachment anxiety and the skills that work for attachment avoidance.* In a way, adapting to a patient with fearful attachment comes down to timing. As it pertains to narrative incoherence, this timing means using the skills that work for attachment anxiety and for attachment avoidance and choosing the moments when they may best apply. Review the recommendations made in the two previous chapters because they may all apply, at least some of the time.

First, *use your observations about incoherence as useful information.* In particular, the way in which a patient with fearful attachment is expressing himself (the quality of his incoherence) gives a useful clue about whether attachment anxiety or attachment avoidance is the leading dimension of insecurity at this point, which will help you to choose an effective mode of response. Next, *use the skills of active listening.* Extensive effort spent on clarifying the story that is being told will help to avoid miscommunication and solidify the therapeutic alliance. Use techniques of reflection and paraphrasing, guess at meanings, and test your intuitions. Finally, *enquire with curiosity.* Look for opportunities to ask a little bit more, to put things in context, or to understand his situation more fully. On the other hand, if his story is disorganized because of excessively vague or partial meanings, you may need to provide some structure (especially through the skills of active listening) from which you can enquire more deeply into his situation.

In relationships that are close and reciprocal, the inner world of one of the participants often becomes mirrored somehow in the inner world of the other. In the relationship between a health care professional and a patient with fearful attachment, this is often apparent in the tension each experiences between approach and withdrawal. The patient lives with a seemingly unresolvable dilemma in which neither opening up to an attachment figure nor withdrawing into independence leads to feeling secure. The professional's mirroring of this dilemma typically comes in the form of experiencing an unpleasant tension between the desire to actively engage the patient in a caring alliance and the urge to reject him. The latter inclination may not be experienced as rejection per se (which would feel hostile and unprofessional) but rather as an acceptance of the patient's retreat or as simply following norms (e.g., "Look, I would have been happy to see you, but you have made an appointment and cancelled it at the last minute twice, and it is not our policy to make a third appointment under those circumstances").

Even within a patient-professional relationship that is fairly well established, the emotional strain of this dilemma is often pronounced. It may be expressed in strategic terms when a professional thinks, "I am damned if I do and damned if I don't. I don't know which signals to pay attention to: her anxiety or her need to keep me at a distance." The patient may well be stuck between these opposite drives, but the professional needs a way to break the impasse.

5. *Focus on reducing attachment anxiety.* In our experience, when the conflicting pressures of a patient's attachment anxiety and attachment avoidance threaten to paralyse progress in a therapeutic relationship, it is usually best to focus on the anxiety first. Unless anxiety is reduced, at least temporarily, it remains too discombobulating for a patient to be able to make any kind of change. If focusing on reducing anxiety means temporarily ignoring a patient's tendency towards maladaptive avoidance or isolation, so be it. The alternative strategy, to reduce avoidance (which we understand as a psychological and behavioural *defence* against feeling anxious), inevitably increases feelings of insecurity in the short run, which is too uncomfortable to tolerate as an impasse-breaking first step.

The feelings of insecurity that arise from attachment anxiety can be partially reduced with some combination of support, predictability, acceptance, and attention to reducing acute discomfort (discussed next). Although the strategies that can be employed to reduce anxiety are familiar at this point, two deserve special emphasis. The first is to teach specific techniques to reduce anxiety, such as imagery and relaxation exercises. The second is this: *If your patient trusts one or two people to support him, use them.* Although the prototype of a person with fearful attachment describes a state of painful isolation, reality is rarely such an all-or-none situation. Most often your patient has a person or two he would count as belonging in his inner circle, at least tentatively. It can go a long way to reducing the anxiety that arises from insecure attachment to find ways to include these others in your patient's health care. A first step is simply to talk about these relationships – who these people are, when their presence is helpful and when not, their importance to your patient, and some of the things that interfere when these relationships don't work well. The goal is not to make any changes, just to demonstrate your appreciation of the value of close connections and to empathize with and accept the frustrations that also (almost inevitably) arise from them. If your patient views the suggestion positively, invite him to bring a supportive person with him to an appointment, perhaps with a specific assigned task, such as taking notes, to avoid the fear that the person will hijack the meeting.

6. *Break up tasks into manageable chunks.* Individuals who are caught between the proximity-seeking pull of attachment anxiety and the mistrustful push of attachment avoidance often adopt a strategy of trying to be cooperative and compliant with care providers, who are perceived to be the ones with all the power. A person with fearful attachment may agree to take on more than he can reasonably expect to accomplish and become stressed and self-blaming when he cannot follow through on the demand. It is helpful to break tasks into much smaller pieces that set the patient up for success. For example, rather than a goal of losing 50 pounds over a year, set a goal walking for 30 minutes at least three days a week until the next appointment. This smaller goal allows for reinforcement of successes and problem solving without blame around unforeseen obstacles.[10]

7. *Try to reduce the acute symptoms that interfere with focusing on other tasks.* Most patients who overcome reluctance to seek medical care have at least one symptom that is either very bothersome or very worrisome. It will serve to build trust and a stronger sense of alliance to offer some effective response to that symptom. Unfortunately, it is in the nature of the impasse the clinician experiences with a patient who has fearful attachment that reassurance about the symptom(s) alone is unlikely to be very effective. What is far more likely to help is to find a way to actually reduce the symptom. As simple as this idea sounds, it introduces a

host of complications. However, in spite of the complications, symptom reduction is often a helpful strategy; it is a real way of demonstrating your good intentions and effectiveness.

The first complication is that treating symptoms without identifying an underlying disorder (or in spite of the likelihood that no identifiable underlying disorder exists) has the reputation of being "bad medicine," and it has this reputation for some very good reasons. Providing symptomatic relief as a *first* step runs all of these risks: (1) masking symptoms that are important clues to a serious medical condition; (2) reinforcing your patient's intolerance of temporary suffering, rather than helping her to overcome it; (3) exposing your patient unnecessarily to the adverse effects of unnecessary treatments; (4) obscuring the fact that the first principle of the medical treatment in this situation is to build a therapeutic alliance; and (5) colluding with the idea that all that is going on is a simple transaction about symptom relief. A health care professional needs to bear all these risks in mind because each is legitimate. Nonetheless, if the suspicion that an acutely serious medical condition is causing the symptoms is low, *and* the care provider is clear and transparent about the goal of symptom relief, *and* the view of symptom relief is as a short-term step towards helping a patient to deal more effectively with her circumstances in their entirety and not as a long-term treatment plan, then it makes sense to proceed in spite of the risks.

The second complication is that some symptoms are more easily treated than others. Often, no simple strategy exists for symptom relief that has an acceptable cost-benefit ratio, or all the easy fixes have been tried and have failed before the patient comes to you. In such a case symptom relief may not be possible as a first step to breaking the anxiety/avoidance impasse.

However, three of the most commonly distressing symptoms are often under-treated in people with severe attachment insecurity: insomnia, symptomatic anxiety, and pain. In each case, non-drug treatments (such as relaxation training, discussed above) can sometimes reduce the symptoms. Unfortunately, when a patient and clinician are facing an anxiety/avoidance impasse, engaging in non-pharmacological strategies to reduce symptoms sometimes requires more trust, patience, and tolerance than are available. That the leading symptomatic treatments of these problems are potentially addictive is no coincidence – addiction and attachment insecurity are intimately interconnected.[11] Because of this complication, and of the nature of an attachment anxiety/avoidance impasse that brings with it a lack of balance and flexibility, in our experience the symptomatic treatment of anxiety, insomnia, and pain in this situation tends to be either excessive or insufficient. As difficult as it may be to find the rational and compassionate middle ground, that should be the goal. It is unnecessarily inflexible for a clinician who is capable of prescribing to refuse to do so just because addiction is a *possibility* (no matter how remote). Nor is it helping a patient in the long run to rely on medications, such as benzodiazepines,[12] when signs of tolerance and dependency have emerged or to the exclusion of attention to core problems. Nonetheless, in an impasse, don't exclude the possibility of something that might work for the sake of an inflexible principle. Often, your effort to help a patient with the problem he has identified is taken as good faith regardless of the actual benefits, and as such it serves the first principle of strengthening the alliance.

Interpersonal troubles for health care providers

Most of health care occurs in the context of treatment teams and collaborative relationships of various kinds. Responding to a patient with fearful attachment can play havoc within those relationships. Often this disruption occurs because each member of the team feels the mirrored experience of the patient's inner world mentioned above. This mirroring means nothing more than that health care workers are empathic and intuitive enough to tune in to some aspects of what the patient is communicating (often non-verbally) and therefore to feel differently than they usually would in such circumstances (more angry or more nervous or more dismissive, for example). However, since the patient's inner world is complex and chaotic, and people differ in the issues to which they are sensitive, different members of the team may tune into and respond to different aspects of the patient's distress. This can lead to clinicians taking sides in unnecessary conflicts over patient care that wouldn't usually arise, which in turn can create other interpersonal problems.[13] The key to getting these working relationships back on track is to recognize that these troubles are not caused by wrong-headed colleagues but are in fact *providing information* about what is going wrong in the difficult interpersonal world of the patient whom the entire team is trying to help. Once this fact is recognized, some simple strategies can move the team towards a constructive outcome, such as identifying a single point person to coordinate communication.

   8. *Think of the patient as troubled rather than troubling.* It is much easier for most health care providers to deal with a patient's emotions when

she is *internalizing* (i.e., when she is afraid, ashamed, sad, or guilty) than when she is *externalizing* (especially when she is hostile). It is helpful to reframe what a patient with fearful attachment expresses as evidence that she is troubled *within* herself, rather than simply being a source of trouble for others. The reframing encourages the team to adopt a more sympathetic and effective approach.

Consider the example given above in which a patient fails to keep regularly scheduled appointments and then repeatedly requests to be fit in for a crisis but fails to attend the crisis appointment. It is easy in this situation for members of the team to disparage the patient as irresponsible, immature, or selfish. How might they respond differently if instead they see a patient who is trying her best to get the help that she needs but who is overcome by fear at the precise moment when she is required to act in her own interests?

Understanding that attachment is a developmental theory can sometimes help with this effort to reframe "bad" behaviour. Many health care providers are able to see that the behaviour of a young child is caused by something other than what it directly expresses (e.g., a tantrum that occurs because of fatigue or children acting angry when they are afraid). The behavioural results of the quandary of a person stuck between the pulls towards attachment anxiety and avoidance is not so different. Use the model of a child's behaviour if it is helpful, but beware of how patronizing it can sound to compare your patient to a child if the analogy is not understood in the manner in which it is intended.

9. Refer to your usual good standard of care. The intense emotions, inconsistent behaviours, and strong unmet interpersonal needs that are often in play when a person with fearful attachment is ill can lead to poor choices by health care providers. For example, it often happens that hospitalized patients are either discharged from hospital far too quickly (to make a problem go away) or far too slowly (because of an exaggerated sense of the patient's incapacity to manage independently or an exaggerated fear of other consequences of discharge – like missing a serious diagnosis or being sued). To avoid *irrational* responses to insecure attachment, it is helpful to refer back to the usual standard of care. Experienced health care providers can remind themselves and each other – explicitly – that they are good at their jobs, that the basics of the current medical situation are familiar to them, and that they have a standard approach to such problems that has become the standard for good reasons. *Rational* adaptations of the standards of care are valuable and crucial for a person with fearful attachment, but each adaptation should be well considered and carefully monitored. When the plan of care is veering too far off course without a clear and sound justification, it is time to be reminded of what you would be doing for anyone else in this situation.

10. Manage the treatment team. Collaboration and communication among members of the team are more important than ever when insecure attachment leads to difficult care. Agreeing on a shared approach to a patient's problems and providing consistent communication about the goals and the plan helps to calm the patient's feelings of insecurity (which are stoked by inconsistent and conflicting messages, even if they are solicited by the patient) and reduce the potential for unnecessary conflict between team members. Consultation and collaboration help to share the burden of care and to keep the care plan more nearly aligned with the usual standards. Furthermore, a team functions more effectively when each of its members is able to work within her field of competence. Clear communication and effective delegation of tasks to those who are best equipped to deal with them helps to keep care on track.

Depression and anxiety

11. Treat mental illness if it is present. People with fearful attachment are at higher risk than the next person for mental health problems, such as major depression and anxiety disorders. This risk is further amplified when they are physically ill. Mental illness both complicates the rest of a person's medical care and substantially increases the burden of being ill. Furthermore, depression or an anxiety disorder is often quite responsive to specific treatment. It is important in a complex and sometimes confusing situation to attend to problems that are familiar and readily treatable. If mental illness is present in addition to whatever else is going on, it should be treated.

Advice to patients

Dealing with the opposing pulls of anxiety and avoidance is a miserable and potentially paralysing experience. Here is what we tell patients about how to minimize the impact of fearful attachment on health.

1. Focus on reducing anxiety.
- If the conflict between the pull to seek contact and the push to isolate yourself feels irresolvable, then you need to choose to

address one or the other of these pulls first. Our suggestion is to give priority to attending to attachment anxiety. It is usually easier to overcome your misgivings about seeking help and accepting the response that is offered than it is to act constructively without help.

- If you have a person whom you trust to provide support and solace, use him or her. The power of feeling the support of one trusted person can be enough to break a seemingly irresolvable stand-off.
- Use every healthy trick that you have learned to control and reduce fear when you feel it. Use whatever techniques work for you to help you to approach others (including professionals) and not to flee when the tension starts to rise.

2. Work on change during the times when your health is not in crisis.

- It is very hard to practise adjusting your approach to health care interactions in the midst of a crisis and much easier to work on overcoming your reluctance to engage in health care during the times when you are feeling healthier. Under those circumstances, when the stakes are lower, try to set up a schedule of regular visits for routine medical care. In this way you can try to find the reassuring rhythm of regular contact. Over time this can start to feel normal – each successful visit makes the next one easier. You can do this in different domains, such as visits to the family doctor and to the dentist, which gives you more opportunities to practise and normalize the experience. Often you can recruit the clinic's help in this, if you feel up to it. You won't be the first person to tell your dentist that you are phobic of dental work, for example, so she may have some suggestions that will help.

3. Encourage yourself to report symptoms and concerns.

- Suffering in silence may be one of the greatest costs of a pattern of fearful attachment. Perhaps past bad experiences with health care professionals make you wary about trying again. Maybe you don't feel entitled to use the time of a busy expert. Maybe you don't want others to think you are a whiner or a wimp. Perhaps you aren't sure if your health concerns are real or substantial enough to merit a professional's time. Whatever your reasons, these inhibitions to speaking your mind all lead to the same unfortunate result: perpetual concern and suffering where instead there could be understanding and the possibility of effective treatment. The way to break this cycle is to find ways to speak up and be heard.

- Learn and practise the skills of assertiveness. Focusing your attention on techniques of speaking and acting serves to sidestep questions of your personal worth and entitlement or what someone else is thinking, which are subjective concerns that are difficult to resolve.
- Pay attention to the response you get from health care workers when you speak up. If they listen to the information that you are providing, ask questions about it, and maybe take some further action, that is a sign that you are being heard and your efforts to speak up are succeeding. If the response is not as positive, it may mean that you need to continue to work on organizing and clarifying your communication or that the match between you and this particular professional is not ideal. If you do have a positive response, see if you can find a time to check out with that person what has worked so you can replicate it. It'll probably also feel good – you may be surprised at how positively others view you.

4. Focus on the present.
- You have this interpersonal style for a reason. The people who acted as models of care in your developmental years may have provided a model of care that created fear or shame rather than comfort or solace. But that was then and this is now. While your history (and your body's reaction to that history) may be shouting that you are walking into an unsafe situation, try to see health care for what it actually is *here and now*. Try to give people a chance to show you what you can expect of them.

5. Watch for depression and anxiety.
- Fearful attachment increases the risk of experiencing illnesses like depression and anxiety disorders. During times when you are seriously ill, your vulnerability to experiencing mental illness is particularly high. It is important to be watchful for signs of a mental illness that merits treatment in itself. Anxiety disorders and depression are often very treatable, so recognizing that one is present can provide an opportunity to markedly improve your level of function and comfort.

Adapting health care to meet the needs of people with fearful attachment is a challenge for all health care professionals. A clinician who understands this in the framework of attachment theory sees that meeting the challenge requires the skills and resources that are useful for adapting to either dimension of insecure attachment on its own. Clinicians without this framework often feel that they have no effective way to respond and are vulnerable to blaming the patient for the difficulty.

15 Changing the System

Methods of providing health care are always in flux, changing in response to new information and circumstances. In the past two hundred years, health care has been shaped by new knowledge about the causes of disease, from the discovery of germs to the mapping of the genome; by social forces that have influenced methods of payment, civil rights, and gender roles; by advances in statistical methods and research methodology; by the rise of multinational corporations that profit from medical advances; by increasing international travel, immigration, and communication; by the increasing role of evidence in medical decision making; and by the Internet, two world wars, and an aging population.

It would be a small thing to add to this list a new awareness that *illness happens between people*, and yet the consequences might be substantial. What would health care look like if the system came to recognize that making people feel insecure is bad for their health? First, we have to recognize that the health care system was not built with patients' feelings of well-being anywhere near its centre. Although things have improved – health care professionals are now trained to recognize that biological, psychological, and social forces are all at play in illness and disease, and health care systems are shifting towards a patient-centred model – that improvement has not extended to understanding the importance of attachment and of feeling secure. Specifically, we are not taught that a sick person, above all else, needs to feel safe and secure or that fear trumps everything. A sick person cannot focus on getting well and cannot distinguish who to trust and collaborate with and what to do and what to avoid while she is afraid.

Attachment theory as a force of change

These things can change. The role of parents in the hospital care of children provides an example. Like most fathers of our generation, we were present for the births of each of our children. During the fortunately few times when they were hospitalized as children, one or both of their parents were with them virtually around the clock. However, it was not that way for our parents' generation. How did it change?

In Chapter 7 we described how attachment theory was born in a hospital, when in 1948 James Robertson went to Central Middlesex Hospital to observe young children who were separated from their parents. It was normal hospital policy at that time for hospitalized children to have only very brief visits with their parents. Most of the day, the sick children were looked after by nurses, doctors, and other hospital staff – which is to say they were looked after by strangers. Robertson observed that although the nurses were caring, little children protested this arrangement vigorously in their first few days in hospital, crying in obvious distress. After a few days, protest gave way to despair and sadness, which in turn gave way to detachment. In the end, these two- and three-year-old children often gave no further indication of any sense of connection or interest in those around them, including their visiting parents. Recognizing that this shift to passivity was not a positive adaptation but the consequence of despair, Robertson went on to become a vocal and effective champion of children's hospital reform. He was a pioneer whose efforts contributed to the completely revised philosophy of modern children's hospitals, where families play together and parents are often encouraged to stay with their young ones throughout the day and the night.

James Robertson was not working alone. He had been hired at the Tavistock Clinic, a centre for psychoanalysis, by John Bowlby. Bowlby was the head of the Department for Children and Parents, the former Children's Department, which he had renamed as soon as he assumed leadership. The name change gives a clue that Bowlby had long recognized the importance of the relationship between parents, especially mothers, and their children. He had worked with troubled youth earlier in his career and had advanced the understanding of antisocial behaviour when he published his observations of how juvenile delinquents had frequently experienced maternal deprivation and separation when they were young. Surprisingly, his psychoanalyst mentors considered Bowlby's view that a child's feelings and attitudes were closely tied to his actual experience with his parents to be heresy. At one point his clinical supervisor, the highly influential psychoanalyst Melanie Klein, forbade him to speak to the mother of a troubled three-year-old that he was seeing in child analysis. Her view was that an analyst needed to understand and interpret the internal psychological drives, fantasies, and conflicts of a child, not the forces of the child's external world. Bowlby opposed that point of view for his entire career.[1]

John Bowlby shared Robertson's interest in the effects of early separation on children and his concern about the harm that was being done by standard hospital practices. Perhaps he was sensitive to the children's troubles because, like so many middle- and upper-class boys of his time in England, he had endured boarding school starting at the age of seven, which he later wrote was something he would not do to a dog.[2] Together, Bowlby and Robertson showed the documentary film *A Two-Year-Old Goes to Hospital* to the British Psychoanalytic Society, and together they faced the fierce opposition to their insistence that the hospitalized child's distress they documented, which was undeniable to anyone who watched the film, was the direct result of her separation from her parents.[3] If their observation seems obvious now, it is only because in the meantime their argument has been won. Through the 1950s and the early 1960s, Bowlby advocated for the well-being of children as a mental health consultant to the World Health Organization, and throughout his life he continued to defend the view that actual experiences in the real world were critical determinants of childhood security.

Since then, children's hospitals in Western countries have changed their attitudes towards the presence of parents. Over the same time policies that used to keep mothers separate from their newborn infants and fathers excluded from the birth process altogether have also gone by the wayside. So well-considered changes are possible, even when they inconvenience health professionals and defy accepted wisdom.

Patient-centred care

It is inevitable that the attachment system will always be on display in clinics and hospitals because these will always be places where people are sick, injured, disabled, and in pain, each of which are triggers of attachment behaviour. On the other hand, the culture of modern health care causes additional fear by adding unnecessary interpersonal stresses to the situation. Health professionals cause fear by not respecting the things that people need to do to maintain feelings of security. An avoidant patient needs to maintain a safe distance, for example, whereas an anxious patient needs the comfort of a reassuring companion. As health professionals, we cause fear by adopting impersonal models of care because they are efficient or convenient to us or our institution instead of providing enduring, trustworthy provider-patient relationships. We also prevent comfort or cause fear by not including partners and family in our care plan.

Many of the changes that we would advocate to help patients feel more secure fit within the mandate of patient- and family-centred care, a movement that has caught the attention of many health care institutions.[4] Patient- and family-centred care has a much broader mandate for increasing collaboration between patients, families, and health care institutions than the view that we are taking – it even includes things like changing the architectural design of hospitals to improve the patient experience. Patient- and family-centred care also emphasizes that interactions between professionals, patients, and families should be collaborative, be respectful, and recognize mutual strengths. These principles are a good fit with what attachment theory would prescribe, but our interests are more specific. We want to promote the types of collaboration that help patients to feel the most secure. In particular, we want to emphasize how that sort of collaborative, respectful interaction should lead to different *kinds* of interaction for different *kinds* of patients.

Health care needs to be tailored to individual relational styles

The health care system should allow people to play to their strengths. That means that we should not force all people to adapt to the same medical environment. People with different patterns of attachment differ in the kinds of interaction with health care professionals that are optimal for their health.

People with a secure pattern favour collaboration, assume personal responsibility for healthy choices, and can identify the exceptional circumstances in which accepting direction and receiving care from others is what the situation demands.

On the other hand, people with high attachment anxiety often respond better to care that is more directive and reassuring and don't do well with an impersonal system. Continuity of care, meaning seeing the same person for the same problem over time, helps to build trust and to reduce anxiety. Since health care that is personal, directive, and reassuring is not too far from the old paternalistic model, we need to be aware of its risks.[5] In particular we need to be sure that a patient's right and need to choose for herself is protected and facilitated, not usurped. The onus is on the health care provider to find the right balance between providing direct support on one hand and encouraging her patient to develop in autonomy, confidence, and assertiveness on the other hand. The implication is that training for health care professions needs to directly and specifically address these challenges. Being a health care professional involves more than knowing what treatment to recommend; it also, crucially, requires knowing how to tailor that treatment to a particular individual. In addition, many patients with high attachment anxiety would feel more comfortable if we routinely included their partners (and sometimes siblings, parents, or children) in the circle of care.

A patient with high attachment avoidance would be likely to recoil from the directive and reassuring care that we just described. Worse yet, it might lead that patient to feel that regaining a sense of personal autonomy was more urgent than making sound health decisions. For such a person self-management strategies might be a better alternative. A movement is growing towards providing patients with education and tools that allow them to manage their illness as their own personal experts. For example, for persons with diabetes, it is considered a cornerstone of medical care that they learn to manage their disease day to day by monitoring their levels of physical activity, food intake, and blood glucose levels,[6] which is getting easier thanks to the development of apps and smart blood glucose monitors. This approach could be crucial to keeping a patient with high attachment avoidance engaged in treatment. It would also likely work well with a secure patient, but it could be much more of a challenge for patients with high attachment anxiety. The latter patient might be better served by being paired with a health care partner.

Care that is adapted to interpersonal style allows each person to use external and internal resources most effectively so that the person can keep the focus and energy directed towards the most important goal: maintaining health. However, it is an enormous demand to ask health care providers to adapt to the style and needs of different patients. It raises some legitimate questions, such as how a health care professional is supposed to recognize patients' patterns of attachment in the first place and which modifications of health care techniques are most effective for particular attachment styles. Very little evidence currently exists to guide this kind of individualized treatment. Providing personalized health care requires a shift in the priorities of health care research so that these questions can be asked and answered by well-funded, high-quality research.

Health care professionals should be interpersonal experts

Health care professionals are trained in a range of skills that include not only being a technical expert but also communicating effectively, being part of a team, advocating for patients, and more. It may be a small further step to say that they should also know something about interpersonal relationships as far as they affect health and illness and should have some skills in managing difficult interpersonal situations. Once gaps in practice are recognized, they can be bridged. We are advocating that bridging the gap in care that results from not identifying interpersonal differences is a goal that is very much in line with the improvements that were advocated by the American Institute of Medicine almost a decade ago to bring North American health care "into the 21st century."[7]

Of course, degrees of expertise are possible. No one expects surgeons to be leading psychotherapy groups. However, it does not take a degree in psychology or a residency in psychiatry to understand the basics. With a modest amount of training, health care providers can recognize prototypical patterns of attachment.[8] It is a short step from there to being able to modify their style in response to the differing needs and strengths of different patients. Many practitioners do this intuitively anyway. All that we are suggesting is that it behooves health care providers to make this implicit adjustment an explicit choice. We should know what we are doing and we should do it because we recognize that it is the right thing to do.

There may also be innovations that can help providers to personalize health care. Paul Ciechanowski piloted a system in which patients filled out a few standard questionnaires at the start of treatment that included a measure of attachment. Clinicians would then be given a brief summary of the patient's individual style, strengths, and vulnerabilities at the start of each appointment – a head start on a more effective and satisfying interaction for both parties.[9] It isn't complicated to turn that sort of information into the start of a transparent and collaborative conversation: "I see you're a very self-reliant person – have I got that right? Okay, then we'll be more successful as a team if we can find ways to help you make the health choices that keep you going on your own without too many visits here getting in your way."

Pushing it even further, health care professionals who have reliable contact with patients over time can use their interpersonal skills to help patients to trust more and fear less. In this way, attachment insecurity becomes another item on the problem list for which a treatment exists, no different in principle from hypertension or asthma.

Of course the time and place to do the most effective teaching of interpersonal principles is in professional schools, before our students even get to the clinics. We think schools do a better job now than they once did. Courses in therapeutic communication are the norm. Still, schools have a long way to go, and the idea that a relational approach is actually good for health is not yet a part of the curriculum.

Health care settings should make people feel secure

Although good health care should help patients to feel more secure, the opposite often happens. Fortunately, small changes can sometimes make a big difference. We have an example from the breast cancer clinic at our hospital.

A focus group at the clinic identified that patients found one particular time in the treatment process to be very stressful – the gap that occurred after frequent visits to the surgeon ended and before visits to the medical oncologist (who would prescribe chemotherapy) started. Although the gap was never longer than two weeks, it felt like a gaping hole in their care, unsurprisingly, although staff didn't realize it until the focus group was held. These women had been diagnosed with breast cancer and had a major operation, both of which were scary events. They were eager to get on with the next phase of treatment both because it worried them and because it held their best chance of a long-term cure. But at this crucial moment, instead of feeling that there was a team looking out for their care, they were given some pamphlets and a future appointment with a stranger. They felt unsure if the delay was compromising their treatment, disconnected from the clinic, and uncertain about whom they could call if they had questions.[10]

The fix was simple, thanks to our hospital having a primary nursing care model in which each patient is assigned to a particular nurse (or pair of nurses) for the delivery of her chemotherapy. Once the need was identified by the focus groups, the assigned chemotherapy nurse, who previously waited to meet the patient at her first medical oncol-ogy appointment, simply made a point of being in contact with the patient at her last surgical appointment. This provided a face, a name, and a phone number for the patient – and more importantly provided her with a relational bridge to the next phase of treatment. When we asked the nurses how they fared with yet another additional work task, they reported that their workload had actually decreased. More often than not, patients who were provided with a bridge were calmer, and so they came to the medical oncology clinic visit in better shape and subsequently made fewer phone calls and were easier to care for. In the new system, women felt more secure and less frightened. It seems likely this frame of mind is better for patients as they approach a six-month course of chemotherapy, and the cost to the system or any indi-vidual nurse was negligible.

Health care providers have attachment styles too

The fundamental unit of human relationship is not an individual but a pair. Talking exclusively about the attachment style of consumers of health care without attending to the providers of care ignores half of the interaction. Only a small amount of research has been done on the effects of the attachment patterns of health professionals, but what has been done suggests that we should be paying closer attention. Here is a sample:

- Among medical students, those who are more secure are more likely to choose careers in family practice and primary care than in other specialties.[11]
- The match between provider and patient makes a difference.[12] When discussing psychotherapy, Jeremy Holmes says that when the therapist and patient are both prone to attachment anxiety, therapy never ends; but when the therapist and patient are both prone to attachment avoidance, therapy never starts.[13] Something similar applies to general medical care. A health care provider who is too concerned about rejection and disapproval may lack the assertiveness and independence that he needs to steer a clear course. A provider who is not open to intimacy and vulnerability has many opportunities to hide behind the white coat, the technology of medicine, and the myth of dispassionate care to the detriment of his patient.

- Patterns of attachment influence the ways that health care providers respond to the stresses of their work. For example, we found that attachment anxiety was a predictor of the amount of stress that hospital workers experienced in difficult circumstances.[14] Similarly, attachment insecurity seems to be one of the driving forces determining how paramedics respond to their inevitable exposure to "critical incidents."[15]
- Some evidence is emerging that physicians who are more secure are also more empathic.[16]

Trying to understand "difficulty" or "miscommunication" or "noncompliance" in health care interactions by exclusively studying patients is like trying to understand marital problems by studying only one partner. We expect the attachment system of a patient to be activated frequently in a health care setting and the attachment system of a provider to be activated less often; nonetheless, a provider-patient relationship is one of vulnerability and intimacy. It isn't a balanced and reciprocal relationship (nor should it be – providers have a fiduciary responsibility to maintain appropriate boundaries and protect the interests of patients, who expose their vulnerabilities in trust), but providers of health care are far from neutral participants in the interpersonal dance of health care. It is hard to get professionals to participate in psychological research as subjects, but it is about time. We health care providers need to know more about ourselves so that we can become better dance partners.

We can't know in advance exactly how health care training and provision will change when the importance of attachment security to health is taken into account. However, we can be sure that one of the results will be that quality will improve. It is a fair bet, beyond that, that health care will become more efficient through reducing the wasted effort and cost that currently result from overuse and underuse.[17] Increasing both quality and efficiency means increasing value and decreasing costs. This alone should be a strong argument for developing personalized medicine for actual people.

16 Becoming More Secure

Patterns of attachment are evidence of our ability as humans to adapt to the circumstances in which we develop. They are part of our normal human psychology, as integral to who we are as individuals as the differences in our personalities. From an evolutionary perspective, our species is strengthened by having a variety of attachment patterns represented in our pool of social behaviours because this diverse behavioural profile makes us more adaptable to a wide range of environments.[1] The evolutionary pressure to maintain this diversity may contribute to the similarity of the relative distribution of secure and insecure attachment patterns across different regions and cultures.[2] The implication of this view is that, at least at the species level, little reason exists to *try* to reduce insecure patterns of attachment and little likelihood exists that such a project would succeed. On the other hand, a core argument of this book is that attachment insecurity contributes to the risk of chronic disease and illness and that finding ways to reduce feelings of insecurity is a valuable and under-exploited path to better health. How do we reconcile these apparently conflicting views?

First, it is important to distinguish between *changing* a person's attachment style from an insecure pattern to a secure pattern versus merely finding ways to help a person with an insecure pattern to *feel* more comfortable more often. The latter is a more modest goal and is the intended outcome of most of the adaptations that we have encouraged for health care providers, patients, and designers of policy and curricula in the previous four chapters. Our main agenda is not to reduce the number of insecure people in our midst but to change how health care works and take insecure patterns of attachment into account. This pragmatic conclusion is inevitable if we are right about evolutionary forces, the length of time required to influence insecurity, and the limited access available in typical health care interactions.

Second, we nonetheless need to distinguish between societal goals and the goals of individuals. Although increasing the number of secure people among us is not necessarily a practical goal at a societal level, it may well be the personal goal of many individuals. Many of the kinds of problems that lead people to seek counselling, psychotherapy, meditation, stress management skills, and the like are problems that result from attachment insecurity. Whether or not it is expressed in these terms, many individuals put a great deal of effort into becoming more secure.

Finally, whatever the effect on patterns of attachment in general, a healthy society should undoubtedly strive to eliminate the most extreme of the developmental conditions that promote insecure attachment. Abuse and neglect of children remains a "silent epidemic."[3] Childhood poverty and hunger should have no place in the affluent societies in which they are still all too common.[4] More subtle sources of the development of insecure attachment are mostly beyond the purview of government and policy,[5] but the grossest sources of harm to children merit all the energy and resources that we can constructively direct at eliminating them – on their own merits, irrespective of the risks they pose for health later in life.

Raising more secure children

Most parents would prefer their children to grow up secure, and parents more than anyone else have the power to facilitate and support attachment security. This is not to say that a child's eventual pattern of attachment is entirely determined by parental attitudes and behaviour because the roles of genetics, other determinants of temperament, and factors beyond parents' control, such as poverty and peer influences, are substantial. (A parent only has to have two children to realize that the power of parenting to shape a child's personality is not as strong as she thought.) Nonetheless, when we look at the many influences on an individual's pattern of attachment, parents are paramount.

Providing guidance and advice about raising children with secure attachment is an industry and a movement currently, but we do not have the expertise to add to the instruction (or the debate about some of the extreme positions that have been adopted within the movement).[6] Some resources, however, have proved useful to parents looking to reduce their inadvertent contribution to their children's vulnerability to feeling insecure. These resources focus on enhancing a parent's ability to intuit a child's mental states and to see things from the child's point of view. This mentalizing of a child's inner world fosters security and reduces the frightening and frightened parental behaviours that lead to insecurity, such as withdrawing from the child when comfort is needed, giving conflicting cues, being "negatively intrusive" (e.g., mocking), or being dazed or disoriented when the child is frightened.[7]

Lisa Berlin, an attachment researcher who is particularly interested in applying what is known about infant attachment to improving public health, suggests that building security in children is best accomplished by helping *parents* to feel more secure (or at least to be more reflective about their models of self and others) and providing parents with specific information about how babies express their needs and how parents' actions can meet those needs or not. Furthermore, she suggests that this work needs to occur within a relationship in which the teacher is able to provide a secure base for the parent-learner; you cannot learn to foster security for your child in a relationship with a teacher that makes you feel insecure.[8]

A sample of some of the resources that have a strong theoretical base or evidence of effectiveness includes the following:

- The *Circle of Security* program teaches parents basic practical attachment theory and poses two tasks to parents: to provide closeness when the child needs it and to facilitate exploration when the child signals a need to explore.[9]
- The *Minding the Baby* program, designed for very high-risk mothers, involves home visitors who help mothers to describe their baby's behaviour and link it to hypothesized mental states – directly practising their skills of mentalizing.[10]
- Our colleague Diane Benoit, one of the researchers responsible for demonstrating that patterns of attachment are passed from generation to generation,[11] focuses on broader targets. She has produced a short video suitable for all parents: *A Simple Gift: Comforting Your Baby*. It teaches parents, for example, that providing comfort teaches trust and does not spoil a baby. She has also produced a video for parents at risk of frightening and frightened behaviour: *A Simple Gift: Ending the Cycle of Hurt*.

Finally, we have often wondered about the impact of providing a very minimal nudge in the direction of security to a very large group of people simply by increasing information and discussion about attachment security in prenatal classes for prospective parents and encouraging reflection about their bonds with their new child (e.g., by talking about how their baby is able to recognize its mother's voice before birth[12]).

Becoming more secure *after* an attachment pattern has developed

Throughout this book we have spoken about patterns of adult attachment as if they never change, which is a fair first approximation because these patterns generally show a substantial amount of stability over time. In this chapter, however, we are interested in the possibility of shifting attachment patterns towards greater security, so we need to look at this more closely.

The first thing to emphasize about fluctuations in attachment behaviour is that even when a pattern of attachment is consistent and stable over time, the behaviour that is characteristic of the pattern is not always evident because the attachment system is not always turned on. The attachment system is triggered only when we detect danger or the sort of isolation that indicates a risk of harm. A stable attachment system produces similar patterns of behaviour from one such episode to the next. Thus the occurrence of attachment behaviour is determined by intermittent events (i.e., it is state dependent), whereas the consistency of attachment behaviour depends on the underlying attachment pattern. In the remainder of the chapter, when we are talking about changes in patterns of attachment, we are not talking about the variability that occurs when the attachment system is turned on and turned off, but rather about the more fundamental change that occurs when a shift takes place in the *type* of attachment behaviour that is triggered by attachment threats.

Patterns of attachment are complex and dynamic social-psychological phenomena. For example, while we often think of an infant as belonging in one category of attachment or another (such as secure or avoidant), observations of infants in the strange situation reveal that it is quite possible for a child to display one category of attachment behaviour towards her mother and another towards her father.[13] Similarly, adults may have more than one attachment relationship and may act differently in different attachment circumstances. Although this observation complicates our descriptions of attachment phenomena, it makes good sense; context-dependent learning is one of our brain's more powerful survival strategies.

Bearing this complexity in mind, what does the evidence tell us about stability and change in patterns of attachment? Overall, quite a bit of evidence shows that attachment patterns are usually stable. Studies of continuity in attachment patterns over long periods or through key periods of developmental transition often report rates of test-retest stability in the range of 60% to 80%.[14]

For the other 20% to 40%, two leading explanations describe why attachment patterns sometimes change. The first is that these patterns change in response to circumstance, life experiences that are sufficiently persistent and powerful force new learning. We can think of a pattern of attachment as a point of balance between two sets of pulls. The first of these is the tension between affiliation and interdependence and self-sufficiency. The second is the tension between expression and suppression of personal vulnerability. Life experiences that are powerful, persistent, and inconsistent with the point of balance represented by a pattern of attachment may shift the balance.[15] According to this view, patterns of attachment will either demonstrate continuity or will change in a way that is logically and predictably associated to circumstances, a process known as *lawful discontinuity*. The second, alternative explanation of change in attachment patterns over time is that the change is the result of individual differences; some people are more prone to change and others are more prone to stability.

The evidence has not yet fully resolved the question of why attachment patterns change. Some studies have found results that are consistent with lawful change. Although the "laws" at work in these studies are open to interpretation, the trends are consistent with the ideas that persistent exposure to adversity exerts some pressure towards attachment avoidance,[16] whereas engagement in a committed relationship favours increasing attachment security (and reduced attachment anxiety).[17] On the other hand, some studies of young adults support the relevance of individual differences, particularly that early exposure to adversity leads to later instability in patterns of attachment[18] or to complex interactions between individual factors and circumstances.[19]

Intentional change in patterns of attachment

People investing time and effort into changing the ways that they relate to others and the way that they feel about themselves is common. The size of the self-help section at your local bookstore is one indicator of how common it is to at least *want* to make big changes. Actually making changes, of course, requires more than reading a book – it takes practice and usually requires working with someone who is not directly involved in the trouble, such as a counsellor, coach, therapist, or teacher. Many of the most common goals for change can be understood as consequences of dissatisfaction with insecure attachment. Marital and relationship troubles, excessive anxiety or depression, and repetitive patterns of problems with coping and self-esteem can all be rooted in attachment insecurity, among their many other causes.

Some of the best evidence that psychotherapy can succeed in reducing attachment insecurity comes from the treatment of one of the more severe and difficult-to-treat psychiatric conditions: borderline personality disorder. This disorder involves very long-standing (almost lifelong) problems with wildly fluctuating emotional states, intense and unstable personal relationships, and impulsive, harmful behaviour. Although the causes of borderline personality disorder are not well understood and are undoubtedly complex, many experts consider that one of its fundamental causes is a disorganized state of attachment. It is certainly true that it is very common for people with borderline personality disorder to have a great deal of trouble mentalizing or inhibiting automatic thoughts and reactions to exercise more reflective thinking. *Mentalization-based therapy*, which is designed to help people with borderline personality disorder to enhance their capacity for slow, reflective thought (among other goals) has demonstrated very impressive success, not only helping patients to stop behaving in ways that are harmful to them but also helping them to improve their ability to regulate their emotions and relationships so much that a large proportion of them can no longer be said to have a personality disorder.[20]

Other forms of psychotherapy have also helped people with borderline personality disorder and other (often less severe) reasons for seeking treatment to reduce attachment insecurity.[21] Whether conducted in groups or in a therapist-patient dyad, the types of psychotherapy that increase attachment security are notable for direct and explicit attention to what is happening in close relationships – either the relationship between the therapist and the patient or the relationship between the patient and his attachment figures, or both.

Most of our attention in this book is directed towards helping individuals and institutions adapt to the patterns of attachment as they occur, rather than to changing those patterns. However, change is possible. It happens naturally, often based on life experiences that allow people to develop more security over time or that teach people to avoid and distance themselves from close attachment to minimize the risk of harm. It can also happen intentionally, when living with the consequences of insecurity is so dissatisfying that the effort and cost of psychotherapy is warranted.

17 Beyond Health Care Relationships: A Wider Attachment Perspective on Health

Put succinctly, what follows is the story we have told about the importance of attachment to human health.

Human beings are social animals. Our survival as a species has depended on our ability to trust our well-being to others and to reciprocate that trust. Our biological and psychological health depends on our capacity to engage constructively with others to provide and to receive support, protection, and soothing. That means our survival and health depend on our ability to love and be loved. We are born into relationships of care and our obligatory developmental dependency shapes our growing brains and bodies and determines how we communicate with others, what we fear, and where we find solace.

Patterns of attachment, including insecure patterns, are an achievement of our profoundly adaptive social brains. They allow us to prepare for, recognize, and accommodate to the social environment in which we are raised. For cultures and societies in which longevity allows the slow accumulation of small health effects over decades, insecure attachment is a weak force with a large and undesirable effect on health at all levels. Insecure patterns of attachment increase the health costs of life stress, increase the number and burden of physical symptoms we experience, increase the incidence of common diseases, decrease years of life, reduce the quality of life, increase the cost of medical care, interfere with health-sustaining relationships, provide obstacles to obtaining medical treatment, interfere with healthy behaviour choices, and contribute to problems with mental health.

Having come to appreciate this story, it seems obvious to us that approaches to health that neglect its interpersonal context will always be deficient. We discover new opportunities to promote health and manage illness more effectively when we take into account the urgent drive to feel secure, which we all experience when circumstances expose our insecurities. In the last few chapters we have given our full attention to opportunities to improve health *within health care relationships* by implementing strategies that are based on sound evidence and many years of experience. In this final chapter, we look towards opportunities to improve health outside of health care relationships. This shift requires a wider lens that surveys the possibility of changes in public policy and other social forces.

In particular, we need new approaches to the public health challenges that are posed by the vexing health care that we described in Chapters 1 and 2. Consider these examples of problems that increase long-term health risks, for which our current approaches to improving lifestyles are not very effective.

- In spite of his knowledge of the risks and some sensible evidence-based steps to reducing his weight, Will's BMI continues to hover around the boundary between overweight and obese.
- At 15, Charlene becomes infected with human papillomavirus, increasing her future risk of cervical cancer. Although she doesn't really enjoy sex with her boyfriend very much, he insists and she doesn't want to lose him. She finds sex easier when they are drunk.
- Jason started smoking as a teenager, and now that he is in his late twenties he has tried to stop twice and failed. He has used a nicotine patch, a pill prescribed by his family doctor, and hypnosis, but he hasn't been able to maintain his abstinence for more than a couple of months. The last relapse occurred when he went out with some friends for a few drinks – it just seemed like second nature to light up as well.
- Angelina joined a gym but stopped going after a few weeks because she felt self-conscious about being heavier than the other clients.
- Rodney and Simone have opted not to have their children vaccinated because they don't trust that the experts really have their best interests in mind.

Eating, drinking, smoking, having sex, exercising, and even driving a car are complex behaviours that tend to be enacted in ways that become habitual. Changing habits is hard and maintaining changes once they are made requires a lot of effort. As a result, the best strategies to improve public health are multifocal, battling the power of inertia on many fronts at once. Such efforts need to go far beyond "just say no."

Our multimodal societal efforts to change habitual health risks such as these tend to hit a floor beyond which further progress is elusive, because the interpersonal context is not adequately taken into account. For example, the prevalence of smoking decreased from more than 50% to about 20% from the early 1960s to the turn of the twenty-first century through a sustained effort that included changes in public policy and pricing of cigarettes, the emergence of irrefutable evidence of harm, public health messaging, and the development of cessation interventions. In the last decade, however, no further progress has been made. Twenty per cent seems to be a floor that isn't going to give way until we find new strategies. Appreciating the interpersonal context in which choices are made to start smoking and the interpersonal levers that may help a smoker to quit (or thwart his efforts) could be the kind of insight that could push the floor lower.[1]

Harry Stack Sullivan, the father of interpersonal psychiatry, once said, "I think it is fairly safe to say that anybody and everybody devotes much of his lifetime, a great deal of his energy ... and a good part of his effort in dealing with others, to avoiding more anxiety than he already has and, if possible, to getting rid of this anxiety. *Many things which seem to be independent entities, processes, and whatnot, are seen to be, from [this] standpoint ... various techniques for minimizing or avoiding anxiety in living.*"[2] What Harry Stack Sullivan called anxiety in his context, we call attachment insecurity. The drive to rid ourselves of insecure feelings is so strong that we are very likely to take the path to feeling less insecure regardless of the other risk that it may pose. This perspective can illuminate many behavioural choices. From this perspective, promoting change is not a question of convincing people that they *should* behave differently – we've reached the limit of the effectiveness of that strategy – but rather is a question of finding ways to align healthy behavioural choices with feeling secure or to align unhealthy choices with feeling more insecure.

One of the great challenges at the core of vexing health care is to find ways to limit the power of interpersonal insecurity to amplify suffering. This challenge has not been understood clearly until now, and so we have little evidence to guide our actions. But answers will come if we can reframe the question in a way that invites them: *How can we use the insights of attachment theory to suggest new approaches to reducing disease and illness in society?*

Although we don't have the answers, we have ideas. Here is a selection of them, intended to start the conversation.

Public health messaging

Working from current theories of health behaviour, such as we reviewed in Chapter 2, public health messages typically aim to increase the perceived risk of behaviours like smoking. It is worth considering whether instead, or in addition, advertisements could take the power of interpersonal forces into account. The message that smoking kills may not have as much power, for example, as the message that your partner will love that you quit or that your children need you around.

On the other hand, a slogan that has appeared on posters and seems designed to increase fear of interpersonal rejection among smokers – "Kissing a smoker is like licking an ashtray" – has not been very effective. Maybe it fails because it isn't true. Or perhaps it fails because it doesn't consider attachment avoidance. The message that smoking increases the risk of rejection plays on attachment anxiety but will have no impact (or perhaps even an unintended reverse impact) on someone who disavows being concerned about rejection.

One size does not fit all

This second point reminds us that one of the fundamental insights of viewing health challenges through an attachment lens is that people need to be treated individually. In particular, what works for a person with high attachment anxiety may have the opposite effect for a person with high attachment avoidance, and vice versa.

In the same way that we have prescribed different (and sometimes opposite) adaptations to patients and clinicians who are dealing with one or the other dimensions of insecure attachment, public health planners may need to take into account that different strategies are required for different members of a group that is targeted for behaviour change. This is inconvenient and may add expense to public health initiatives. In the end, the fact that the same message has a very different motivational effect on people with different attachment styles may limit the potential effectiveness of mass market messaging. On the other hand, as evidence emerges that some risky behaviours are more closely linked to attachment anxiety and others to attachment avoidance, some of these strategic choices will be clarified.

Using interpersonal leverage

One approach to the public health dilemma would be to focus on the leverage that is found in actual relationships rather than just trying to get the content of the message right in mass communication strategies. By way of example, Atul Gawande wanted to tackle the infant mortality rate in rural India because he knew that some very simple manoeuvres, like swaddling a neonate to protect against hypothermia, could increase survival. He found that the overworked and under-resourced practitioners could make these changes – when these changes were suggested by individuals with whom the practitioners had developed a relationship. The knowledge by itself failed to change practice, but when introduced and followed-up by someone the nurse practitioners had come to know, and respect, and whom they understood appreciated their circumstances, the changes could take root. Relationships are crucial for creating a context in which behaviour can change.[3]

So the content of the message is dependent on the messenger. How can we import this lesson to other public health tasks? Could a primary care provider meet with both a patient and a person from his inner (attachment) circle to work out an individualized, dyadic strategy to take on very resistant habits like smoking or overeating? The intervention here would be with the person who was the source of the patient's attachment security, giving her ways to help her loved one make and sustain a change. Would Will control his weight more effectively if his partner promoted Will's adoption of new diet and exercise routines?[4] Even if Will's partner was willing to take on this role (which a reasonable person could certainly decline), what strategy would work: Encouragement? Pressure? Joining in with the change? Perhaps we need to be giving as much thought to resources for partners as we do to resources for patients.[5]

Enhancing reflective thought

Gains can be made on many fronts by enhancing the slow, reflective thought that inhibits and modifies automatic reactions. Reflective thinking allows a person to consider and reconsider what is going on in her own mind and in the minds of others; to put off immediate pleasure in the service of long-term gain; to resist automatic conditioned actions, such as reaching for a cookie or a cigarette; and to tolerate temporary discomfort that would only get worse if she reacted instead of waiting it out. As a result, reflective thought is a major contributor to regulating emotional stress and distress, to managing interpersonal relations and minimizing interpersonal injury, and to overcoming unhealthy habits. Reflection is also a skill that can be taught and practised.

- Meditation practices, such as mindfulness meditation, increase reflective thought and have been demonstrated to be useful for many health outcomes.[6]
- Interpersonal interventions to increase a person's capacity to mentalize that have been developed for psychotherapy[7] could be adapted to incorporate into other kinds of treatment, such as the education and support that is provided in smoking-cessation clinics.
- Since the face-to-face interventions that improve reflection can be quite resource intensive, we developed an interactive e-learning computer course designed to achieve that outcome much more cheaply and flexibly.[8] *The Stress Vaccine* is designed to help health care workers reduce stress and build resilience by enhancing interpersonal skills and reflective capacity through virtual interpersonal interactions and coaching. Its first version succeeded in reducing interpersonal problems, increasing self-efficacy, increasing the perception of being supported by the employer, and improving coping.[9] This could be a model of more widely applicable and accessible resources.

Bolstering social support

The value of social support for health is widely understood but hasn't really been incorporated into health care very effectively, let alone into preventive medicine. What attachment theory adds is the insight that support from attachment figures – typically marital or romantic partners but sometimes others as well (especially for those who are not living with partners) – is far more protective of health than practical or emotional support from non-attachment figures.

If preserving and facilitating support within attachment relationships is understood as serving to improve public health, then public initiatives that make it easier for individuals to provide such support to their loved ones may be seen as more valuable. Practical public endorsement and support of same-sex marriage and adoption is an example of an opportunity for the state to reduce impediments to individuals forming health-supporting attachments. Providing practical assistance to family members who care for loved ones with dementia and mental illness is another way in which public policy can be directed towards enabling attachment support to do work that cannot be accomplished as effectively (or as cheaply) through other means.

The positive power of small changes and weak forces

In Chapter 6 we discussed the potential for a weak force of adversity to have a large negative impact on health over time. The same can apply on the positive side of the ledger. Especially if we are thinking about the health of our entire population rather than individual health, very small increments of benefit to individuals can add up to very large improvements in societal health – and lower costs of disease and illness.

The implication is that we don't always have to be thinking on a grand scale when we consider how to improve population health. A little nudge in the right direction can make a big difference if it is something that can be applied to a phenomenon, such as attachment insecurity, that is very common in very large groups of people.

Is it possible to build a secure society?

As a society, we could do more to reduce interpersonal insecurity and its long-term burden and costs. We won't be able to eliminate insecurity, but many parents face unnecessary obstacles to providing consistent, responsive, and safe care for their children. Poverty, a lack of resources for parents with addictions and mental illness, and family violence demand community advocacy and effective public policy. At a societal level, the possibility of optimal parenting in the earliest weeks of life requires support in policies for such things as statutory paid parental leave. Ensuring young parents have a decent income while their children are babies might accomplish much for the security of the next generation.

Furthermore, parents need access to good-quality health care for both their infants and themselves. A parent cannot feel confident responding to the needs of an infant unless she knows that she can get help when she thinks the child is sick and is able to maintain her own health. The reassuring presence of a resource that can provide authoritative (and appropriately limited) medical advice over the telephone, for example, can reduce anxiety and avoid unnecessary and expensive visits to the emergency department. It is the kind of resource that we think could make a world of difference for the security of some parents and their children.

We also advocate investing in early childhood education that is affordable, consistent, child centred, and focused at least as much on emotional and social development as on cognitive or academic development. Good-quality group-based daycare outside the home is not bad for children's security and may actually be protective for some children from unusually risky homes. To provide that, as a society we should be prepared to pay well-trained early childhood educators a wage that is commensurate with the importance of their task.[10]

These are just suggestions for strategies. However, the business maxim that "culture eats strategy for lunch" has the ring of truth. We know that the strategies that we think could be most useful to our health as individuals will succeed only to the extent that they are consistent with the values of families, communities, businesses, and governments. Much work remains for advocates of relational health, but we have every reason to believe it will be worth it.

Afterword

A few final words. In this book, we have followed many paths to reach some simple conclusions:

- We can understand much about human relationships by appreciating how we manage our closest attachments with others to avoid fear.
- The strategies that individuals use to minimize fear and feel secure (their patterns of attachment) tend to be consistent over time and are a fundamental source of individual differences that need to be taken into account for optimal health.
- Attachment insecurity is a force that contributes to cumulative risks for a range of chronic diseases over a lifetime.
- It is not difficult to recognize individual differences in patterns of attachment.
- Recognizing individual patterns of attachment provides the information that is required to adapt health care practices to the strengths and needs of individual patients.
- We could be healthier and medical care could be more effective if we took these lessons to heart and attended more closely to what happens between people in health and in illness.

This list is what we mean when we say that health happens *between* people. Indeed, we are advocating that recognizing how health and illness emerge from our closest relationships is the key to truly individualized health care. In the end, and for almost all aspects of health, we are better together.

Notes

Introduction

1 *Breathing with Sandra*, a documentary by Aziza Sindhu, was presented on the CBC 1 radio show *The Current* on October 11, 2011.

2 A myocardial infarction, or MI, refers to the death of muscle cells in the heart that occurs when blood flow in the arteries that serve the heart is blocked and the cells do not receive enough oxygen.

3 A stent is a tube that keeps an artery open so that blood can flow and feed oxygen to the muscle in the wall of the heart.

4 Bowlby, 1969; Bretherton, 1995.

5 Harlow, 1958; Harlow & Harlow, 1962; van der Horst, LeRoy, & van der Veer, 2008.

6 The patterns of attachment displayed by infants were first classified scientifically by Mary Ainsworth (1978).

7 Bartholomew & Horowitz, 1991; Hazan & Shaver, 1987; Main, Kaplan, & Cassidy, 1985; Mikulincer & Shaver, 2007.

8 Groves, 1978.

9 House, Landis, & Umberson, 1988.

10 Feeney, 1995; Feeney & Raphael, 1992; Feeney & Ryan, 1994.

11 Feeney & Kirkpatrick, 1996.

12 Hunter & Maunder, 2001; Maunder & Hunter, 2001.

13 Ciechanowski, Walker, Katon, & Russo, 2001; Ciechanowski, Katon, Russo, & Walker, 2002.

14 Since the initial correspondence of John Bowlby and Harry Harlow (van der Horst et al., 2008), attachment theory has always benefited from observations of mother-infant interactions in non-human species. The path from Bowlby to recent investigations of human attachment and health that

we have very briefly summarized is complemented by a parallel story of extraordinary advances in understanding the biology of attachment in other species, especially the work of Myron Hofer (1984, 1995, 2004), Gary Kraemer (1992), Stephen Suomi (1995, 2006), and Michael Meaney (2001). Although we have avoided much discussion of animal research in this book, the work of Hofer and Meaney is so central to the story that we are telling in this book that it is described in some detail later.

15 Fricchione, 2011.

1. What Is Health Care?

1 Although our intent is to understand health care, broadly defined, the cultural prototypes that we are referring to are about *medicine*, which has a narrower, physician-centric connotation.

2 Bloom et al., 2011.

3 This number is very hard to get your head around. The Global Economic Forum and Harvard School of Public Health, which provided the projection, put it in context like this: $47 trillion represents "75% of *global* GDP in 2010" (our italics) or "enough money to eradicate two-dollar-a-day poverty among the 2.5 billion people in that state for more than half a century" (Bloom et al., 2011).

4 World Health Organization, 2009.

5 Elfhag & Rossner, 2005; Wing & Hill, 2001.

6 Cokkinides, Bandi, Ward, Jemal, & Thun, 2006.

7 Statistics Canada, 2008.

8 Our friend and colleague, Gary Newton, who heads the division of cardiology at two major teaching hospitals, sums this up by saying that in medicine we define success as taking an imminently fatal disease and "turning it into diabetes."

9 The Institute of Medicine is American. Given the large differences between the health care systems in the United States and in other countries, including Canada, we use its findings cautiously. The problem of high health care use, however, is driven by forces that transcend the differences between our health care systems. The Institute of Medicine talks about "overuse" rather than high use, which introduces an assumption about the optimal degree of use that we would like to avoid for the time being (Committee on the Quality of Health in America, 2001).

10 Ovens & Chan, 2001.

11 Alexander et al., 1998; Barsky, Orav, & Bates, 2005; Hahn et al., 1996; Kroenke, 2003; Nagel, McGrady, Lynch, & Wahl, 2003; Simon, Ormel, Vonkorff, & Barlow, 1995.

12 Groves, 1978.

13 The true cost of managing a chronic disease while underusing medical resources is hard to know because the answer depends on doing research with people who are not likely to be willing or able to participate in research.

14 Elliott, 2003.

15 Ciechanowski, Hirsch, & Katon, 2002.

2. Why Else Do We Get Sick?

1 The distinction between illness and disease is important. Disease is a biological concept; it refers to the consequences of abnormal physiological processes. Illness is a subjective and social thing; it refers to feeling sick and acting like a sick person. Obviously, disease is an important cause of illness, but it isn't the only one. In this chapter we are focused on disease, but when we turn our lens more broadly on what is troubling about vexing health care and how a relational point of view illuminates the issues, we will need to think about illness as well.

2 Minino, Xu, Kochanek, & Tejada-Vera, 2009.

3 Rappaport, 2012.

4 The nucleotide sequence in this sentence is the beginning of the gene that codes for human insulin.

5 For yet another layer of (somewhat mind-bending) complexity, we also have genes that code for proteins that influence epigenetic changes – so some of the influence of the environment on our genes is *inherited*. That's GxExG if you are keeping score (Fraga et al., 2005).

6 Cohen, Janicki-Deverts, & Miller, 2007.

7 Sapolsky, 2004.

8 Studies of stress may investigate any of those components (stressor → appraisal → stress response) but not usually all of them, so different kinds of stress research are not always easy to reconcile.

9 This is sometimes expanded to "fight, flight, or freeze," because each of these responses is common in nature when an organism detects that it is in peril.

10 Taylor et al., 2000.

11 Joels & Baram, 2009.

12 Sympathetic and vagal nerves' autonomy from the control of the brain's cortex, their capacity to self-govern, is the reason that this system is called the autonomic (i.e., independent) nervous system. People who have problems that are directly controlled by the ANS and *not open to direct voluntary control*, such as increased bowel motility, sometimes benefit a

great deal from realizing the distinction – it allows them to stop blaming themselves for failing to control something that is not actually under their control.

13 McEwen & Wingfield, 2003.

14 An example drawn from recent research is the evidence that excess sympathetic drive makes it easier for some cancers to spread beyond their primary site, a crucial step in their progress from acute, but curable, to fatal disease (Cohen et al., 2012; Moreno-Smith, Lutgendorf, & Sood, 2010).

15 Rozanski, Blumenthal, & Kaplan, 1999; Sapolsky, Uno, Rebert, & Finch, 1990.

16 Dr Michael Lauer defines normal recovery as a decrease of 15 to 25 beats/minute with two minutes of rest after exercise. A bigger decrease is a sign of very good cardiovascular health. A smaller decrease is associated with health risks, including increased mortality (Nishime, Cole, Blackstone, Pashkow, & Lauer, 2000).

17 Kodama et al., 2009.

18 A substantial difference in fitness is associated with about a 50% difference in multi-year mortality – depending on the duration of the study, how fitness is measured, and so forth (Kodama et al., 2009).

19 Goldsmith, Bigger, Bloomfield, & Steinman, 1997; Tulppo et al., 2003.

20 Rats that are licked and groomed less as pups also behave differently when they are stressed. They are more fearful, which is expressed by exploring less or by being more defensive (Liu et al., 1997).

21 Bagot & Meaney, 2010.

22 The leap from rats to humans is shorter than you may think. Steve Cole has shown that social isolation in humans is very consistently linked with changes in the expression of a coordinated cluster of genes that turn up gene expression in genes that drive our basic inflammatory responses and turn down the systems that protect us against viral illness (Cole et al., 2007).

23 Norris, 1992.

24 Kessler, Sonnega, Bromet, Hughes, & Nelson, 1995.

25 Yehuda, 2004.

26 Yehuda & Bierer, 2007. Presumably, some evolutionary advantage of having a blunted stress response exists for the offspring of highly stressed parents. Maybe it provides children with a head start on environmental exposure, in effect preparing them in utero for a high-stress environment.

27 Yehuda et al., 2007.

28 Janz & Becker, 1984.

29 Madden, Ellen, & Ajzen, 1992.

30 Bandura, 1977, 2004.

31 It is far from an arithmetic certainty that Will will die of heart disease; in fact, it is more likely to not occur. This is just math: doubling the probability of a somewhat unlikely outcome (which is a huge increase in risk from a public health point of view) does not turn the risk into an inevitability.

32 When we were in medical school, our class newsletter featured a comic strip that starred Brainstem Man, whose superpowers were restricted to shivering and vomiting.

33 In the central nervous system, evolutionary age corresponds roughly to anatomical location such that moving higher reveals functions that have emerged more recently.

34 Kahneman, 2011.

35 This distinction between fast, automatic thoughts and slow, reflective ones is analogous to the distinction between two of our memory processes. Declarative memory is slow and thoughtful. It concerns things that we remember and can then describe, such as the answers to exam questions. Procedural memory refers to remembering how to do something, like driving a car. Procedural memory is not the subject of reflection.

36 As a cognitive psychologist, Kahneman has explored fast and slow neural processes by using problem solving. Take a question that has an intuitive, but incorrect, answer: *A ball and a bat together cost $1.10. The bat costs $1 more than the ball. How much does the ball cost?* A person answering this question will reveal which cognitive system she is using by answering either 10¢ (the appealing but wrong answer generated by the fast system) or 5¢ (the correct answer, which takes considerably more effort to determine). Don't worry, by far most people get this wrong – it isn't about intelligence; it is about the way we are built to make rapid assessments that are close enough to true most of the time.

37 Psychologists of emotion make a technical distinction between the words *affect, emotion,* and *feeling.* Although those distinctions are important to their work, they don't concern us here. We will use these words as synonyms.

38 Mischel, Ebbesen, & Raskoff Zeiss, 1972.

39 Mischel, Shoda, & Peake, 1988.

3. Health Happens between Us

1 Christakis & Allison, 2006; this was a study of heterosexual couples. Although we are not aware of similar research on same-sex couples, we

have no reason to think the results would be different. The same principle applies to most of the couple research reported in this book.

2 Lachman, 2003.

3 Pinquart & Sorensen, 2003.

4 We will have more to say later in this book about the important effects of weak forces that influence the health of very large groups of people because it is a recurrent theme in the story of attachment and health (Pinquart & Sorensen, 2007; Vitaliano, Zhang, & Scanlan, 2003).

5 Kiecolt-Glaser, Marucha, Mercado, Malarkey, & Glaser, 1995.

6 Doyle, 1997.

7 Coryell et al., 1999; Hoover et al., 2011.

8 Well-designed studies of various communities yield surprisingly consistent results. Although it matters how the questions are posed and how abuse is defined, in spite of that complexity we can be fairly sure that almost one in three children experiences physical or sexual abuse while growing up. Sexual abuse is more commonly experienced by girls, and physical abuse is more commonly experienced by boys, but many children experience both. The prevalence is even higher when emotional abuse and various forms of neglect are included (Afifi et al., 2014; Felitti et al., 1998; Koenen, Roberts, Stone, & Dunn, 2010; MacMillan et al., 1997).

9 Finkelhor, Ormrod, & Turner, 2007.

10 Marmot et al., 1991.

11 The Whitehall Study was first conducted in the late 1960s and repeated in the 1980s with essentially the same results. It demonstrates a robust and reliable effect.

12 Sapolsky, 2005.

13 Kivimaki et al., 2004.

14 Berkman & Syme, 1979.

15 Hemingway & Marmot, 1999. A meta-analysis of good studies that have looked at the links between various measures of social connection and decreased mortality in life-threatening diseases found that the benefits of social support and integration are on par with or stronger than the effects of things like quitting smoking, abstaining from alcohol, exercising, going to cardiac rehab, and getting a flu shot (Holt-Lunstad, Smith, & Layton, 2010).

16 One mark each for at least biweekly contact with a person in each of these categories: spouse, parents, parents-in-law, children, other close relationships, close neighbours, friends, workmates, students, fellow volunteers, members of recreational groups, and members of religious groups.

17 Cohen, Doyle, Skoner, Rabin, & Gwaltney, 1997; Cohen, Doyle, Turner, Alper, & Skoner, 2003.
18 Maunsell, Brisson, & Deschenes, 1995.
19 Cole et al., 2007.
20 Brown, Bhrolchain, & Harris, 1975; Brown & Harris, 1978.
21 West, Livesley, Reiffer, & Sheldon, 1986.
22 Although most of our examples of disease and illness in this book are physical, depression is no less of a health concern. It is as biological as any of the diseases that are conventionally thought of as physical diseases and one of the most burdensome illnesses worldwide.
23 Sinha, 2012.
24 Stroebe, Stroebe, Abakoumkin, & Schut 1996.

4. What Is Attachment?

1 Laughlin, de Ruyter van Steveninck, & Anderson, 1998; Leonard, Robertson, Snodgrass, & Kuzawa, 2003.
2 We are using "mother" here rather than "parent" because we are talking about human evolutionary history, in which we are not aware of much evidence of shared parenting with respect to continuous parent-infant interactions. We will revert to "parent" when we get back to the contemporary world.
3 Fonagy, Gergely, Jurist, & Target, 2005; Fonagy & Target, 1997.
4 Evolutionary explanations sometimes sound like just-so stories. The explanations that we are reviewing here are widely held to be plausible and likely, but they are far from certain. It is beyond our scope to provide a critique – it is enough to set a plausible context in which to understand the emergence of the attachment system.
5 Bowlby, 1969, 1973, 1980; Bowlby, Robertson, & Rosenbluth, 1952.
6 Winnicott, 1957.
7 Although what it means to feel secure may seem to be self-evident, the question sometimes arises. We are referring to feeling safe, comfortable, and unafraid. It is a pleasant state.
8 In attachment theory, the cognitive-emotional schemas that guide expectations and behaviour are called the internal working model, which consists of a model of the self and a model of others. The model of the self includes attributions of the extent to which one is loveable or worth helping, resilient, and capable. The model of others includes attributions of the extent to which attachment figures are responsive, reliable, and caring (Bowlby, 1969).

9 In attachment theory the word *secure* refers to two different things. First, it refers to the feeling of being safe, comfortable, and unafraid. Second, it is the name of a particular pattern of attachment: the pattern Janice is displaying.

10 We refer to patterns of attachment and styles of attachment interchangeably, simply for variety of usage.

11 We are not going to put much stress on the nomenclature of infant attachment because our emphasis in this book is on patterns of attachment in adults, which are described somewhat differently (see Chapter 6).

12 Sroufe & Waters, 1977.

13 Jon Allen (2013) describes the two prototypical categories of attachment insecurity as being stuck at either end of the attachment spectrum – either stuck clinging to one's secure base or stuck exploring.

14 Harlow & Harlow, 1962.

15 The rat pup–dam interactions that we are describing here were all discovered and described by Myron Hofer (1995).

16 Depue & Morrone-Strupinsky, 2005; Machin & Dunbar, 2011.

17 Eisenberger, Lieberman, & Williams, 2003.

18 The game, Cyberball, was developed by Kipling Williams and colleagues (Zadro, Williams, & Richardson, 2004).

19 The experience that we are referring to here inevitably involves GxE interactions, where the most important element of the environment (E) concerns typical behaviours and attitudes of the adults who have most responsibility for parenting a child. A wealth of research exists on the particular aspects of parental behaviour that are most important to determining patterns of attachment, as well as on the relative balance of genetic and environmental contributions to those patterns. Since our concern is mostly with adult health rather than parenting, we are not reviewing that research here. For the record, we don't think a thoughtful reading of the research that is currently available on human attachment is compatible with the view that the concepts of attachment justify blaming parents for their children's ills – even if that attitude was historically true of some of attachment theory's proponents.

5. Attachment Sculpts the Brain

1 Frith & Frith, 1999; Frith & Frith, 2003.

2 Perner & Wimmer, 1985.

3 Lieberman, 2007.

4 Lieberman, 2007; Satpute & Lieberman, 2006.

5 Frith & Frith, 2003.

6 Lieberman, 2007.

7 Mitchell, Macrae, & Banaji, 2004.

8 Mentalizing does not have to be explicitly thoughtful. It can also be less conscious, or implicit, as when we make a determination without explicit reflection about what the leader of the pack is intending when he dashes at us across the field. Mentalizing is a special class of thinking that is defined by the subject of the thoughts.

9 Lieberman, 2007.

10 Taylor, Phan, Decker, & Liberzon, 2003.

11 Dolan, 2007.

12 Ragozzino, 2007.

13 The OFC also serves as a brake on the adrenalin-driven arousal that accompanies fight-flight reactions. In this role the OFC allows us to calm down and tune into another person's non-verbal signals.

14 Jacobsen, Huss, Fendrich, Kruesi, & Ziegenhain, 1997.

15 Even exceptionally accurate mirroring is not enough in itself. What makes all the difference is the feedback (like marking) that subtly communicates to Tyler that he has been processed by Carol's brain (Stern, 1985).

16 Schore, 1994, 2002.

17 The strengthening occurs through the growth of more synapses (the connections that allow communication between nerves cells) between cells that communicate often and the pruning of synapses between cells that don't. As psychologist Donald Hebb declared long before the physiology of neural plasticity was understood, "Nerves that fire together, wire together."

18 Torsten Wiesel and David Hubel won a Nobel Prize for demonstrating how visual experiences during critical periods of development permanently alter the visual cortex of kittens.

19 Karl Kim and his colleagues (Kim, Relkin, Lee, & Hirsch, 1997) used functional magnetic resonance imaging (fMRI) to study a language-related area of the cortex called Broca's area. Children who learned two languages in early childhood used the same part of Broca's area for both languages. On the other hand, if the second language was learned as an adult, the fMRI revealed that the second language was served by a distinct, segregated part of Broca's area.

20 Fonagy, Steele, Moran, Steele, & Higgitt, 1991.

6. All Grown Up and Still Attached

1 A great deal of research has accumulated in support of Bowlby's assertion that the attachment system remains functional and influential throughout

life (Bowlby, 1969; Doherty & Feeney, 2004; Friedlmeier & Granqvist, 2006; Mayseless, 2004; Nickerson & Nagle, 2005; Pitman & Scharfe, 2010; Trinke & Bartholomew, 1997; Zeifman & Hazan, 2008). See also the discussion of stability and change in attachment over the lifespan in Chapter 16.

2 Diamond & Fagundes, 2010; Puig, Englund, Simpson, & Collins, 2013.

3 Carter, 2003; Carter, Williams, Witt, & Insel, 1992; Light, Grewen, & Amico, 2005; Nelson & Panksepp, 1998.

4 Buchheim et al., 2009; Kosfeld, Heinrichs, Zak, Fischbacher, & Fehr, 2005.

5 Carter, Lederhendler, & Kirkpatrick, 1997; Heinrichs, Baumgartner, Kirschbaum, & Ehlert, 2003; McCabe et al., 2002; McCabe, Paredes, Szeto, & Schneiderman, 2006; Rodrigues, Saslow, Garcia, John, & Keltner, 2009.

6 Allen, Stein, Fonagy, Fultz, & Target, 2005.

7 West & Sheldon-Kellor, 1994.

8 The researchers who developed the questions in this section were Hazan and Zeifman (1999; Zeifman & Hazan, 2008). See also Hazan, Gur-Yaish, and Campa (2004).

9 Proximity seeking is a little more complicated than this simple description, because its effects depend on a person's attachment style – described later in this chapter. Proximity (even the idea of proximity) to Lynn allows Bob to feel secure because Bob is able to obtain this feeling readily – he has a secure pattern of attachment. A person who is high in attachment anxiety experiences a very pronounced urge to *seek* proximity and to protest against separation but is often frustrated that closeness only brings modest or temporary relief from feeling insecure. A person who is high in attachment avoidance defends himself against the possibility of injury by disavowing the need for proximity (and thus it is difficult to get clear information about how proximity makes him feel).

10 Zeifman & Hazan, 2008.

11 Zeifman & Hazan, 2008; Hazan, Gur-Yaish, & Campa, 2004. This timing (two years) varies across couples and depends on patterns of attachment. In our experience, it is typical of persons with high attachment anxiety to attribute the characteristics of an attachment figure to others quite quickly (prematurely) and to be disappointed by the results. At least two studies show that young adults who are high in attachment avoidance and low in attachment anxiety tend to transfer attachment functions to peers earlier than those with other attachment patterns, and this transfer is associated with greater resilience to stress (Mayseless, 2004; Pitman & Scharfe, 2010).

12 Fraley & Davis, 1997; Zeifman & Hazan, 2008.
13 Our assertion is that a health care provider can temporarily serve the function of safe haven in spite of not being an attachment figure (i.e., not the person who is the provider or target of *all* attachment functions: proximity seeking, separation protest, safe haven, and secure base; and not the consistent provider of any of them). The assertion is somewhat controversial. The alternative view is that patients under stress behave towards their health care providers as they would behave towards one of their attachment figures because patients' behaviour is guided by their internal working model in this circumstance; patients are not using the health care provider as a safe haven – they are just trying to cope with the stressful situation, guided by their internal working model. In this view, when Bob was comforted by the nurse, he was unconsciously reminded of the comfort his attachment figures had provided him in the past, but the nurse did not actually serve any attachment function for him. The differences between these perspectives may be semantic. Emerging research is attempting to measure the degree to which patients receiving psychotherapy are attached to their therapists (Lilliengren et al., 2014) but there is little other empirical study of this question to date.
14 "You're a Whole Different Person When You're Scared" is a song written by Hunter S. Thompson and Warren Zevon and recorded on Zevon's album *My Ride's Here* (2002).
15 Maunder & Hunter, 2012.
16 Jeremy Holmes (personal communication, November 2003). For further discussion of this idea see Holmes (2006).
17 This system of nomenclature divides people by body shape into endomorphs (round in the middle), mesomorphs (square and muscular), and ectomorphs (tall and thin). Like most systems of classification it leads us to wonder how to classify intermediate cases.
18 Maunder & Hunter, 2012.
19 Bowlby (1969) described the internal working model, which is a cognitive-emotional schema of close relationships that is based on interactions between a child and his or her primary caregiver(s). The internal working model includes two components: a model of the self and a model of others. The two primary dimensions of adult attachment insecurity correspond to a negative model of the self (attachment anxiety) and a negative model of others (attachment avoidance). See Bartholomew and Horowitz (1991). These models are linked to common patterns of attachment behaviour as follows. A negative model of the self manifests as a sense of low self-worth, unloveability, fragility, and likely rejection. If this negative

model of the self is combined with a positive model of others, it leads to overemphasis on seeking contact with others and clinging. On the other hand, a negative model of others manifests as mistrust and the expectation of disappointment or harm. If this model is combined with a positive model of the self, it leads to overemphasis on self-reliance and a devaluing of the importance of interdependency. The combination of negative models of both the self and the other leads to patterns of behaviour that combine distress and distancing, such as fearful withdrawal or angry withdrawal.

20 In Bartholomew and Horowitz's (1991) influential model of adult attachment patterns, the four prototypes we are describing are called secure, preoccupied (high attachment anxiety and low attachment avoidance), dismissing-avoidant (high attachment avoidance and low attachment anxiety) and fearful-avoidant (high attachment anxiety and high attachment avoidance).

21 To minimize jargon we are not going to use the name of the prototypical style that is characterized by high attachment anxiety and low attachment avoidance. However, in other sources you will find it called *preoccupied attachment*.

22 This is an interesting variant of mentalizing. Susan thinks *a lot* about what other people are thinking, and her intuitions about their negative responses to her are often accurate. However, she does not really mentalize effectively because her ability to imagine their positive and neutral responses is much more limited. She has learned to use a highly sensitive and inflexible ability to mentalize as a kind of danger detector.

23 West et al., 1986.

24 Mikulincer, Florian, & Weller, 1993.

25 This part of the anecdote, the nurse's no-win responses in particular, is based on a case described by Jeremy Holmes (2001).

26 Collins & Feeney, 2000.

27 The prototypical style that is characterized by high attachment avoidance is named *dismissing attachment*.

28 George & West, 2001.

29 Simpson, Rholes, & Nelligan, 1992.

30 The fearful pattern was first described by Bartholomew and Horowitz (1991). This description of avoidance as a defence that fails in the face of stress is from Shaver and Mikulincer (2002).

31 This pattern draws on different schemes of understanding adult attachment, where it may be referred to as fearful-avoidant, disorganized, or unresolved for trauma.

32 Ciechanowski, Katon, Russo, & Dwight-Johnson, 2002; Ciechanowski, Walker, et al., 2002.

33 Maunder et al., 2006.

34 This pattern was called disorganized/disoriented by Main and Solomon (1986), who first described it.

35 Schore, 2001.

36 Lyons-Ruth & Jacobvitz, 2008.

37 It is a further complication that "unresolved attachment" and "disorganized attachment" are constructs that are strongly linked to observer-rated methods of assessing attachment (the unresolved category emerging from the Adult Attachment Interview and disorganized attachment from the strange situation), whereas the four categories of organized attachment that we describe emerge from self-report methods. The two methods of measurement are not completely compatible with each other (and some experts would say are not compatible at all), and so the categories cannot be reconciled into one neat scheme. We have argued for a scheme that incorporates insights and observations from both of these approaches to attachment into one system of description (see Maunder & Hunter, 2012), but the effort at reconciliation has not yet prevailed. The description of attachment patterns in this book attempts to sidestep these complications because we think they are not a great concern for most of our readers. Those who are interested in this dilemma should read Shaver and Mikulincer (2002). The Adult Attachment Interview is well described in Hesse (2008) and the strange situation in Ainsworth, Blehar, Waters, and Wall (1978), and self-report measures are well reviewed in Mikulincer and Shaver (2007). The links between insecure attachment and psychiatric disorder (and its treatment) are further elaborated in Patricia Crittenden's dynamic-maturational model of attachment (Crittenden, 2006).

38 Mickelson, Kessler, & Shaver, 1997.

39 van Ijzendoorn & Sagi-Schwartz, 2008.

40 The various tools that are used to measure attachment styles and the evidence for their validity is reviewed in Ravitz, Maunder, Hunter, Sthankiya, and Lancee (2010).

41 The URL leads to Chris Fraley's attachment website and the online "Close Relationships Questionnaire," which is identical to the research instrument known as the "Experience in Close Relationships-Revised" or ECR-R (Fraley, Waller, & Brennan, 2000). Many attachment researchers consider the Adult Attachment Interview (AAI) to be the gold standard of assessing adult attachment (Hesse, 2008; Main et al., 1985). The AAI requires expert analysis of the transcript of a structured interview about attachment experiences (particularly in childhood) and classifies adults according to their "state of mind with respect to attachment." The AAI is a powerful tool but an impractical one for most of our readers.

42 Hunter & Maunder, 2001; Maunder & Hunter, 2001, 2008.

43 Sapolsky, 2004.

44 Belsky, 1997.

45 A third way that a weak force can exert a large effect is as a trigger when other forces have brought a system to the brink of a big change (a tipping point). We are not aware of any circumstance in which insecure attachment works in this way.

46 A longitudinal prospective study that followed children who had been assessed in the strange situation and surveyed their health 30 years later found that insecure attachment was most strongly linked to inflammatory disease. On the other hand, a very large epidemiological study of the link between adult attachment and health found that attachment insecurity was most strongly linked to cardiovascular disease (McWilliams & Bailey, 2010; Puig et al., 2013).

7. Depression

1 Wells et al., 1989.

2 Evans et al., 2005; Katon, 1996.

3 Blumenthal et al., 2003; Frasure-Smith, Lesperance, & Talajic, 1993; Hemingway & Marmot, 1999.

4 Beyond these effects, depression is often accompanied by changes in the immune system. In particular, depressed people tend to have high levels of molecules called cytokines in their blood (even when depression occurs without any accompanying physical illness). Some of these cytokines act on the brain to cause sickness behaviour. If you have a fever because of an infection, your cytokines cause lethargy, depressed appetite, sleepiness, and a loss of motivation to care for yourself. To some extent, major depression is like experiencing sickness behaviour in the absence of a fever, and so some people have wondered if depression is sometimes the result of circulating cytokines. The main job of cytokines in the body is not to cause sickness behaviour but to fight foreign invaders by increasing inflammation (if the inflammatory cells that fight against infections and other threats from the environment are like soldiers, cytokines signal the need for a troop escalation). This fact has led to speculation that one of the reasons that depression and many other diseases occur together so often, is that once one has a disease that pumps up the flow of cytokines, depression is simply another manifestation of the resulting hyper-inflammatory state. Alternatively, it is possible that both depression and an inflammatory disease are caused by some unknown factor X further up the

causal stream that kick-starts the flow of cytokines. In that case, depression and the other disease are not causally related to each other; they are just coincident consequences of a common cause.

5 Bruce, Leaf, Rozal, & Hoff, 1994.
6 Lyness, King, Cox, Yoediono, & Caine, 1999.
7 Barry, Allore, Bruce, & Gill, 2009.
8 Barefoot et al., 1996; Kubzansky, Davidson, & Rozanski, 2005; Penninx et al., 2001.
9 Harris, Brown, & Bifulco, 1990.
10 Tennant, 1988.
11 Breier et al., 1988.
12 Seligman & Maier, 1967.
13 Simpson, Rholes, Campbell, Tran, & Wilson, 2003; Wei, Mallinckrodt, Russell, & Abraham, 2004; Wei, Russell, & Zakalik, 2005.
14 Bifulco, Moran, Ball, & Bernazzani, 2002; Bifulco, Moran, Ball, & Lillie, 2002; Carnelley, Pietromonaco, & Jaffe, 1994; Scharfe, 2007.
15 Bowlby et al., 1952; Robertson, 1952.
16 Panksepp & Solms, 2008.
17 Writing Committee for the ENRICHD Investigators, 2003; Frasure-Smith et al., 2006; Glassman et al., 2002; Joynt & O'Connor, 2005; Lespérance et al., 2007; Sheps, Freedland, Golden, & McMahon, 2003.

8. Attachment Is a Response to Stress

1 Porges, 2003.
2 The amygdala in the mesolimbic area of the brain is the main centre for fast detection of possible threats.
3 Jia's reflection and re-evaluation occurred in her prefrontal cortex in areas that we labelled the C-system in Chapter 5.
4 Sethi, Mischel, Aber, Shoda, & Rodriguez, 2000.
5 Champoux, Hwang, Lang, & Levine, 2001; De Bellis et al., 1999.
6 Boyce & Ellis, 2005; Ellis, Essex, & Boyce, 2005.
7 Selye, 1979.
8 Joels & Baram, 2009.
9 Roy, Steptoe, & Kirschbaum, 1998.
10 Sroufe & Waters, 1977.
11 Luecken, 1998.
12 Maunder, Lancee, Nolan, Hunter, & Tannenbaum, 2006.
13 Mikulincer et al., 1993.
14 Maunder, Lancee, et al., 2006.

15 Attachment avoidance is associated with a discrepancy between subjective and objective measures of stress response. While attachment avoidance is consistently linked to either no increase in reports of subjective stress or to under-reporting during exposure to stressors, it is nonetheless linked with exaggerated blood pressure and electrodermal reactivity (Carpenter & Kirkpatrick, 1996; Diamond, Hicks, & Otter-Henderson, 2006; Feeney & Kirkpatrick, 1996; Kim, 2006; Roisman, 2007), greater cortisol reactivity (Laurent & Powers, 2007; Powers, Pietromonaco, Gunlicks, & Sayer, 2006; Rifkin-Graboi, 2008), and lower vagal tone (Maunder, Lancee, et al., 2006).

16 Halpern, Maunder, Schwartz, & Gurevich, 2011.

17 Halpern, Maunder, Schwartz, & Gurevich, 2012.

18 Branco, Atalaia, & Paiva, 1994; Harding, 1998.

19 The study referred to is by Sloan, Maunder, Hunter, and Moldofsky (2007). Beyond that study, the evidence that attachment insecurity is linked to aspects of sleep is diverse. Toddlers with sleeping problems are much more likely to have mothers with insecure attachment than toddlers without sleeping problems (Benoit, Zeanah, Boucher, & Minde, 1992) and to have an insecure pattern of attachment themselves (Beijers, Jansen, Riksen-Walraven, & de Weerth, 2011). In adults, attachment anxiety is associated with daytime napping and using sleep medication (Verdecias, Jean-Louis, Zizi, Casimir, & Browne, 2009). With respect to sleep physiology, another study (in addition to our paper with Eileen Sloan) found a link between attachment patterns and EEG patterns: in military veterans with sleep disturbances, attachment anxiety was associated with reduced stage 3 and 4 sleep, whereas attachment avoidance was associated with more delta power during REM sleep (Troxel & Germain, 2011). Attachment patterns are also linked to dreaming: one study found more dream recall and more intense dream images associated with higher attachment anxiety (McNamara, Andresen, Clark, Zborowski, & Duffy, 2001), while others have found that the themes that emerge in dreams are consistent with the waking relationship wishes and representations associated with the dreamers' patterns of attachment (Mikulincer, Shaver, & Avihou-Kanza, 2011).

20 For example, when securely attached children first make the transition to daycare, their cortisol levels double in the absence of their mothers (Ahnert, Gunnar, Lamb, & Barthel, 2004).

21 Gunnar, Larson, Hertsgaard, Harris, & Brodersen, 1992.

22 Gunnar, Brodersen, Nachmias, Buss, & Rigatuso, 1996; Gunnar & Donzella, 2002.

23 For infants who are inhibited about approaching novel stimuli, parents of kids with insecure attachment seem to actively interfere with the children's

efforts to cope by intrusively insisting on the children confronting the thing they are afraid of, resulting in increased HPA activity (Nachmias, Gunnar, Mangelsdorf, & Parritz, 1996).

24 Fraley & Shaver, 1998.

25 Collins & Feeney, 2004.

26 Ditzen et al., 2008; Feeney & Kirkpatrick, 1996.

27 At first, we thought this must be about the perception of events rather than the actual occurrence of events, so we went back to look at the checklist we had used. We had asked the participants in the study to check off every event that had happened in the previous six months from a long list, which included things like "there was a serious accident in the family," "I got fired," "I had an increase in my net income," and so on. We thought perhaps the apparent excess of events among insecure people was due to some items on the list that require more interpretation, where differences in appraisal might lead to false differences in total counts of events. These are items like "I found my partner to be unsupportive," where one person's assessment of their partner's supportiveness might not be the same as another person's assessment of the same behaviour, for example. However, these subjective items were in the minority on the life events checklist that we used, and we found that even when they were removed altogether, it makes no difference to the result: people with insecure attachment still report more events. We then considered that differences in memory might account for the difference, but it doesn't seem very plausible – six months is not very long to remember that there was a serious accident in the family or that you moved in with someone new.

28 Others had already figured out something similar to this long before the question occurred to us. Over 20 years before, Kenneth Kendler and his colleagues had looked at the effects of genes versus luck in explaining the relationship between stressful life events and depression in twins. He found that both luck and genes were important, but it was the events that were not caused by luck but depended instead on some characteristics of the person that were far more likely to cause depression (Kendler, Karkowski, & Prescott, 1999).

29 It was our friend and colleague Bill Lancee who pointed this out to us.

9. Why Are So Many of Us Fat, Drunk, Stationary Smokers?

1 Statistics Canada, 2012.

2 Obesity is defined as a body mass index (BMI) greater than 30. Overweight is defined as a BMI greater than 25. BMI is weight in kilograms divided by

height in metres squared. BMI calculators are easy to find online. Statistics are from Shields and Carroll (2011).

3 Heavy drinking is defined as drinking five or more drinks on one occasion at least monthly for the last year. Statistics are from Mazzuca (2002) and Statistics Canada (2013).

4 Inactivity in these statistics is defined by Statistics Canada as endorsing activities that account for an energy expenditure of less than 1.5 kcal/kg/day (Statistics Canada, 2011).

5 Slovic, 1987.

6 Hofer, 1995.

7 Insel, 1997.

8 Although they are representative of the clinic, they are not representative of the surrounding community. Most were white (74%) and well educated (67% had a university degree). We think this emphasizes the importance of her findings – in socio-economic terms this was an *advantaged* group. It is fair to assume that the situation is worse for those who are less advantaged.

9 The high threshold counts only (1) drinking that is likely to have *already caused* harm according to the World Health Organization's Alcohol Use Disorders Identification Test (i.e., an AUDIT score > 8); (2) a BMI > 30 (i.e., obesity), or (3) *current* cigarette smoking. The AUDIT is described by Babor, Higgins-Biddle, Saunders, and Monteiro (2001).

10 Canadian Centre on Substance Abuse, 2013.

11 Of course Thao Lan Le is not the only one who has found that these behaviours tend to co-occur (ever seen someone holding a beer and a cigarette at the same time?), but her data are very helpful in illustrating the links between attachment and health behaviour.

12 Department of Health and Human Services Public Health Service Office on Smoking and Health, 1994.

13 Anda et al., 1999.

14 This view is consistent with the health relief model and the theory of reasoned action, which we reviewed in Chapter 2.

15 Petraitis, Flay, & Miller, 1995.

16 Bahr, Hoffmann, & Yang, 2005; Eitle, 2005; Fleming, Kim, Harachi, & Catalano, 2002; Henry, 2008; Karcher & Finn, 2005; Scragg, Reeder, Wong, Glover, & Nosa, 2008; Sokol-Katz, Dunham, & Zimmerman, 1997.

17 Statistics are from Scragg et al. (2008). Talking about weak and strong attachment, which is the language of this body of research, is not really the same as talking about secure and insecure attachment. So, the available evidence seems to support the attachment hypothesis and certainly

does nothing to refute it, but research that was explicitly focused on the attachment hypothesis would clarify things.

18 Fraley & Davis, 1997.

19 Bahr et al., 2005; Henry, 2008; Karcher & Finn, 2005.

20 Support is more effective in helping people to quit smoking when it comes from a marital or common-law partner – more evidence for the specificity of attachment over generic support (Park, Tudiver, Schultz, & Campbell, 2004).

21 Currently, no research evaluates whether attachment security leads to smokers in withdrawal having stronger or weaker cravings, but it is a good question to test.

22 Huebner et al., 2005.

23 In her survey about 50% of the people had smoked at least 100 cigarettes in their lives, and of these 40% (or about 20% overall) continued to smoke. Attachment avoidance was much more weakly linked to smoking status than attachment anxiety.

24 Dube et al., 2006.

25 Hodson, Newcomb, Locke, & Goodyear, 2006.

26 Bahr et al., 2005; Droomers, Schrijvers, Casswell, & Mackenbach, 2003; Hahm, Lahiff, & Guterman, 2003; Henry, 2008; Hoffmann & Su, 1998; Kuendig & Kuntsche, 2006; Sokol-Katz et al., 1997.

27 Link, 2008.

28 Bahr et al., 2005; Eitle, 2005; Henry, 2008; Link, 2008.

29 Hoffmann & Su, 1998.

30 Daily and weekly limits from Canada's *Low-Risk Drinking Guidelines*: 10 drinks a week for women, with no more than 2 drinks a day most days; 15 drinks a week for men, with no more than 3 drinks a day most days (Canadian Centre on Substance Abuse, 2013).

31 Davis, Shaver, & Vernon, 2003.

32 Davis et al., 2003; McNally, Palfai, Levine, & Moore, 2003.

33 Remember, these are mostly high socio-economic status, highly educated family practice patients, not a high-risk inner-city population.

34 The most direct effects are the effects of drinking itself (as opposed to the increased risk that is posed for other diseases, like ulcers and cirrhosis). In Thao Lan Le's study the rate of harmful drinking (i.e., a lifetime history of probable alcoholism) was found in 3% of those who drank nothing in the last month, 2% of those who drank within low-risk limits, and 36% of those drinking above low-risk guidelines.

35 For example, looking just at physical abuse, a BMI ≥ 30 is found in 23% of people who report no physical abuse, in 26% of people who were hit but

not injured, in 28% of people who were hit and sometimes injured, and in 36% of people who were hit and often injured.

36 D'Argenio et al., 2009; Williamson, Thompson, Anda, Dietz, & Felitti, 2002.

37 Hintsanen, Jokela, Pulkki-Raback, Viikari, & Keltikangas-Jarvinen, 2010. Waist-to-hip ratio is particularly important because midline fat contributes more to disease than fat distributed elsewhere in your body.

38 Bosmans, Goossens, & Braet, 2009; Javo & Sorlie, 2009; Mayer, Muris, Meesters, & Zimmermann-van Beuningen, 2009.

39 Gjerdingen et al., 2009.

40 Wilkinson, Rowe, Bishop, & Brunstrom, 2010.

41 Colton, Olmsted, Daneman, Rydall, & Rodin, 2007.

42 Morse, Ciechanowski, Katon, & Hirsch, 2006.

43 Ward et al., 2001.

44 Actually, Hazan and Shaver's hypotheses referred to categories of insecure attachment, preoccupied and dismissing, rather than dimensions of attachment anxiety and attachment avoidance (Shaver & Hazan, 1988), but it is easy to translate one to the other and the difference needn't bog us down. The relationship between categories and dimensions of attachment is addressed in Chapter 6.

45 Feeney, Noller, & Patty, 1993.

46 Davis, Shaver, & Vernon, 2004.

47 Kalichman et al., 1994; Tracy, Shaver, Albino, & Cooper, 2003.

48 Brennan & Shaver, 1995; Gentzler & Kerns, 2004; Schachner & Shaver, 2004.

49 Feeney et al., 1993.

50 Birnbaum, Reis, Mikulincer, Gillath, & Orpaz, 2006.

51 Tracy et al., 2003.

52 Feeney et al., 1993.

53 Feeney, Kelly, Gallois, Peterson, & Terry, 1999.

54 Hillis, Anda, Felitti, & Marchbanks, 2001; Hillis, Anda, Felitti, Nordenberg, & Marchbanks, 2000.

55 As a further challenge to healthy choices, young people with insecure attachment patterns are more likely to be intoxicated during sex. Obviously, lack of assertiveness and intoxication are major impediments to making prudent choices, such as using condoms.

10. I Don't Know What You Have, but I've Seen It Before and You Have It Bad

1 Jon's reaction to the Dustins of the world is to feel hopeless and fatigued, as if the oxygen had been sucked out of the room. We mention this because

of how differently people can affect one another; just because a patient has a consistent manner with different professionals doesn't mean he will evoke exactly the same reaction from each of them. Nonetheless, both Jon's and Bob's reactions share a disinclination to engage with Dustin. Clinicians are better prepared to understand and work around the reactions that can interfere with care if they know themselves and what their reactions tell them about the person in front of them.

2 Surveys of people in the community consistently demonstrate that, on average, new symptoms emerge more frequently than weekly (Demers, Altamore, Mustin, Kleinman, & Leonardi, 1980; White, Williams, & Greenberg, 1961).

3 Cherry, Hing, Woodwell, & Rechtsteiner, 2008.

4 The prevalence of symptoms that are unexplained by medical investigations depends on the setting, with reports ranging from 35% (Kroenke, 2003) to 80% (Kroenke & Mangelsdorff, 1989).

5 Ciechanowski, Katon, et al., 2002; Ciechanowski, Walker, et al., 2002; Taylor, Mann, White, & Goldberg, 2000; Waller, Scheidt, & Hartmann, 2004.

6 Ciechanowski, Walker, et al., 2002.

7 Ciechanowski, Katon, et al., 2002; Ciechanowski, Walker, et al., 2002; Costa-Martins et al., 2014; Meredith, Strong, & Feeney, 2006.

8 Ordering tests that are expected to have negative results for the purpose of reassurance is a strategy that often fails (Rolfe & Burton, 2013) and in the case of attachment anxiety may backfire because the test provides a new source of anxiety-provoking uncertainty.

9 For a caveat to the suggestion that a health care provider can provide safe haven to Dustin, see footnote 13 from Chapter 6.

10 Meredith, Strong, & Feeney, 2005; Meredith et al., 2006.

11 Couprie, Wijdicks, Rooijmans, & van Gijn, 1995; Crimlisk et al., 1998; Stone, Sharpe, Rothwell, & Warlow, 2003.

12 Many factors bias medical diagnosis, help-seeking, and patterns of referral, not just attachment anxiety. Specialists also see more women and see more individuals with psychiatric illness, for example.

13 Ciechanowski, Katon, et al., 2002.

14 Ciechanowski, Sullivan, Jensen, Romano, & Summers, 2003.

15 McWilliams & Bailey, 2010.

16 Winnicott, 1989.

17 Rhoades, McFarland, Finch, & Johnson, 2001.

18 Marvel, Epstein, Flowers, & Beckman, 1999.

19 Ong, de Haes, Hoos, & Lammes, 1995.

20 McCarthy et al., 2012.

21 Main, 2000. Grice's maxims inform the analysis of the structure of discourse that is used to identify attachment types in the Adult Attachment Interview (Hesse, 2008).
22 Groves, 1978.
23 So far we have spoken of difficult, unexplained symptoms as if they form a homogeneous group, but this is far from the case. For starters, virtually every medical specialty includes at least one *functional syndrome* that has symptoms that are typical of its other diseases without any of the usual physical causes (e.g., irritable bowel syndrome in gastroenterology, non-cardiac chest pain in cardiology, chronic fatigue syndrome and fibromyalgia in rheumatology, and so on). It is not clear that these functional syndromes are as distinct as the diagnostic labels imply. For example, if you ask the right questions, you will find that people who have one functional syndrome are quite likely to also have others (Aaron & Buchwald, 2001; Kim & Chang, 2012). Furthermore, the traditional distinction between *organic* (symptoms that result from visible or measurable pathological changes in tissue) and *functional* (symptoms that arise in spite of an absence of those physical changes) is inaccurate – research has demonstrated physiological abnormalities associated with most functional syndromes (Sharpe & Carson, 2001); they are just not as consistent or obvious as the changes in organic diseases. Chronic pain syndromes are a good example. They are notoriously resistant to being described as simply physical or simply psychological; they are always both.

In this chapter, we give diagnosis short shrift because we find the relational dynamics of help seeking and fear to be similar across the various possible diagnoses and far more helpful in trying to manage the suffering that results from unexplained symptoms. Furthermore, we should not fool ourselves into believing that we know with any precision what is actually going on with difficult unexplained symptoms. Nonetheless, diagnosis is important to patients and health care providers alike. Patients with chronic unexplained symptoms often feel invalidated by others' reactions to their suffering, when they are treated as whiners and fakers. Invalidating present-day experiences may echo invalidating developmental interactions that are linked emotionally to feelings of insecurity. A diagnosis signals that a person is suffering from something real and is not alone. Often the person received further validation from advocacy groups that form in support of a particular diagnosis and from blogs and websites that create a virtual community. Validation, community, and support have powerful benefits.

11. Trouble in the Patient-Provider Relationship

1 Spurgeon, 2001.
2 College of Physicians and Surgeons of Canada, 2008.
3 Groves, 1978.
4 Salmon & Young, 2009. For a caveat to the suggestion that a health care provider can provide safe haven to Dustin, see footnote 13 from Chapter 6.
5 Winnicott, 1957.
6 Note that the link between insecure attachment, impaired mentalizing, and difficult provider-patient interactions was well described early in the history of adult attachment theory by Fonagy (1998).
7 They used a standard definition of a difficult interaction, using a scale that asks doctors to rate questions such as "How frustrating do you find this patient?" and "How difficult is it to communicate with this patient?" At the time of this assessment, physicians were blind to the measure that was used to assess the patients' attachment style.
8 Maunder, Panzer, et al., 2006. The nature of the difficulties in the exchange between a health care provider and a patient with insecure attachment were explored by Liotti (1991) as they play out in cognitive psychotherapy.
9 Hillen, de Haes, & Smets, 2011.
10 Pegman, Beesley, Holcombe, Mendick, & Salmon, 2011.
11 Clark, Beesley, Holcombe, & Salmon, 2011; Hinnen et al., 2014; Holwerda et al., 2013; Pegman et al., 2011.
12 Groopman, 2007.
13 Rolfe & Burton, 2013.
14 Longer-term control of diabetes is reliably measured with a blood test, hemoglobin A1C (the percentage of hemoglobin that is glycosylated by high circulating levels of glucose over several weeks), so much of the effort that a patient like Linda and her medical team put into controlling diabetes is translated into the goal of reducing A1C. People without diabetes usually have A1C levels below 6%. Although guidelines change over time, recent recommendations are for people with diabetes to aim to keep A1C below 7% (Canadian Diabetes Association Clinical Practice Guidelines Expert Committee, 2008). As an example of the impact of tight control of diabetes, reducing A1C levels from 8% to 7.2% results in a 40% to 50% reduction in the incidence of damage to the small arteries in the retina of the eye. However, it is a difficult goal. Reducing A1C levels below 7% requires frequent monitoring of blood glucose levels and intensive treatment. Poor control of diabetes, as indicated by A1C levels > 8% occurs almost twice as often among people with diabetes who are

high in attachment avoidance than among insecure people with diabetes (Ciechanowski, Hirsch, & Katon, 2002). The interaction between patient attachment avoidance and provider communication style is discussed in Ciechanowski et al. (2004).

15 Ciechanowski, Russo, et al., 2006.

16 Ciechanowski & Katon, 2006.

12. How Health Care Providers Can Adapt When Attachment Anxiety Interferes

1 The combination of high attachment anxiety and low attachment avoidance that is the topic of this chapter is also known as preoccupied attachment.

2 Ciechanowski, Walker, et al., 2002.

3 The effect of relaxation training is to bolster the anxious person's vagal brake (see Chapter 2). Evidence suggests that this has direct health benefits, such as regulating inflammation (Nolan, Reid, Seidelin, & Lau, 2007) and reducing the anxiety that is acting as an impediment to health care.

4 Ciechanowski, Walker, et al., 2002.

5 Committee on the Quality of Health in America, 2001.

6 An important part of the therapeutic work that ended up being very helpful for Susan (the patient who was introduced in Chapter 6) was simply repeating to her that she had to finish her sentences, as she habitually dropped them without a clear conclusion. Instead of responding to the implied invitation for Jon to finish the sentences as if he knew what was in her mind, she needed to learn that she had to tell the other person her thought in its entirety if she was going to be understood.

7 George & West, 2001.

8 Bifulco, Moran, Ball, & Bernazzani, 2002; Bifulco, Moran, Ball, & Lillie, 2002; Maunder & Hunter, 2012.

9 Our advice to patients is presented in the second person, addressing patients directly. As a care provider, you may find it useful to use these examples when considering how to guide your own patients.

13. How Health Care Providers Can Adapt When Attachment Avoidance Interferes

1 The combination of high attachment avoidance and low attachment anxiety that is the topic of the chapter, is also known as dismissing attachment.

2 Ciechanowski, Katon, et al., 2002; Ciechanowski, Walker, et al., 2002.

3 Maunder & Greenberg, 2004.

4 The link between high attachment avoidance and non-adherence to directions has been confirmed as it applies to self-managing diabetes (Ciechanowski et al., 2004), wearing seat belts (Ahrens, Ciechanowski, & Katon, 2012), screening for prostate cancer (Consedine, Tuck, & Fiori, 2013), and taking medication for hepatitis C (Sockalingam, Blank, Abdelhamid, Abbey, & Hirschfield, 2012). Attachment avoidance is also associated with being late to attend a dentist (Graetz et al., 2013).

5 Chen, Creedy, Lin, & Wollin, 2012.

6 Rollnick, Miller, & Butler, 2008.

7 A practical guide to the essentials of motivational interviewing for beginners and for those with some experience is available (Skinner & Cooper, 2013).

8 Disconfirming negative interpersonal expectations in this way was once called providing a "corrective emotional experience" by Franz Alexander, a pioneer in treating difficulties that lie at the interface of medicine and psychology (Alexander & French, 1946, Chapter 2).

9 Our point is not to discount the legitimate complaints of health care consumers but to suggest that this mode of expression is particularly attractive to some patients with high attachment avoidance.

10 See, for example, Lorig, Holman, Sobel, and Laurent (2006). Obviously, self-management is not an alternative to face-to-face care by health professionals; it is a tool to integrate into an overall health strategy. It is too soon to know how effective this type of integrated care is compared with traditional health care methods. However, even in the absence of definitive evidence, it is a good bet that self-management is better than neglect.

11 Maunder & Greenberg, 2004.

14. How Health Care Providers Can Adapt When Fearful Attachment Interferes

1 *I Hate You – Don't Leave Me* is the title of a book that captures a hostile version of this ambivalence perfectly (Kreisman & Straus, 2010). The book is about borderline personality disorder rather than insecure attachment. The links between borderline personality disorder and fearful attachment are important but largely beyond the scope of this text. The most important commonalities are the severe disorder of affect regulation and the intense and unstable interpersonal relationships that are found in both borderline personality and attachment that is *disorganized* or *unresolved for*

loss or trauma, designations from the attachment literature that sometimes, but not always, occur with the fearful pattern. Attachment theory may provide insight into the genetic and environmental origins of borderline personality disorder.

2 Maunder, Panzer, et al., 2006.

3 Madigan, Moran, & Pederson, 2006.

4 Ciechanowski, Walker, et al., 2002.

5 This is in stark contrast to secure attachment, for which a health care professional can essentially assume a therapeutic alliance and proceed with the work tasks.

6 As health care professionals, we often expect that our ability to provide solutions will be one of the main ways in which we earn the trust of patients. In this case, solutions that are offered prematurely (regardless of whether or not they are good ideas) can impair trust. The solution that feels like an intrusion on the patient's personal control activates ambivalence and fear. So premature solutions are not only unproductive but actually counterproductive.

7 Ciechanowski, Katon, et al., 2002; Ciechanowski, Walker, et al., 2002.

8 Ciechanowski & Katon, 2006, p. 3072.

9 Fearful attachment is often associated with narrative incoherence but not always. Sometimes fearful individuals tell quite coherent stories about their distressing relationships.

10 We are indebted to an anonymous peer reviewer for this example.

11 As discussed in Chapter 4, the feeling of security is promoted at least in part by endogenous opioids, which implies that addiction to opioid analgesic drugs is a greater risk among persons with insecure attachment. Furthermore alterations in dopaminergic "wanting" (i.e., reward-seeking) may increase the risk of addictions of all types for insecure persons.

12 The benzodiazepines are drugs, such as lorazepam, clonazepam, and diazepam, that are commonly used to treat anxiety and insomnia.

13 Those trained in mental illness will likely recognize this as a simplified description of the interpersonal problems that result from defensive processes, such as *projective identification* and *splitting*. However, the psychoanalytic terminology and its theoretical foundation are not necessary for understanding and sorting out the troubles that emerge.

15. Changing the System

1 Bretherton, 1995.

2 van der Horst, 2011.

3 Bowlby et al., 1952; Robertson, 1952.
4 Bergeson & Dean, 2006; Mead & Bower, 2000.
5 Although the recommendations from an attachment model align with old-fashioned paternalism to some extent in this case, in general they don't. The idea that a health care professional doesn't just get to do things the way she wants and instead must change her practice for different patients is the antithesis of the paternalistic perspective.
6 Mensing et al., 2007.
7 Committee on the Quality of Health in America, 2001.
8 Maunder & Hunter, 2009.
9 Personal communication with Paul Ciechanowski.
10 Of course, this transition would be most difficult for women who are high in attachment anxiety.
11 Ciechanowski, Worley, Russo, & Katon, 2006.
12 Dozier, Cue, & Barnett, 1994.
13 Holmes, 2001.
14 Maunder et al., 2004; Maunder, Peladeau, Savage, & Lancee, 2010.
15 Halpern et al., 2012.
16 We are referring to a personal communication from Christina Maar Andersen, a PhD student in Denmark, about data that are not yet published (April 2014).
17 Committee on the Quality of Health in America, 2001; Porter & Teisberg, 2006.

16. Becoming More Secure

1 Ein-Dor, Mikulincer, Doron, & Shaver, 2010.
2 van Ijzendoorn & Sagi-Schwartz, 2008.
3 Koenen et al., 2010.
4 In 2009, close to one million Canadian children lived in low-income households (Cool, 2009).
5 Mostly, but not entirely. Providing support for high-quality daycare so that parents, especially mothers, are not forced to choose between working and providing an excellent daytime environment for their children would improve the lives of children and the health of society.
6 We are referring to the movement of *attachment parenting*.
7 Bronfman, Parsons, & Lyons-Ruth, 1993; Lyons-Ruth & Jacobvitz, 2008.
8 Berlin, Zeanah, & Lieberman, 2008. This is an important point that applies to other forms of learning as well – including teaching health care professionals to be more responsive and adaptive to their patients' needs.

9 Hoffman, Marvin, Cooper, & Powell, 2006.
10 Slade et al., 2005.
11 Benoit & Parker, 1994.
12 Kisilevsky et al., 2003; Kisilevsky et al., 2009.
13 Goossens & van Ijzendoorn, 1990. Although multiple attachments are typical, infants identify one primary attachment figure, who is the person they prefer when in distress and whose separation they protest most vigorously (Zeifman & Hazan, 2008).
14 Concordance of infant attachment was 82% with classification at age six in a study of German children (Wartner, Grossmann, Fremmer-Bombik, & Suess, 1994), 84% over the same period for attachment to mothers in a middle-class American cohort (Main & Cassidy, 1988), and 77% (for secure versus insecure) with classification in adolescence for a sample that was mixed for two-parent and single-parent American families (Hamilton, 2000). Considerable stability of attachment patterns also exists over two to four years in adolescents (Zimmermann & Becker-Stoll, 2002; Ammaniti, Van Ijzendoorn, Speranza, & Tambelli, 2000) and college students (Rice, FitzGerald, Whaley, & Gibbs, 1995). One study has even shown consistency of attachment patterns over three generations: grandmothers, mothers, and infants (Benoit & Parker, 1994). In adults, Kirkpatrick and Hazan (1994) showed high test-retest stability over four years. Using multiple methods of assessment, Klohnen and Bera (1998) found evidence for stability of attachment avoidance and security over 31 years. Crowell, Treboux, and Waters (2002) found that attachment representations were stable from pre-marriage to 18 months post-wedding in 78% of young adults.
15 We are referring to the internal working model changing in response to life circumstances. A modified model of the self or model of others will lead to new expectations in future circumstances that trigger the attachment system.
16 For example, a 20-year study that compared the attachment patterns of infants with the patterns found in those same individuals once they had grown to university age found that over 70% of those young adults had the same classifications as adults that were observable when they were toddlers. Of those whose pattern had changed, the discontinuity was attributable to very substantial family experiences: abuse, parental death or divorce, or a parent with a life-threatening disease or a mental illness (Waters, Merrick, Treboux, Crowell, & Albersheim, 2000). The relatively high degree of predictability in this group contrasts with another study of attachment patterns over time that found that attachment patterns

were mostly *discontinuous* from childhood to young adulthood, with only 39% having the same pattern at both times (Weinfield, Sroufe, & Egeland, 2000). The major difference between these studies was that they were observing children growing up in very different circumstances. In the first cohort, children were growing up in middle-class two-parent families. In the second, most children had young single mothers with low income, little education, poor social support, and unplanned pregnancies – an environment for raising children that comes with a substantially higher risk of various kinds of adversity. In addition, the changes in patterns of attachment from childhood to young adulthood in the higher-risk group were not random – they were largely children who started classified as secure but who, by young adulthood, had developed a much more avoidant (dismissing) pattern of attachment. We interpret this to be the result of living a life with enough adverse experiences that a child or an adolescent learns that self-reliance and suppression of vulnerability or distress is the safest course. The finding that attachment avoidance is more prevalent in older adults (Magai et al., 2001; Magai, 2008) is also consistent with the idea that life experience can nudge people towards attachment avoidance, although other explanations are just as plausible (such as cohort effects that result from differences in circumstances or in parenting practices in different historical periods, or the possibility that non-avoidant people die younger).

17 Couples in the first year and a half of marriage have shown increased attachment security (Davila, Karney, & Bradbury, 1999), and women who were initially high in attachment anxiety have shown increased security over decades (Klohnen & Bera, 1998; Klohnen & John, 1998).

18 Davila, Burge, & Hammen, 1997; Davila, 2003. The latter study also suggests the further complication that patterns of stability and change are different depending on how attachment is measured.

19 Davila et al., 1999.

20 Bateman & Fonagy, 2009, 2010.

21 Kinley & Reyno, 2013; Levy et al., 2006; Ravitz, Maunder, & McBride, 2008.

17. Beyond Health Care Relationships: A Wider Attachment Perspective on Health

1 Of course, we aren't arguing that interpersonal dynamics account for all the unhealthy behaviour that is not addressed by conventional approaches, just that they are among the important unaddressed forces.

2 Sullivan, 1953, p. 11 (emphasis added)

3 Gawande, 2013.

4 See Rusbult, Kumashiro, Kubacka, and Finkel (2009) for a discussion of the Michelangelo effect, by which our partners bring out the best in us.

5 Unfortunately, the people who are at the highest risk for these risky behaviours, at least from an attachment perspective, are the ones who are least likely to have a partner who provides effective support. This problem may limit the potential power of the strategy of leveraging interpersonal relationships for their public health benefit, but it still leaves many people (maybe the majority) for whom interpersonal leverage could provide a nudge in the right direction.

6 Astin, 1997; Fjorback, Arendt, Ornbol, Fink, & Walach, 2011; Kabat-Zinn, 1990; Reiner, Tibi, & Lipsitz, 2013; Teasdale et al., 2000.

7 Bateman & Fonagy, 2009, 2010.

8 The team that developed *The Stress Vaccine* was led by Bob Maunder and Bill Lancee and included Jon Hunter, Molyn Leszcz, Reet Mae, Nathalie Peladeau, and Leslie Vincent.

9 Maunder et al., 2010.

10 Although these initiatives are expensive, we shouldn't assume that we currently have our priorities right when distributing health resources. The costs of investing in parental postnatal leaves and good-quality daycare, although very large, would pale in comparison to the current costs of the health care provided during the last 12 months of our lives – which have been estimated at 20% to 25% of health care expenditures (Hoover, Crystal, Kumar, Sambamoorthi, & Cantor, 2002). As a society we are heroic, beyond reason, in trying to keep dying people alive and negligent, beyond excuse, in trying to give our young their best chance.

References

Aaron, L. A., & Buchwald, D. (2001). A review of the evidence for overlap among unexplained clinical conditions. *Annals of Internal Medicine, 134*(9_Part_2), 868–81. http://dx.doi.org/10.7326/0003-4819-134-9_Part_2-200105011-00011

Afifi, T. O., MacMillan, H. L., Boyle, M., Taillieu, T., Cheung, K., & Sareen, J. (2014). Child abuse and mental disorders in Canada. *Canadian Medical Association Journal, 186*(9), E324–32. http://dx.doi.org/10.1503/cmaj.131792

Ahnert, L., Gunnar, M. R., Lamb, M. E., & Barthel, M. (2004). Transition to child care: Associations with infant-mother attachment, infant negative emotion, and cortisol elevations. *Child Development, 75*(3), 639–50. http://dx.doi.org/10.1111/j.1467-8624.2004.00698.x

Ahrens, K. R., Ciechanowski, P., & Katon, W. (2012). Associations between adult attachment style and health risk behaviors in an adult female primary care population. *Journal of Psychosomatic Research, 72*(5), 364–70. http://dx.doi.org/10.1016/j.jpsychores.2012.02.002

Ainsworth, M., Blehar, M., Waters, E., & Wall, S. (1978). *Patterns of attachment: A psychological study of the strange situation.* Hillsdale, NJ: Erlbaum.

Alexander, F., & French, T. M. (1946). *Psychoanalytic therapy: Principles and application.* New York, NY: Ronald Press.

Alexander, R. W., Aaron, L. A., Alberts, K. R., Martin, M. Y., Stewart, K. E., Bradley, L. A., ... Triana-Alexander, M. (1998). Sexual and physical abuse in women with fibromyalgia: Association with outpatient health care utilization and pain medication usage. *Arthritis Care and Research, 11*(2), 102–15. http://dx.doi.org/10.1002/art.1790110206

Allen, J. G. (2013). *Restoring mentalizing in attachment relationships: Treating trauma with plain old therapy.* Washington, DC: American Psychiatric Publishing.

Allen, J. G., Stein, H., Fonagy, P., Fultz, J., & Target, M. (2005). Rethinking adult attachment: A study of expert consensus. *Bulletin of the Menninger Clinic, 69*(1), 59–80. http://dx.doi.org/10.1521/bumc.69.1.59.62266

Ammaniti, M., Van Ijzendoorn, M. H., Speranza, A. M., & Tambelli, R. (2000). Internal working models of attachment during late childhood and early adolescence: An exploration of stability and change. *Attachment & Human Development, 2*(3), 328–46. http://dx.doi.org/10.1080/14616730010001587

Anda, R. F., Brown, D. W., Felitti, V. J., Dube, S. R., & Giles, W. H. (2008). Adverse childhood experiences and prescription drug use in a cohort study of adult HMO patients. *BMC Public Health, 8*(1), 198. http://dx.doi.org/10.1186/1471-2458-8-198

Anda, R. F., Croft, J. B., Felitti, V. J., Nordenberg, D., Giles, W. H., Williamson, D. F., & Giovino, G. A. (1999). Adverse childhood experiences and smoking during adolescence and adulthood. *Journal of the American Medical Association, 282*(17), 1652–8. http://dx.doi.org/10.1001/jama.282.17.1652

Astin, J. A. (1997). Stress reduction through mindfulness meditation. *Psychotherapy and Psychosomatics, 66*(2), 97–106. http://dx.doi.org/10.1159/000289116

Babor, T. F., Higgins-Biddle, J. C., Saunders, J. B., & Monteiro, M. G. (2001). *The alcohol use disorders identification test: Guidelines for use in primary care world health organization* (2nd ed.). Retrieved from the World Health Organization website: http://whqlibdoc.who.int/hq/2001/who_msd_msb_01.6a.pdf

Bagot, R. C., & Meaney, M. J. (2010). Epigenetics and the biological basis of gene x environment interactions. *Journal of the American Academy of Child and Adolescent Psychiatry, 49*(8), 752–71. http://dx.doi.org/10.1016/j.jaac.2010.06.001

Bahr, S. J., Hoffmann, J. P., & Yang, X. (2005). Parental and peer influences on the risk of adolescent drug use. *Journal of Primary Prevention, 26*(6), 529–51. http://dx.doi.org/10.1007/s10935-005-0014-8

Bandura, A. (1977). *Social learning theory.* Upper Saddle River, NJ: Prentice-Hall.

Bandura, A. (2004). Health promotion by social cognitive means. *Health Education & Behavior, 31*(2), 143–64. http://dx.doi.org/10.1177/1090198104263660

Barefoot, J. C., Helms, M. J., Mark, D. B., Blumenthal, J. A., Califf, R. M., Haney, T. L., ... Williams, R. B. (1996). Depression and long-term mortality risk in patients with coronary artery disease. *American Journal of Cardiology, 78*(6), 613–17. http://dx.doi.org/10.1016/S0002-9149(96)00380-3

Barry, L. C., Allore, H. G., Bruce, M. L., & Gill, T. M. (2009). Longitudinal association between depressive symptoms and disability burden among older persons. *Journals of Gerontology. Series A, Biological Sciences and Medical Sciences, 64A*(12), 1325–32. http://dx.doi.org/10.1093/gerona/glp135

Barsky, A. J., Orav, E. J., & Bates, D. W. (2005). Somatization increases medical utilization and costs independent of psychiatric and medical comorbidity. *Archives of General Psychiatry, 62*(8), 903–10. http://dx.doi.org/10.1001/archpsyc.62.8.903

Bartholomew, K., & Horowitz, L. M. (1991). Attachment styles among young adults: A test of a four-category model. *Journal of Personality and Social Psychology, 61*(2), 226–44. http://dx.doi.org/10.1037/0022-3514.61.2.226

Bateman, A., & Fonagy, P. (2009). Randomized controlled trial of outpatient mentalization-based treatment versus structured clinical management for borderline personality disorder. *American Journal of Psychiatry, 166*(12), 1355–64. http://dx.doi.org/10.1176/appi.ajp.2009.09040539

Bateman, A., & Fonagy, P. (2010). Mentalization based treatment for borderline personality disorder. *World Psychiatry, 9*, 11–15.

Beijers, R., Jansen, J., Riksen-Walraven, M., & de Weerth, C. (2011). Attachment and infant night waking: A longitudinal study from birth through the first year of life. *Journal of Developmental and Behavioral Pediatrics, 32*(9), 635–43. http://dx.doi.org/10.1097/DBP.0b013e318228888d

Belsky, J. (1997). Attachment, mating and parenting. *Human Nature, 8*(4), 361–81. http://dx.doi.org/10.1007/BF02913039

Benoit, D., & Parker, K. C. (1994). Stability and transmission of attachment across three generations. *Child Development, 65*(5), 1444–56. http://dx.doi.org/10.2307/1131510

Benoit, D., Zeanah, C. H., Boucher, C., & Minde, K. K. (1992). Sleep disorders in early childhood: Association with insecure maternal attachment. *Journal of the American Academy of Child and Adolescent Psychiatry, 31*(1), 86–93. http://dx.doi.org/10.1097/00004583-199201000-00013

Bergeson, S. C., & Dean, J. D. (2006). A systems approach to patient-centered care. *Journal of the American Medical Association, 296*(23), 2848–51. http://dx.doi.org/10.1001/jama.296.23.2848

Berkman, L. F., & Syme, S. L. (1979). Social networks, host resistance, and mortality: A nine-year follow-up study of Alameda County residents. *American Journal of Epidemiology, 109*, 186–204.

Berlin, L., Zeanah, C. H., & Lieberman, A. F. (2008). Prevention and intervention programs for supporting early attachment security. In J. Cassidy & P. R. Shaver (Eds.), *Handbook of attachment: Theory, research and clinal applications* (2nd ed., pp. 745–61). New York, NY: Guilford Press.

Bifulco, A., Moran, P. M., Ball, C., & Bernazzani, O. (2002). Adult attachment style. I: Its relationship to clinical depression. *Social Psychiatry and Psychiatric Epidemiology, 37*(2), 50–9. http://dx.doi.org/10.1007/s127-002-8215-0

Bifulco, A., Moran, P. M., Ball, C., & Lillie, A. (2002). Adult attachment style. II: Its relationship to psychosocial depressive-vulnerability. *Social Psychiatry and Psychiatric Epidemiology*, 37(2), 60–7. http://dx.doi.org/10.1007/ s127-002-8216-x

Birnbaum, G. E., Reis, H. T., Mikulincer, M., Gillath, O., & Orpaz, A. (2006). When sex is more than just sex: Attachment orientations, sexual experience, and relationship quality. *Journal of Personality and Social Psychology*, 91(5), 929–43. http://dx.doi.org/10.1037/0022-3514.91.5.929

Bloom, D. E., Cafiero, E. T., Jané-Llopis, E., Abrahams-Gessel, S., Bloom, L. R., Fathima, S., ... Weinstein, C. (2011). *The global economic burden of noncommunicable diseases*. Geneva, Switzerland: World Economic Forum.

Blumenthal, J. A., Lett, H. S., Babyak, M. A., White, W., Smith, P. K., Mark, D. B., ... Newman, M. F. (2003). Depression as a risk factor for mortality after coronary artery bypass surgery. *Lancet*, 362(9384), 604–9. http://dx.doi.org/10.1016/S0140-6736(03)14190-6

Bosmans, G., Goossens, L., & Braet, C. (2009). Attachment and weight and shape concerns in inpatient overweight youngsters. *Appetite*, 53(3), 454–6. http://dx.doi.org/10.1016/j.appet.2009.08.011

Bowlby, J. (1969). Attachment and loss (Vol. 1). *Attachment*. New York, NY: Basic Books.

Bowlby, J. (1973). Attachment and loss (Vol. 2). *Separation: Anxiety and anger*. New York, NY: Basic Books.

Bowlby, J. (1980). Attachment and loss (Vol. 3). *Loss: Sadness and depression*. New York, NY: Basic Books.

Bowlby, J., Robertson, J., & Rosenbluth, D. (1952). A two-year-old goes to hospital. *Psychoanalytic Study of the Child*, 7, 82–94.

Boyce, W. T., & Ellis, B. J. (2005). Biological sensitivity to context: I. An evolutionary-developmental theory of the origins and functions of stress reactivity. *Development and Psychopathology*, 17(02), 271–301. http://dx.doi. org/10.1017/S0954579405050145

Branco, J., Atalaia, A., & Paiva, T. (1994). Sleep cycles and alpha-delta sleep in fibromyalgia syndrome. *Journal of Rheumatology*, 24(6), 1113–17.

Breier, A., Kelsoe, J. R., Jr., Kirwin, P. D., Beller, S. A., Wolkowitz, O. M., & Pickar, D. (1988). Early parental loss and development of adult psychopathology. *Archives of General Psychiatry*, 45(11), 987–93. http:// dx.doi.org/10.1001/archpsyc.1988.01800350021003

Brennan, K. A., & Shaver, P. R. (1995). Dimensions of adult attachment, affect regulation and romantic relationship functioning. *Personality and Social Psychology Bulletin*, 21(3), 267–83. http://dx.doi.org/10.1177/01461672 95213008

Bretherton, I. (1995). The origins of attachment theory: John Bowlby and Mary Ainsworth. In S. Goldberg, R. Muir, & J. Kerr (Eds.), *Attachment theory:*

Social, developmental and clinical perspectives (pp. 45–84). Hillsdale, NJ: The Analytic Press.

Bronfman, E., Parsons, E., & Lyons-Ruth, K. (1993). *Atypical maternal behavior instrument for assessment and classification (AMBIANCE): Manual for coding disrupted affective communication.* Cambridge, MA: Author.

Brown, G. W., Bhrolchain, M. N., & Harris, T. (1975). Social class and psychiatric disturbance among women in an urban population. *Sociology, 9*(2), 225–54. http://dx.doi.org/10.1177/003803857500900203

Brown, G. W., & Harris, T. O. (1978). *Social origins of depression: A study of psychiatric disorder in women.* London, England: Tavistock.

Bruce, M. L., Leaf, P. J., Rozal, G. P., Florio, L., & Hoff, R. A. (1994). Psychiatric status and 9-year mortality data in the New Haven epidemiologic catchment area study. *American Journal of Psychiatry, 151*(5), 716–21. http://dx.doi.org/10.1176/ajp.151.5.716

Buchheim, A., Heinrichs, M., George, C., Pokorny, D., Koops, E., Henningsen, P., ... Gündel, H. (2009). Oxytocin enhances the experience of attachment security. *Psychoneuroendocrinology, 34*(9), 1417–22. http://dx.doi.org/10.1016/j.psyneuen.2009.04.002

Canadian Centre on Substance Abuse. (2013). *Low-risk alcohol drinking guidelines.* Retrieved from http://www.ccsa.ca/Resource%20Library/2012-Canada-Low-Risk-Alcohol-Drinking-Guidelines-Brochure-en.pdf

Canadian Diabetes Association Clinical Practice Guidelines Expert Committee. (2008). Canadian Diabetes Association 2008 clinical practice guidelines for the prevention and management of diabetes in Canada. *Canadian Journal of Diabetes, 32*(Suppl. 1), S1–S201.

Carnelley, K. B., Pietromonaco, P. R., & Jaffe, K. (1994). Depression, working models of others, and relationship functioning. *Journal of Personality and Social Psychology, 66*(1), 127–40. http://dx.doi.org/10.1037/0022-3514.66.1.127

Carpenter, E. M., & Kirkpatrick, L. A. (1996). Attachment style and presence of a romantic partner as moderators of psychophysiological responses to a stressful laboratory situation. *Personal Relationships, 3*(4), 351–67. http://dx.doi.org/10.1111/j.1475-6811.1996.tb00121.x

Carter, C. S. (2003). Developmental consequences of oxytocin. *Physiology & Behavior, 79*(3), 383–97. http://dx.doi.org/10.1016/S0031-9384(03)00151-3

Carter, C. S., Lederhendler, I. I., & Kirkpatrick, B. (1997). The integrative neurobiology of affiliation. *Annals of the New York Academy of Sciences, 807,* 469–71

Carter, C. S., Williams, J. R., Witt, D. M., & Insel, T. R. (1992). Oxytocin and social bonding. *Annals of the New York Academy of Sciences, 652*(1), 204–11. http://dx.doi.org/10.1111/j.1749-6632.1992.tb34356.x

Champoux, M., Hwang, L., Lang, O., & Levine, S. (2001). Feeding demand conditions and plasma cortisol in socially-housed squirrel monkey mother-infant dyads. *Psychoneuroendocrinology, 26*(5), 461–77. http://dx.doi.org/10.1016/S0306-4530(01)00006-3

Chen, S. M., Creedy, D., Lin, H. S., & Wollin, J. (2012). Effects of motivational interviewing intervention on self-management, psychological and glycemic outcomes in type 2 diabetes: A randomized controlled trial. *International Journal of Nursing Studies, 49*(6), 637–44. http://dx.doi.org/10.1016/j.ijnurstu.2011.11.011

Cherry, D. K., Hing, E., Woodwell, D. A., & Rechtsteiner, E. A. (2008). National ambulatory medical care survey: 2006 summary. *National Health Statistics Reports, 3*, 1–39. Retrieved from Centers for Disease Control and Prevention website: http://www.cdc.gov/nchs/data/nhsr/nhsr003.pdf

Christakis, N. A., & Allison, P. D. (2006). Mortality after the hospitalization of a spouse. *New England Journal of Medicine, 354*(7), 719–30. http://dx.doi.org/10.1056/NEJMsa050196

Ciechanowski, P., Hirsch, I. B., & Katon, W. J. (2002). Interpersonal predictors of HbA(1c) in patients with type 1 diabetes. *Diabetes Care, 25*(4), 731–6. http://dx.doi.org/10.2337/diacare.25.4.731

Ciechanowski, P., & Katon, W. J. (2006). The interpersonal experience of health care through the eyes of patients with diabetes. *Social Science & Medicine, 63*(12), 3067–79. http://dx.doi.org/10.1016/j.socscimed.2006.08.002

Ciechanowski, P., Katon, W. J., Russo, J. E., & Dwight-Johnson, M. M. (2002). Association of attachment style to medically unexplained symptoms in patients with hepatitis C. *Psychosomatics, 43*(3), 206–12. http://dx.doi.org/10.1176/appi.psy.43.3.206

Ciechanowski, P., Russo, J., Katon, W., Simon, G., Ludman, E., Von Korff, M., ... Lin, E. (2006). Where is the patient? The association of psychosocial factors and missed primary care appointments in patients with diabetes. *General Hospital Psychiatry, 28*(1), 9–17. http://dx.doi.org/10.1016/j.genhosppsych.2005.07.004

Ciechanowski, P., Russo, J., Katon, W., Von Korff, M., Ludman, E., Lin, E., ... Bush, T. (2004). Influence of patient attachment style on self-care and outcomes in diabetes. *Psychosomatic Medicine, 66*(5), 720–8. http://dx.doi.org/10.1097/01.psy.0000138125.59122.23

Ciechanowski, P., Sullivan, M., Jensen, M., Romano, J., & Summers, H. (2003). The relationship of attachment style to depression, catastrophizing and health care utilization in patients with chronic pain. *Pain, 104*(3), 627–37. http://dx.doi.org/10.1016/S0304-3959(03)00120-9

Ciechanowski, P., Walker, E. A., Katon, W. J., & Russo, J. E. (2002). Attachment theory: A model for health care utilization and somatization. *Psychosomatic Medicine, 64,* 660–7.

Ciechanowski, P. S., Katon, W. J., Russo, J. E., & Walker, E. A. (2001). The patient-provider relationship: Attachment theory and adherence to treatment in diabetes. *American Journal of Psychiatry, 158*(1), 29–35. http://dx.doi.org/10.1176/appi.ajp.158.1.29

Ciechanowski, P. S., Worley, L. L., Russo, J. E., & Katon, W. J. (2006). Using relationship styles based on attachment theory to improve understanding of specialty choice in medicine. *BMC Medical Education, 6*(1), 3. http://dx.doi.org/10.1186/1472-6920-6-3

Clark, L., Beesley, H., Holcombe, C., & Salmon, P. (2011). The influence of childhood abuse and adult attachment style on clinical relationships in breast cancer care. *General Hospital Psychiatry, 33*(6), 579–86. http://dx.doi.org/10.1016/j.genhosppsych.2011.07.007

Cohen, L., Cole, S. W., Sood, A. K., Prinsloo, S., Kirschbaum, C., Arevalo, J. M., ... Pisters, L. (2012). Depressive symptoms and cortisol rhythmicity predict survival in patients with renal cell carcinoma: Role of inflammatory signaling. *PLoS ONE, 7*(8), e42324. http://dx.doi.org/10.1371/journal.pone.0042324

Cohen, S., Doyle, W. J., Skoner, D. P., Rabin, B. S., & Gwaltney, J. M., Jr. (1997). Social ties and susceptibility to the common cold. *Journal of the American Medical Association, 277*(24), 1940–4. http://dx.doi.org/10.1001/jama.1997.03540480040036

Cohen, S., Doyle, W. J., Turner, R., Alper, C. M., & Skoner, D. P. (2003). Sociability and susceptibility to the common cold. *Psychological Science, 14*(5), 389–95. http://dx.doi.org/10.1111/1467-9280.01452

Cohen, S., Janicki-Deverts, D., & Miller, G. E. (2007). Psychological stress and disease. *Journal of the American Medical Association, 298*(14), 1685–7. http://dx.doi.org/10.1001/jama.298.14.1685

Cokkinides, V., Bandi, P., Ward, E., Jemal, A., & Thun, M. (2006). Progress and opportunities in tobacco control. *CA: A Cancer Journal for Clinicians, 56*(3), 135–42. http://dx.doi.org/10.3322/canjclin.56.3.135

Cole, S. W., Hawkley, L. C., Arevalo, J. M., Sung, C. Y., Rose, R. M., & Cacioppo, J. T. (2007). Social regulation of gene expression in human leukocytes. *Genome Biology, 8*(9), R189. http://dx.doi.org/10.1186/gb-2007-8-9-r189

College of Physicians and Surgeons of Canada. (2008, December 25). Difficult encounters with patients [Blog post]. Retrieved from http://www.cpso.on.ca

Collins, N. L., & Feeney, B. C. (2000). A safe haven: An attachment theory perspective on support seeking and caregiving in intimate relationships.

Journal of Personality and Social Psychology, 78(6), 1053–73. http://dx.doi.org/10.1037/0022-3514.78.6.1053

Collins, N. L., & Feeney, B. C. (2004). Working models of attachment shape perceptions of social support: Evidence from experimental and observational studies. *Journal of Personality and Social Psychology, 87*(3), 363–83. http://dx.doi.org/10.1037/0022-3514.87.3.363

Colton, P. A., Olmsted, M. P., Daneman, D., Rydall, A. C., & Rodin, G. M. (2007). Natural history and predictors of disturbed eating behaviour in girls with Type 1 diabetes. *Diabetic Medicine, 24*(4), 424–9. http://dx.doi.org/10.1111/j.1464-5491.2007.02099.x

Committee on the Quality of Health in America. (2001). *Crossing the quality chasm: A new health system for the 21st century.* Washington, DC: National Academies Press.

Considine, N. S., Tuck, N. L., & Fiori, K. L. (2013). Attachment and health care utilization among middle-aged and older African-descent men: Dismissiveness predicts less frequent digital rectal examination and prostate-specific antigen screening. *American Journal of Men's Health, 7*(5), 382–93. http://dx.doi.org/10.1177/1557988312474838

Cool, J. (2009). *Child poverty in Canada (Research Report No. PRB 08-62E).* Retrieved from Library of Parliament website: http://www.parl.gc.ca/Content/LOP/ResearchPublications/prb0862-e.pdf

Coryell, W., Turvey, C., Leon, A., Maser, J. D., Solomon, D., Endicott, J., ... Keller, M. (1999). Persistence of depressive symptoms and cardiovascular death among patients with affective disorder. *Psychosomatic Medicine, 61*(6), 755–61. http://dx.doi.org/10.1097/00006842-199911000-00006

Costa-Martins, J. M., Pereira, M., Martins, H., Moura-Ramos, M., Coelho, R., & Tavares, J. (2014). The role of maternal attachment in the experience of labor pain. *Psychosomatic Medicine, 76*(3), 221–8. http://dx.doi.org/10.1097/PSY.0000000000000040

Couprie, W., Wijdicks, E. F., Rooijmans, H. G., & van Gijn, J. (1995). Outcome in conversion disorder: A follow up study. *Journal of Neurology, Neurosurgery, and Psychiatry, 58*(6), 750–2. http://dx.doi.org/10.1136/jnnp.58.6.750

Crimlisk, H. L., Bhatia, K., Cope, H., David, A., Marsden, C. D., & Ron, M. A. (1998). Slater revisited: 6 year follow up study of patients with medically unexplained motor symptoms. *BMJ, 316*(7131), 582–6. http://dx.doi.org/10.1136/bmj.316.7131.582

Crittenden, P. M. (2006). A dynamic-maturational model of attachment. *Australian and New Zealand Journal of Family Therapy, 27*(2), 105–15. http://dx.doi.org/10.1002/j.1467-8438.2006.tb00704.x

Crowell, J. A., Treboux, D., & Waters, E. (2002). Stability of attachment representations: The transition to marriage. *Developmental Psychology*, *38*(4), 467–79. http://dx.doi.org/10.1037/0012-1649.38.4.467

D'Argenio, A., Mazzi, C., Pecchioli, L., Di Lorenzo, G., Siracusano, A., & Troisi, A. (2009). Early trauma and adult obesity: Is psychological dysfunction the mediating mechanism? *Physiology & Behavior*, *98*(5), 543–6. http://dx.doi.org/10.1016/j.physbeh.2009.08.010

Davila, J., Burge, D., & Hammen, C. (1997). Why does attachment style change? *Journal of Personality and Social Psychology*, *73*(4), 826–38. http://dx.doi.org/10.1037/0022-3514.73.4.826

Davila, J., Karney, B. R., & Bradbury, T. N. (1999). Attachment change processes in the early years of marriage. *Journal of Personality and Social Psychology*, *76*(5), 783–802. http://dx.doi.org/10.1037/0022-3514.76.5.783

Davis, D., Shaver, P. R., & Vernon, M. L. (2003). Physical, emotional, and behavioral reactions to breaking up: The roles of gender, age, emotional involvement, and attachment style. *Personality and Social Psychology Bulletin*, *29*(7), 871–84. http://dx.doi.org/10.1177/0146167203029007006

Davis, D., Shaver, P. R., & Vernon, M. L. (2004). Attachment style and subjective motivations for sex. *Personality and Social Psychology Bulletin*, *30*(8), 1076–90. http://dx.doi.org/10.1177/0146167204264794

De Bellis, M. D., Baum, A. S., Birmaher, B., Keshavan, M. S., Eccard, C. H., Boring, A. M., ... Ryan, N. D. (1999). Developmental traumatology part 1: Biological stress systems. *Biological Psychiatry*, *45*(10), 1259–70. http://dx.doi.org/10.1016/S0006-3223(99)00044-X

Demers, R. Y., Altamore, R., Mustin, H., Kleinman, A., & Leonardi, D. (1980). An exploration of the dimensions of illness behavior. *Journal of Family Practice*, *11*, 1085–92.

Department of Health and Human Services Public Health Service Office on Smoking and Health. (1994). *Preventing tobacco use among young people: A report of the surgeon general*. Washington, DC: Government Printing Office.

Depue, R. A., & Morrone-Strupinsky, J. V. (2005). A neurobehavioral model of affiliative bonding: Implications for conceptualizing a human trait of affiliation. *Behavioral and Brain Sciences*, *28*(03), 313–50. http://dx.doi.org/10.1017/S0140525X05000063

Diamond, L. M., & Fagundes, C. P. (2010). Psychobiological research on attachment. *Journal of Social and Personal Relationships*, *27*(2), 218–25. http://dx.doi.org/10.1177/0265407509360906

Diamond, L. M., Hicks, A. M., & Otter-Henderson, K. (2006). Physiological evidence for repressive coping among avoidantly attached adults.

Journal of Social and Personal Relationships, 23(2), 205–29. http://dx.doi. org/10.1177/0265407506062470

Ditzen, B., Schmidt, S., Strauss, B., Nater, U. M., Ehlert, U., & Heinrichs, M. (2008). Adult attachment and social support interact to reduce psychological but not cortisol responses to stress. Journal of Psychosomatic Research, 64(5), 479–86. http://dx.doi.org/10.1016/j.jpsychores.2007.11.011

Doherty, N. A., & Feeney, J. A. (2004). The composition of attachment networks throughout the adult years. Personal Relationships, 11(4), 469–88. http://dx.doi.org/10.1111/j.1475-6811.2004.00093.x

Dolan, R. J. (2007). The human amygdala and orbital prefrontal cortex in behavioural regulation. Philosophical Transactions of the Royal Society of London. Series B, Biological Sciences, 362(1481), 787–99. http://dx.doi. org/10.1098/rstb.2007.2088

Doyle, J. K. (1997). Judging cumulative risk. Journal of Applied Social Psychology, 27(6), 500–24. http://dx.doi.org/10.1111/j.1559-1816.1997.tb00644.x

Dozier, M., Cue, K. L., & Barnett, L. (1994). Clinicians as caregivers: Role of attachment organization in treatment. Journal of Consulting and Clinical Psychology, 62(4), 793–800. http://dx.doi.org/10.1037/0022-006X.62.4.793

Droomers, M., Schrijvers, C. T., Casswell, S., & Mackenbach, J. P. (2003). Occupational level of the father and alcohol consumption during adolescence; patterns and predictors. Journal of Epidemiology and Community Health, 57(9), 704–10. http://dx.doi.org/10.1136/jech.57.9.704

Dube, S. R., Anda, R. F., Felitti, V. J., Edwards, V. J., & Croft, J. B. (2002). Adverse childhood experiences and personal alcohol abuse as an adult. Addictive Behaviors, 27(5), 713–25. http://dx.doi.org/10.1016/ S0306-4603(01)00204-0

Dube, S. R., Miller, J. W., Brown, D. W., Giles, W. H., Felitti, V. J., Dong, M., & Anda, R. F. (2006). Adverse childhood experiences and the association with ever using alcohol and initiating alcohol use during adolescence. Journal of Adolescent Health, 38(4), 444.e1–444.e10. http://dx.doi.org/10.1016/j. jadohealth.2005.06.006

Ein-Dor, T., Mikulincer, M., Doron, G., & Shaver, P. (2010). The attachment paradox: How can so many of us (the insecure ones) have no adaptive advantages? Perspectives on Psychological Science, 5(2), 123–41. http://dx.doi. org/10.1177/1745691610362349

Eisenberger, N. I., Lieberman, M. D., & Williams, K. D. (2003). Does rejection hurt? An FMRI study of social exclusion. Science, 302(5643), 290–2. http:// dx.doi.org/10.1126/science.1089134

Eitle, D. (2005). The moderating effects of peer substance use on the family structure-adolescent substance use association: Quantity versus quality of

parenting. *Addictive Behaviors, 30*(5), 963–80. http://dx.doi.org/10.1016/j.
addbeh.2004.09.015

Elfhag, K., & Rossner, S. (2005). Who succeeds in maintaining weight loss?
A conceptual review of factors associated with weight loss maintenance
and weight regain. *Obesity Reviews, 6*(1), 67–85. http://dx.doi.
org/10.1111/j.1467-789X.2005.00170.x

Elliott, W. J. (2003). The economic impact of hypertension. *Journal of Clinical
Hypertension, 5*(3), 3–13. http://dx.doi.org/10.1111/j.1524-6175.2003.02463.x

Ellis, B. J., Essex, M. J., & Boyce, W. T. (2005). Biological sensitivity to
context: II. Empirical explorations of an evolutionary-developmental theory.
Development and Psychopathology, 17(02), 303–28. http://dx.doi.org/10.1017/
S0954579405050157

Evans, D. L., Charney, D. S., Lewis, L., Golden, R. N., Gorman, J. M., Krishnan,
K. R., ... Valvo, W. J. (2005). Mood disorders in the medically ill: Scientific
review and recommendations. *Biological Psychiatry, 58*(3), 175–89. http://
dx.doi.org/10.1016/j.biopsych.2005.05.001

Feeney, B. C., & Kirkpatrick, L. A. (1996). Effects of adult attachment and
presence of romantic partners on physiological responses to stress.
Journal of Personality and Social Psychology, 70(2), 255–70. http://dx.doi.
org/10.1037/0022-3514.70.2.255

Feeney, J. A. (1995). Adult attachment, coping style and health locus of control
as predictors of health behavior. *Australian Journal of Psychology, 47*(3),
171–7. http://dx.doi.org/10.1080/00049539508257520

Feeney, J. A., Kelly, L., Gallois, C., Peterson, C., & Terry, D. J. (1999).
Attachment style, assertive communication, and safer sex behavior. *Journal
of Applied Social Psychology, 29*(9), 1964–83. http://dx.doi.org/10.1111/j.1559-
1816.1999.tb00159.x

Feeney, J. A., Noller, P., & Patty, J. (1993). Adolescents' interactions with
the opposite sex: Influence of attachment style and gender. *Journal of
Adolescence, 16*(2), 169–86. http://dx.doi.org/10.1006/jado.1993.1015

Feeney, J. A., & Raphael, B. (1992). Adult attachments and sexuality:
Implications for understanding risk behaviours for HIV infection. *Australian
and New Zealand Journal of Psychiatry, 26*(3), 399–407. http://dx.doi.
org/10.3109/00048679209072062

Feeney, J. A., & Ryan, S. M. (1994). Attachment style and affect regulation:
Relationships with health behavior and family experiences of illness
in a student sample. *Health Psychology, 13*(4), 334–45. http://dx.doi.
org/10.1037/0278-6133.13.4.334

Felitti, V. J., Anda, R. F., Nordenberg, D., Williamson, D. F., Spitz, A. M.,
Edwards, V., ... Marks, J. S. (1998). Relationship of childhood abuse and

household dysfunction to many of the leading causes of deaths in adults. *American Journal of Preventive Medicine, 14*(4), 245–58. http://dx.doi.org/10.1016/S0749-3797(98)00017-8

Finkelhor, D., Ormrod, R. K., & Turner, H. A. (2007). Poly-victimization: A neglected component in child victimization. *Child Abuse & Neglect, 31*(1), 7–26. http://dx.doi.org/10.1016/j.chiabu.2006.06.008

Fjorback, L. O., Arendt, M., Ornbol, E., Fink, P., & Walach, H. (2011). Mindfulness-based stress reduction and mindfulness-based cognitive therapy: A systematic review of randomized controlled trials. *Acta Psychiatrica Scandinavica, 124*(2), 102–19. http://dx.doi.org/10.1111/j.1600-0447.2011.01704.x

Fleming, C. B., Kim, H., Harachi, T. W., & Catalano, R. F. (2002). Family processes for children in early elementary school as predictors of smoking initiation. *Journal of Adolescent Health, 30*(3), 184–9. http://dx.doi.org/10.1016/S1054-139X(01)00327-5

Fonagy, P. (1998). An attachment theory approach to treatment of the difficult patient. *Bulletin of the Menninger Clinic, 62*, 147–69.

Fonagy, P., Gergely, G., Jurist, E., & Target, M. (2005). *Affect regulation, mentalization, and the development of the self.* New York, NY: Other Press.

Fonagy, P., Steele, H., Moran, G., Steele, M., & Higgitt, A. (1991). The capacity for understanding mental states: The reflective self in parent and child and its significance for security of attachment. *Infant Mental Health Journal, 13*, 200–17.

Fonagy, P., & Target, M. (1997). Attachment and reflective function: Their role in self-organization. *Development and Psychopathology, 9*(04), 679–700. http://dx.doi.org/10.1017/S0954579497001399

Fraga, M. F., Ballestar, E., Paz, M. F., Ropero, S., Setien, F., Ballestar, M. L., ... Esteller, M. (2005). Epigenetic differences arise during the lifetime of monozygotic twins. *Proceedings of the National Academy of Sciences of the United States of America, 102*(30), 10604–9. http://dx.doi.org/10.1073/pnas.0500398102

Fraley, R. C., & Davis, K. E. (1997). Attachment formation and transfer in young adults' close friendships and romantic relationships. *Personal Relationships, 4*(2), 131–44. http://dx.doi.org/10.1111/j.1475-6811.1997.tb00135.x

Fraley, R. C., & Shaver, P. R. (1998). Airport separations: A naturalistic study of adult attachment dynamics in separating couples. *Journal of Personality and Social Psychology, 75*(5), 1198–1212. http://dx.doi.org/10.1037/0022-3514.75.5.1198

Fraley, R. C., Waller, N. G., & Brennan, K. A. (2000). An item response theory analysis of self-report measures of adult attachment. *Journal of Personality and Social Psychology, 78*(2), 350–65. http://dx.doi. org/10.1037/0022-3514.78.2.350

Frasure-Smith, N., Koszycki, D., Swenson, J. R., Baker, B., van Zyl, L. T., Laliberte, M. A., ... Lespérance, F. (2006). Design and rationale for a randomized, controlled trial of interpersonal psychotherapy and citalopram for depression in coronary artery disease (CREATE). *Psychosomatic Medicine, 68*(1), 87–93. http://dx.doi.org/10.1097/01.psy.0000195833.68482.27

Frasure-Smith, N., Lesperance, F., & Talajic, M. (1993). Depression following myocardial infarction. Impact on 6-month survival. *Journal of the American Medical Association, 270*(15), 1819–25. http://dx.doi.org/10.1001/jama.1993.03510150053029

Fricchione, G. L. (2011). *Compassion and healing in medicine and society: On the nature and use of attachment solutions to separation challenges.* Baltimore, MD: Johns Hopkins University Press.

Friedlmeier, W., & Granqvist, P. (2006). Attachment transfer among Swedish and German adolescents: A prospective longitudinal study. *Personal Relationships, 13*(3), 261–79. http://dx.doi. org/10.1111/j.1475-6811.2006.00117.x

Frith, C. D., & Frith, U. (1999). Interacting minds – A biological basis. *Science, 286*(5445), 1692–5. http://dx.doi.org/10.1126/science.286.5445.1692

Frith, U., & Frith, C. D. (2003). Development and neurophysiology of mentalizing. *Philosophical Transactions of the Royal Society of London. Series B, Biological Sciences, 358*(1431), 459–73. http://dx.doi.org/10.1098/rstb.2002.1218

Gawande, A. (2013, July 29). Slow ideas. *The New Yorker.* Retrieved from http://www.newyorker.com/magazine/2013/07/29/slow-ideas

Gentzler, A. L., & Kerns, K. A. (2004). Associations between insecure attachment and sexual experiences. *Personal Relationships, 11*(2), 249–65. http://dx.doi.org/10.1111/j.1475-6811.2004.00081.x

George, C., & West, M. (2001). The development and preliminary validation of a new measure of adult attachment: The adult attachment projective. *Attachment & Human Development, 3*(1), 30–61. http://dx.doi. org/10.1080/14616730010024771

Gjerdingen, D., Fontaine, P., Crow, S., McGovern, P., Center, B., & Miner, M. (2009). Predictors of mothers' postpartum body dissatisfaction. *Women & Health, 49*(6-7), 491–504. http://dx.doi.org/10.1080/03630240903423998

Glassman, A. H., O'Connor, C. M., Califf, R. M., Swedberg, K., Schwartz, P., Bigger, J. T., Jr., ... Harrison, W. M. (2002). Sertraline treatment of major depression in patients with acute MI or unstable angina. *Journal of the American Medical Association, 288*(6), 701–9. http://dx.doi.org/10.1001/jama.288.6.701

Goldsmith, R. L., Bigger, J. T., Jr., Bloomfield, D. M., & Steinman, R. C. (1997). Physical fitness as a determinant of vagal modulation. *Medicine and Science in Sports and Exercise, 29*(6), 812–17. http://dx.doi.org/10.1097/00005768-199706000-00012

Goossens, F. A., & van Ijzendoorn, M. H. (1990). Quality of infants' attachments to professional caregivers: Relation to infant-parent attachment and day-care characteristics. *Child Development, 61*(3), 832–7. http://dx.doi.org/10.2307/1130967

Graetz, C., Ehrenthal, J. C., Senf, D., Semar, K., Herzog, W., & Dorfer, C. E. (2013). Influence of psychological attachment patterns on periodontal disease – A pilot study with 310 compliant patients. *Journal of Clinical Periodontology, 40*(12), 1087–94. http://dx.doi.org/10.1111/jcpe.12159

Groopman, J. (2007). *How doctors think.* New York, NY: Houghton Mifflin.

Groves, J. E. (1978). Taking care of the hateful patient. *New England Journal of Medicine, 298*(16), 883–7. http://dx.doi.org/10.1056/NEJM197804202981605

Gunnar, M. R., Brodersen, L., Nachmias, M., Buss, K., & Rigatuso, R. (1996). Stress reactivity and attachment security. *Developmental Psychobiology, 29*(3), 191–204. http://dx.doi.org/10.1002/(SICI)1098-2302(199604)29:3<191::AID-DEV1>3.0.CO;2-M

Gunnar, M. R., & Donzella, B. (2002). Social regulation of the cortisol levels in early human development. *Psychoneuroendocrinology, 27*(1–2), 199–220. http://dx.doi.org/10.1016/S0306-4530(01)00045-2

Gunnar, M. R., Larson, M., Hertsgaard, L., Harris, M., & Brodersen, L. (1992). The stressfulness of separation among 9-month old infants: Effects of social context variables and infant temperament. *Child Development, 63*(2), 290–303. http://dx.doi.org/10.2307/1131479

Hahm, H. C., Lahiff, M., & Guterman, N. B. (2003). Acculturation and parental attachment in Asian-American adolescents' alcohol use. *Journal of Adolescent Health, 33*(2), 119–29. http://dx.doi.org/10.1016/S1054-139X(03)00058-2

Hahn, S. R., Kroenke, K., Spitzer, R. L., Brody, D., Williams, J. B., Linzer, M., & deGruy, F. V., III. (1996). The difficult patient. *Journal of General Internal Medicine, 11*(1), 1–8. http://dx.doi.org/10.1007/BF02603477

Halpern, J., Maunder, R. G., Schwartz, B., & Gurevich, M. (2011). Identifying risk of emotional sequelae after critical incidents. *Emergency Medicine Journal, 28*(1), 51–6. http://dx.doi.org/10.1136/emj.2009.082982

Halpern, J., Maunder, R. G., Schwartz, B., & Gurevich, M. (2012). Responses to critical incident distress, and current emotional symptoms in ambulance workers. *Stress and Health, 28*(1), 51–60. http://dx.doi.org/10.1002/smi.1401

Hamilton, C. E. (2000). Continuity and discontinuity of attachment from infancy through adolescence. *Child Development, 71*(3), 690–4. http://dx.doi.org/10.1111/1467-8624.00177

Harding, S. M. (1998). Sleep in fibromyalgia patients: Subjective and objective findings. *American Journal of the Medical Sciences, 315*(6), 367–76. http://dx.doi.org/10.1097/00000441-199806000-00005

Harlow, H. F. (1958). The nature of love. *American Psychologist, 13*(12), 673–85. http://dx.doi.org/10.1037/h0047884

Harlow, H. F., & Harlow, M. K. (1962). Social deprivation in monkeys. *Scientific American, 207*(5), 136–47. http://dx.doi.org/10.1038/scientificamerican1162-136

Harris, T. O., Brown, G. W., & Bifulco, A. T. (1990). Depression and situational helplessness/mastery in a sample selected to study childhood parental loss. *Journal of Affective Disorders, 20*(1), 27–41. http://dx.doi.org/10.1016/0165-0327(90)90047-C

Hazan, C., Gur-Yaish, N., & Campa, M. (2004). What does it mean to be attached? In W. S. Rholes & J. A. Simpson (Eds.), *Adult attachment: Theory, research and clinical implications* [Kindle version]. Retrieved from http://www.amazon.ca

Hazan, C., & Shaver, P. R. (1987). Romantic love conceptualized as an attachment process. *Journal of Personality and Social Psychology, 52*(3), 511–24. http://dx.doi.org/10.1037/0022-3514.52.3.511

Hazan, C., & Zeifman, D. (1999). Pair bonds as attachments: Evaluating the evidence. In J. Cassidy & P. R. Shaver (Eds.), *Handbook of attachment* (pp. 336–54). New York, NY: Guilford Press.

Heinrichs, M., Baumgartner, T., Kirschbaum, C., & Ehlert, U. (2003). Social support and oxytocin interact to suppress cortisol and subjective responses to psychosocial stress. *Biological Psychiatry, 54*(12), 1389–98. http://dx.doi.org/10.1016/S0006-3223(03)00465-7

Hemingway, H., & Marmot, M. (1999). Evidence based cardiology: Psychosocial factors in the aetiology and prognosis of coronary heart disease. Systematic review of prospective cohort studies. *BMJ (Clinical Research Ed.), 318*(7196), 1460–7. http://dx.doi.org/10.1136/bmj.318.7196.1460

Henry, K. L. (2008). Low prosocial attachment, involvement with drug-using peers, and adolescent drug use: A longitudinal examination of mediational mechanisms. *Psychology of Addictive Behaviors, 22*(2), 302–8. http://dx.doi.org/10.1037/0893-164X.22.2.302

Hesse, E. (2008). The adult attachment interview: Protocol, method of analysis, and empirical studies. In J. Cassidy & P. R. Shaver (Eds.), *Handbook of attachment: Theory, research and clinical applications* (2nd ed., pp. 552–98). New York, NY: Guilford Press.

Hillen, M. A., de Haes, H. C., & Smets, E. M. (2011). Cancer patients' trust in their physician-a review. *Psycho-Oncology, 20*(3), 227–41. http://dx.doi.org/10.1002/pon.1745

Hillis, S. D., Anda, R. F., Felitti, V. J., & Marchbanks, P. A. (2001). Adverse childhood experiences and sexual risk behaviors in women: A retrospective cohort study. *Family Planning Perspectives, 33*(5), 206–11. http://dx.doi.org/10.2307/2673783

Hillis, S. D., Anda, R. F., Felitti, V. J., Nordenberg, D., & Marchbanks, P. A. (2000). Adverse childhood experiences and sexually transmitted diseases in men and women: A retrospective study. *Pediatrics, 106*(1), e11. http://dx.doi.org/10.1542/peds.106.1.e11

Hinnen, C., Pool, G., Holwerda, N., Sprangers, M. A., Sanderman, R., & Hagedoorn, M. (2014). Lower level of trust in one's physician is associated with more distress over time in more anxiously attached individuals with cancer. *General Hospital Psychiatry, 36*(4), 382–7. http://dx.doi.org/10.1016/j.genhosppsych.2014.03.005

Hintsanen, M., Jokela, M., Pulkki-Raback, L., Viikari, J. S. A., & Keltikangas-Jarvinen, L. (2010). Associations of youth and adulthood body-mass index and waist-hip ratio with attachment styles and dimensions. *Current Psychology (New Brunswick, N. J.), 29*(3), 257–71. http://dx.doi.org/10.1007/s12144-010-9084-8

Hodson, C., Newcomb, M. D., Locke, T. F., & Goodyear, R. K. (2006). Childhood adversity, poly-substance use, and disordered eating in adolescent Latinas: Mediated and indirect paths in a community sample. *Child Abuse & Neglect, 30*(9), 1017–36. http://dx.doi.org/10.1016/j.chiabu.2005.10.017

Hofer, M. A. (1984). Relationships as regulators: A psychobiological perspective. *Psychosomatic Medicine, 46*(3), 183–97. http://dx.doi.org/10.1097/00006842-198405000-00001

Hofer, M. A. (1995). Hidden regulators: Implications for a new understanding of attachment, separation and loss. In S. Goldberg, R. Muir, & J. Kerr (Eds.), *Attachment theory: Social developmental, and clinical perspectives* (pp. 203–30). Hillsdale, NJ: Analytic Press.

Hofer, M. A. (2004). Developmental psychobiology of early attachment. In B. J. Casey (Ed.), *Developmental psychobiology* (pp. 1–28). Washington, DC: American Psychiatric Publishing.

Hoffman, K. T., Marvin, R. S., Cooper, G., & Powell, B. (2006). Changing toddlers' and preschoolers' attachment classifications: The circle of security intervention. *Journal of Consulting and Clinical Psychology, 74*(6), 1017–26. http://dx.doi.org/10.1037/0022-006X.74.6.1017

Hoffmann, J. P., & Su, S. S. (1998). Parental substance use disorder, mediating variables and adolescent drug use: A non-recursive model. *Addiction, 93*(9), 1351–64. http://dx.doi.org/10.1046/j.1360-0443.1998.93913516.x

Holmes, J. (2001). *The search for the secure base: Attachment theory and psychotherapy.* East Sussex, London: Brunner-Routledge.

Holmes, J. (2006). Mentalization from a psychoanalytic perspective: What's new? In J. G. Allen & P. Fonagy (Eds.), *Handbook of mentalization-based treatment* [Kindle version]. Retrieved from http://www.amazon.ca

Holt-Lunstad, J., Smith, T. B., & Layton, J. B. (2010). Social relationships and mortality risk: A meta-analytic review. *PLoS Medicine, 7*(7), e1000316. http://dx.doi.org/10.1371/journal.pmed.1000316

Holwerda, N., Sanderman, R., Pool, G., Hinnen, C., Langendijk, J. A., Bemelman, W. A., ... Sprangers, M. A. G. (2013). Do patients trust their physician? The role of attachment style in the patient-physician relationship within one year after a cancer diagnosis. *Acta Oncologica, 52*(1), 110–17. http://dx.doi.org/10.3109/0284186X.2012.689856

Hoover, D. R., Crystal, S., Kumar, R., Sambamoorthi, U., & Cantor, J. C. (2002). Medical expenditures during the last year of life: Findings from the 1992–1996 Medicare current beneficiary survey. *Health Services Research, 37*(6), 1625–42. http://dx.doi.org/10.1111/1475-6773.01113

Hoover, R. N., Hyer, M., Pfeiffer, R. M., Adam, E., Bond, B., Cheville, A. L., ... Troisi, R. (2011). Adverse health outcomes in women exposed in utero to diethylstilbestrol. *New England Journal of Medicine, 365*(14), 1304–14. http://dx.doi.org/10.1056/NEJMoa1013961

House, J. S., Landis, K. R., & Umberson, D. (1988). Social relationships and health. *Science, 241*(4865), 540–5. http://dx.doi.org/10.1126/science.33 99889

Huebner, A. J., Shettler, L., Matheson, J. L., Meszaros, P. S., Piercy, F. P., & Davis, S. D. (2005). Factors associated with former smokers among female adolescents in rural Virginia. *Addictive Behaviors, 30*(1), 167–73. http://dx.doi.org/10.1016/j.addbeh.2004.04.004

Hunter, J. J., & Maunder, R. G. (2001). Using attachment theory to understand illness behavior. *General Hospital Psychiatry, 23*(4), 177–82. http://dx.doi.org/10.1016/S0163-8343(01)00141-4

Insel, T. R. (1997). A neurobiological basis of social attachment. *American Journal of Psychiatry, 154*(6), 726–35. http://dx.doi.org/10.1176/ajp.154.6.726

Jacobsen, T., Huss, M., Fendrich, M., Kruesi, M. J., & Ziegenhain, U. (1997). Children's ability to delay gratification: Longitudinal relations to mother-child attachment. *Journal of Genetic Psychology, 158*(4), 411–26. http://dx.doi.org/10.1080/00221329709596679

Janz, N. K., & Becker, M. H. (1984). The health belief model: A decade later. *Health Education Quarterly, 11*(1), 1–47. http://dx.doi.org/10.1177/109019818401100101

Javo, I. M., & Sorlie, T. (2009). Psychosocial predictors of an interest in cosmetic surgery among young Norwegian women: A population-based study. *Plastic and Reconstructive Surgery, 124,* 2142–8.

Joels, M., & Baram, T. Z. (2009). The neuro-symphony of stress. *Nature Reviews. Neuroscience, 10,* 459–66.

Joynt, K. E., & O'Connor, C. M. (2005). Lessons from SADHART, ENRICHD, and other trials. *Psychosomatic Medicine, 67*(Suppl. 1), S63–6. http://dx.doi.org/10.1097/01.psy.0000163454.25036.fc

Kabat-Zinn, J. (1990). *Full catastrophe living: Using the wisdom of your body and mind to face stress, pain and illness.* New York, NY: Delta Books.

Kahneman, D. (2011). *Thinking, fast and slow.* New York, NY: Doubleday.

Kalichman, S. C., Sarwer, D. B., Johnson, J. R., Ali, S. A., Early, J., & Tuten, J. T. (1994). Sexually coercive behavior and love styles: A replication and extension. *Journal of Psychology & Human Sexuality, 6*(1), 93–106. http://dx.doi.org/10.1300/J056v06n01_06

Karcher, M. J., & Finn, L. (2005). How connectedness contributes to experimental smoking among rural youth: Developmental and ecological analyses. *Journal of Primary Prevention, 26*(1), 25–36. http://dx.doi.org/10.1007/s10935-004-0989-6

Katon, W. (1996). The impact of major depression on chronic medical illness. *General Hospital Psychiatry, 18*(4), 215–19. http://dx.doi.org/10.1016/0163-8343(96)00065-5

Kendler, K. S., Karkowski, L. M., & Prescott, C. A. (1999). Causal relationship between stressful life events and the onset of major depression. *American Journal of Psychiatry, 156*(6), 837–41. http://dx.doi.org/10.1176/ajp.156.6.837

Kessler, R. C., Sonnega, A., Bromet, E., Hughes, M., & Nelson, C. B. (1995). Posttraumatic stress disorder in the national comorbidity survey. *Archives of General Psychiatry, 52*(12), 1048–60. http://dx.doi.org/10.1001/archpsyc.1995.03950240066012

Kiecolt-Glaser, J. K., Marucha, P. T., Mercado, A. M., Malarkey, W. B., & Glaser, R. (1995). Slowing of wound healing by psychological stress. *Lancet, 346*(8984), 1194–6. http://dx.doi.org/10.1016/S0140-6736(95)92899-5

Kim, K. H. S., Relkin, N. R., Lee, K.-M., & Hirsch, J. (1997). Distinct cortical areas associated with native and second languages. *Nature, 388*(6638), 171–4. http://dx.doi.org/10.1038/40623

Kim, S. E., & Chang, L. (2012). Overlap between functional GI disorders and other functional syndromes: What are the underlying mechanisms? *Neurogastroenterology and Motility, 24*(10), 895–913. http://dx.doi.org/10.1111/j.1365-2982.2012.01993.x

Kim, Y. (2006). Gender, attachment, and relationship duration on cardiovascular reactivity to stress in a laboratory study of dating couples. *Personal Relationships, 13*(1), 103–14. http://dx.doi.org/10.1111/j.1475-6811.2006.00107.x

Kinley, J. L., & Reyno, S. M. (2013). Attachment style changes following intensive short-term group psychotherapy. *International Journal of Group Psychotherapy, 63*(1), 53–75. http://dx.doi.org/10.1521/ijgp.2013.63.1.53

Kirkpatrick, L. A., & Hazan, C. (1994). Attachment styles and close relationships: A four-year prospective study. *Personal Relationships, 1*(2), 123–42. http://dx.doi.org/10.1111/j.1475-6811.1994.tb00058.x

Kisilevsky, B. S., Hains, S. M., Brown, C. A., Lee, C. T., Cowperthwaite, B., Stutzman, S. S., ... Wang, Z. (2009). Fetal sensitivity to properties of maternal speech and language. *Infant Behavior and Development, 32*(1), 59–71. http://dx.doi.org/10.1016/j.infbeh.2008.10.002

Kisilevsky, B. S., Hains, S. M., Lee, K., Xie, X., Huang, H., Ye, H. H., ... Wang, Z. (2003). Effects of experience on fetal voice recognition. *Psychological Science, 14*(3), 220–4. http://dx.doi.org/10.1111/1467-9280.02435

Kivimaki, M., Ferrie, J. E., Head, J., Shipley, M. J., Vahtera, J., & Marmot, M. G. (2004). Organisational justice and change in justice as predictors of employee health: The Whitehall II study. *Journal of Epidemiology and Community Health, 58*(11), 931–7. http://dx.doi.org/10.1136/jech.2003.019026

Klohnen, E. C., & Bera, S. (1998). Behavioral and experiential patterns of avoidantly and securely attached women across adulthood: A 31-year longitudinal perspective. *Journal of Personality and Social Psychology, 74*(1), 211–3. http://dx.doi.org/10.1037/0022-3514.74.1.211

Klohnen, E. C., & John, O. P. (1998). Working models of attachment: A theory-based prototype approach. In J. A. Simpson & W. S. Rholes (Eds.), *Attachment theory and close relationships* (pp. 115–40). New York, NY: Guilford Press.

Kodama, S., Saito, K., Tanaka, S., Maki, M., Yachi, Y., Asumi, M., ... Sone, H. (2009). Cardiorespiratory fitness as a quantitative predictor of all-cause mortality and cardiovascular events in healthy men and women: A meta-analysis. *Journal of the American Medical Association, 301*(19), 2024–35. http://dx.doi.org/10.1001/jama.2009.681

Koenen, K. C., Roberts, A. L., Stone, D. M., & Dunn, E. C. (2010). The epidemiology of early childhood trauma. In R. A. Lanius, E. Vermetten, & C. Pain (Eds.), *The impact of early life trauma on health and disease* (pp. 13–24).

Cambridge, England: Cambridge University Press. http://dx.doi.org/10. 1017/CBO9780511777042.003

Kosfeld, M., Heinrichs, M., Zak, P. J., Fischbacher, U., & Fehr, E. (2005). Oxytocin increases trust in humans. *Nature, 435*(7042), 673–6. http://dx.doi. org/10.1038/nature03701

Kraemer, G. W. (1992). A psychobiological theory of attachment. *Behavioral and Brain Sciences, 15*(03), 493–511. http://dx.doi.org/10.1017/S0140525X000 69752

Kreisman, J. J., & Straus, H. (2010). *I hate you – Don't leave me: Understanding the borderline personality*. New York, NY: Penguin.

Kroenke, K. (2003). Patients presenting with somatic complaints: Epidemiology, psychiatric comorbidity and management. *International Journal of Methods in Psychiatric Research, 12*(1), 34–43. http://dx.doi. org/10.1002/mpr.140

Kroenke, K., & Mangelsdorff, A. D. (1989). Common symptoms in ambulatory care: Incidence, evaluation, therapy and outcome. *American Journal of Medicine, 86*(3), 262–6. http://dx.doi.org/10.1016/0002-9343(89)90293-3

Kubzansky, L. D., Davidson, K. W., & Rozanski, A. (2005). The clinical impact of negative psychological states: Expanding the spectrum of risk for coronary artery disease. *Psychosomatic Medicine, 67*(Suppl. 1), S10–14. http://dx.doi.org/10.1097/01.psy.0000164012.88829.41

Kuendig, H., & Kuntsche, E. (2006). Family bonding and adolescent alcohol use: Moderating effect of living with excessive drinking parents. *Alcohol and Alcoholism, 41*(4), 464–71. http://dx.doi.org/10.1093/alcalc/agl018

Lachman, M. E. (2003). Negative interactions in close relationships: Introduction to a special section. *Journals of Gerontology. Series B, Psychological Sciences and Social Sciences, 58*(2), P69. http://dx.doi. org/10.1093/geronb/58.2.P69

Laughlin, S. B., de Ruyter van Steveninck, R. R., & Anderson, J. C. (1998). The metabolic cost of neural information. *Nature Neuroscience, 1*(1), 36–41. http://dx.doi.org/10.1038/236

Laurent, H., & Powers, S. (2007). Emotion regulation in emerging adult couples: Temperament, attachment, and HPA response to conflict. *Biological Psychology, 76*(1-2), 61–71. http://dx.doi.org/10.1016/j.biopsycho.2007. 06.002

Leonard, W. R., Robertson, M. L., Snodgrass, J. J., & Kuzawa, C. W. (2003). Metabolic correlates of hominid brain evolution. *Comparative Biochemistry and Physiology. Part A, Molecular & Integrative Physiology, 136*(1), 5–15. http://dx.doi.org/10.1016/S1095-6433(03)00132-6

Lespérance, F., Frasure-Smith, N., Koszycki, D., Laliberte, M. A., van Zyl, L.T., Baker, B., ... CREATE Investigators. (2007). Effects of citalopram and interpersonal psychotherapy on depression in patients with coronary artery disease: The Canadian cardiac randomized evaluation of antidepressant and psychotherapy efficacy (CREATE) trial. *Journal of the American Medical Association, 297*(4), 367–79. http://dx.doi.org/10.1001/jama.297.4.367

Levy, K. N., Meehan, K. B., Kelly, K. M., Reynoso, J. S., Weber, M., Clarkin, J. F., & Kernberg, O. F. (2006). Change in attachment patterns and reflective function in a randomized control trial of transference-focused psychotherapy for borderline personality disorder. *Journal of Consulting and Clinical Psychology, 74*(6), 1027–40. http://dx.doi.org/10.1037/0022-006X.74.6.1027

Lieberman, M. D. (2007). Social cognitive neuroscience: A review of core processes. *Annual Review of Psychology, 58*(1), 259–89. http://dx.doi.org/10.1146/annurev.psych.58.110405.085654

Light, K. C., Grewen, K. M., & Amico, J. A. (2005). More frequent partner hugs and higher oxytocin levels are linked to lower blood pressure and heart rate in premenopausal women. *Biological Psychology, 69*(1), 5–21. http://dx.doi.org/10.1016/j.biopsycho.2004.11.002

Lilliengren, P., Werbart, A., Mothander, P. R., Ekstrom, A., Sjogren, S., & Ogren, M. L. (2014). Patient attachment to therapist rating scale: Development and psychometric properties. *Psychotherapy Research, 24*(2), 184–201. http://dx.doi.org/10.1080/10503307.2013.867462

Link, T. C. (2008). Youthful intoxication: A cross-cultural study of drinking among German and American adolescents. *Journal of Studies on Alcohol and Drugs, 69*, 362–70.

Liotti, G. (1991). Patterns of attachments and the assessment of interpersonal schemata: Understanding and changing difficult patient-therapist relationships in cognitive psychotherapy. *Journal of Cognitive Psychotherapy, 5*, 105–14.

Liu, D., Diorio, J., Tannenbaum, B., Caldji, C., Francis, D., Freedman, A., ... Meaney, M. J. (1997). Maternal care, hippocampal glucocorticoid receptors, and the hypothalamic-pituitary-adrenal responses to stress. *Science, 277*(5332), 1659–62. http://dx.doi.org/10.1126/science.277.5332.1659

Lorig, K., Holman, H., Sobel, D., & Laurent, D. (2006). *Living a healthy life with chronic conditions: Self-management of heart disease, fatigue, arthritis, worry, diabetes, frustration, asthma, pain, emphysema, and others* (3rd ed.). Boulder, CO: Bull Publishing.

Luecken, L. J. (1998). Childhood attachment and loss experiences affect adult cardiovascular and cortisol function. *Psychosomatic Medicine, 60*(6), 765–72. http://dx.doi.org/10.1097/00006842-199811000-00021

Lyness, J. M., King, D. A., Cox, C., Yoediono, Z., & Caine, E. D. (1999). The importance of subsyndromal depression in older primary care patients:

Prevalence and associated functional disability. *Journal of the American Geriatrics Society, 47*, 647–52.

Lyons-Ruth, K., & Jacobvitz, D. (2008). Attachment disorganization: Genetic factors, parenting contexts, and developmental transformation from infancy to adulthood. In J. Cassidy & P. R. Shaver (Eds.), *Handbook of attachment: Theory, research and clinical applications* (2nd ed., pp. 666–97). New York, NY: Guilford Press.

Machin, A. J., & Dunbar, R. I. M. (2011). The brain opioid theory of social attachment: A review of the evidence. *Behaviour, 148*(9), 985–1025. http://dx.doi.org/10.1163/000579511X596624

MacMillan, H. L., Fleming, J. E., Trocmé, N., Boyle, M. H., Wong, M., Racine, Y. A., ... Offord, D. R. (1997). Prevalence of child physical and sexual abuse in the community. *Journal of the American Medical Association, 278*(2), 131–5. http://dx.doi.org/10.1001/jama.1997.03550020063039

Madden, T. J., Ellen, P. S., & Ajzen, I. (1992). A comparison of the theory of planned behavior and the theory of reasoned action. *Personality and Social Psychology Bulletin, 18*(1), 3–9. http://dx.doi.org/10.1177/0146167292181001

Madigan, S., Moran, G., & Pederson, D. R. (2006). Unresolved states of mind, disorganized attachment relationships, and disrupted interactions of adolescent mothers and their infants. *Developmental Psychology, 42*(2), 293–304. http://dx.doi.org/10.1037/0012-1649.42.2.293

Magai, C. (2008). Attachment in middle and later life. In J. Cassidy & P. R. Shaver (Eds.), *Handbook of attachment: Theory, research and clinical applications* (2nd ed., pp. 532–551). New York, NY: Guilford Press.

Magai, C., Cohen, C., Milburn, N., Thorpe, B., McPherson, R., & Peralta, D. (2001). Attachment styles in older European American and African American adults. *Journals of Gerontology. Series B, Psychological Sciences and Social Sciences, 56*(1), S28–S35. http://dx.doi.org/10.1093/geronb/56.1.S28

Main, M., & Cassidy, J. (1988). Categories of response to reunion with the parent at age 6: Predictable from infant attachment classifications and stable over a 1-month period. *Developmental Psychology, 24*(3), 415–26. http://dx.doi.org/10.1037/0012-1649.24.3.415

Main, M., & Solomon, J. (1986). Discovery of a new, insecure-disorganized/disoriented attachment pattern. In T. B. Brazelton & M. Yogman (Eds.), *Affective development in infancy* (pp. 95–124). Norwood, NJ: Ablex.

Main, M. (2000). The organized categories of infant, child, and adult attachment: Flexible vs. inflexible attention under attachment-related stress. *Journal of the American Psychoanalytic Association, 48*(4), 1055–96. http://dx.doi.org/10.1177/00030651000480041801

Main, M., Kaplan, N., & Cassidy, J. (1985). Security in infancy, childhood, and adulthood: A move to the level of representation. *Monographs of the Society for Research in Child Development, 50*(1/2), 66–104. http://dx.doi.org/10.2307/3333827

Marmot, M. G., Stansfeld, S., Patel, C., North, F., Head, J., White, I., ... Smith, G. D. (1991). Health inequalities among British civil servants: The Whitehall II study. *Lancet, 337*(8754), 1387–93. http://dx.doi.org/10.1016/0140-6736(91)93068-K

Marvel, M. K., Epstein, R. M., Flowers, K., & Beckman, H. B. (1999). Soliciting the patient's agenda: Have we improved? *Journal of the American Medical Association, 281*(3), 283–7. http://dx.doi.org/10.1001/jama.281.3.283

Maunder, R. G., & Greenberg, G. R. (2004). Comparison of a disease activity index and patients' self-reported symptom severity in ulcerative colitis. *Inflammatory Bowel Diseases, 10*(5), 632–6. http://dx.doi.org/10.1097/00054725-200409000-00020

Maunder, R. G., & Hunter, J. J. (2001). Attachment and psychosomatic medicine: Developmental contributions to stress and disease. *Psychosomatic Medicine, 63*(4), 556–67. http://dx.doi.org/10.1097/00006842-200107000-00006

Maunder, R. G., & Hunter, J. J. (2008). Attachment relationships as determinants of physical health. *Journal of the American Academy of Psychoanalysis and Dynamic Psychiatry, 36*(1), 11–32. http://dx.doi.org/10.1521/jaap.2008.36.1.11

Maunder, R. G., & Hunter, J. J. (2009). Assessing patterns of adult attachment in medical patients. *General Hospital Psychiatry, 31*(2), 123–30. http://dx.doi.org/10.1016/j.genhosppsych.2008.10.007

Maunder, R. G., & Hunter, J. J. (2012). A prototype-based model of adult attachment for clinicians. *Psychodynamic Psychiatry, 40*(4), 549–73. http://dx.doi.org/10.1521/pdps.2012.40.4.549

Maunder, R. G., Lancee, W. J., Mae, R., Vincent, L., Peladeau, N., Beduz, M. A., ... Leszcz, M. (2010). Computer-assisted resilience training to prepare healthcare workers for pandemic influenza: A randomized trial of the optimal dose of training. *BMC Health Services Research, 10*(1), 72. http://dx.doi.org/10.1186/1472-6963-10-72

Maunder, R. G., Lancee, W. J., Nolan, R. P., Hunter, J. J., & Tannenbaum, D. W. (2006). The relationship of attachment insecurity to subjective stress and autonomic function during standardized acute stress in healthy adults. *Journal of Psychosomatic Research, 60*(3), 283–90. http://dx.doi.org/10.1016/j.jpsychores.2005.08.013

Maunder, R. G., Lancee, W. J., Rourke, S., Hunter, J. J., Goldbloom, D., Balderson, K., ... Fones, C. S. L. (2004). Factors associated with the psychological impact of severe acute respiratory syndrome on nurses and other hospital workers in Toronto. *Psychosomatic Medicine, 66*(6), 938–42. http://dx.doi.org/10.1097/01.psy.0000145673.84698.18

Maunder, R. G., Panzer, A., Viljoen, M., Owen, J., Human, S., & Hunter, J. J. (2006). Physicians' difficulty with emergency department patients is related to patients' attachment style. *Social Science & Medicine, 63*(2), 552–62. http://dx.doi.org/10.1016/j.socscimed.2006.01.001

Maunder, R. G., Peladeau, N., Savage, D., & Lancee, W. J. (2010). The prevalence of childhood adversity among healthcare workers and its relationship to adult life events, distress and impairment. *Child Abuse & Neglect, 34*(2), 114–23. http://dx.doi.org/10.1016/j.chiabu.2009.04.008

Maunsell, E., Brisson, J., & Deschenes, L. (1995). Social support and survival among women with breast cancer. *Cancer, 76*(4), 631–7. http://dx.doi.org/10.1002/1097-0142(19950815)76:4<631::AID-CNCR2820760414>3.0.CO;2-9

Mayer, B., Muris, P., Meesters, C., & Zimmermann-van Beuningen, R. (2009). Brief report: Direct and indirect relations of risk factors with eating behavior problems in late adolescent females. *Journal of Adolescence, 32*(3), 741–5. http://dx.doi.org/10.1016/j.adolescence.2008.12.002

Mayseless, O. (2004). Home leaving to military service: Attachment concerns, transfer of attachment functions from parent to peers, and adjustment. *Journal of Adolescent Research, 19*(5), 533–58. http://dx.doi.org/10.1177/0743558403260000

Mazzuca, J. (2002). *Bottoms up: Drinking trends in U. S., Canada.* Retrieved from Gallup website: http://www.gallup.com/poll/7141/bottoms-up-drinking-trends-us-canada.aspx

McCabe, P. M., Gonzales, J. A., Zaias, J., Szeto, A., Kumar, M., Herron, A. J., & Schneiderman, N. (2002). Social environment influences the progression of atherosclerosis in the watanabe heritable hyperlipidemic rabbit. *Circulation, 105*(3), 354–9. http://dx.doi.org/10.1161/hc0302.102144

McCabe, P. M., Paredes, J. P., Szeto, A., & Schneiderman, N. (2006). The role of central and peripheral oxytocin in the progression of atherosclerosis in the Watanabe Heritable Hyperlipidemic Rabbit. *Psychosomatic Medicine, 68,* A3–A4.

McCarthy, D. M., Waite, K. R., Curtis, L. M., Engel, K. G., Baker, D. W., & Wolf, M. S. (2012). What did the doctor say? Health literacy and recall of medical instructions. *Medical Care, 50*(4), 277–82. http://dx.doi.org/10.1097/MLR.0b013e318241e8e1

McEwen, B. S., & Wingfield, J. C. (2003). The concept of allostasis in biology and biomedicine. *Hormones and Behavior, 43*(1), 2–15. http://dx.doi.org/10.1016/S0018-506X(02)00024-7

McNally, A. M., Palfai, T. P., Levine, R. V., & Moore, B. M. (2003). Attachment dimensions and drinking-related problems among young adults. *Addictive Behaviors, 28*(6), 1115–27. http://dx.doi.org/10.1016/S0306-4603(02)00224-1

McNamara, P., Andresen, J., Clark, J., Zborowski, M., & Duffy, C. A. (2001). Impact of attachment styles on dream recall and dream content: A test of the attachment hypothesis of REM sleep. *Journal of Sleep Research, 10*(2), 117–27. http://dx.doi.org/10.1046/j.1365-2869.2001.00244.x

McWilliams, L. A., & Bailey, S. J. (2010). Associations between adult attachment ratings and health conditions: Evidence from the national comorbidity survey replication. *Health Psychology, 29*(4), 446–53. http://dx.doi.org/10.1037/a0020061

Mead, N., & Bower, P. (2000). Patient-centredness: A conceptual framework and review of the empirical literature. *Social Science & Medicine, 51*(7), 1087–110. http://dx.doi.org/10.1016/S0277-9536(00)00098-8

Meaney, M. J. (2001). Maternal care, gene expression, and the transmission of individual differences in stress reactivity across generations. *Annual Review of Neuroscience, 24*(1), 1161–92. http://dx.doi.org/10.1146/annurev.neuro.24.1.1161

Mensing, C., Boucher, J., Cypress, M., Weinger, K., Mulcahy, K., Barta, P., ... Adams, C. (2007). National standards for diabetes self-management education. *Diabetes Care, 30*(Suppl. 1), S96–S103. http://dx.doi.org/10.2337/dc07-S096

Meredith, P. J., Strong, J., & Feeney, J. A. (2005). Evidence of a relationship between adult attachment variables and appraisals of chronic pain. *Pain Research & Management, 10*, 191–200.

Meredith, P. J., Strong, J., & Feeney, J. A. (2006). The relationship of adult attachment to emotion, catastrophizing, control, threshold and tolerance, in experimentally-induced pain. *Pain, 120*(1–2), 44–52. http://dx.doi.org/10.1016/j.pain.2005.10.008

Mickelson, K. D., Kessler, R. C., & Shaver, P. R. (1997). Adult attachment in a nationally representative sample. *Journal of Personality and Social Psychology, 73*(5), 1092–106. http://dx.doi.org/10.1037/0022-3514.73.5.1092

Mikulincer, M., & Shaver, P. R. (2007). *Attachment in adulthood: Structure, dynamics, and change*. New York, NY: Guilford Press.

Mikulincer, M., Florian, V., & Weller, A. (1993). Attachment styles, coping strategies, and posttraumatic psychological distress: The impact of the Gulf War in Israel. *Journal of Personality and Social Psychology, 64*(5), 817–26. http://dx.doi.org/10.1037/0022-3514.64.5.817

Mikulincer, M., Shaver, P. R., & Avihou-Kanza, N. (2011). Individual differences in adult attachment are systematically related to dream narratives. *Attachment & Human Development, 13*(2), 105–23. http://dx.doi. org/10.1080/14616734.2011.553918

Minino, A. M., Xu, J., Kochanek, K. D., & Tejada-Vera, B. (2009). *Death in the United States, 2007* (NCHS Data Brief No. 26). Atlanta, GA: Centers for Disease Control and Prevention.

Mischel, W., Ebbesen, E. B., & Raskoff Zeiss, A. (1972). Cognitive and attentional mechanisms in delay of gratification. *Journal of Personality and Social Psychology, 21*(2), 204–18. http://dx.doi.org/10.1037/h0032198

Mischel, W., Shoda, Y., & Peake, P. K. (1988). The nature of adolescent competencies predicted by preschool delay of gratification. *Journal of Personality and Social Psychology, 54*(4), 687–96. http://dx.doi.org/10.1037/0022-3514.54.4.687

Mitchell, J. P., Macrae, C. N., & Banaji, M. R. (2004). Encoding-specific effects of social cognition on the neural correlates of subsequent memory. *Journal of Neuroscience, 24*(21), 4912–17. http://dx.doi.org/10.1523/JNEUROSCI.0481-04.2004

Moreno-Smith, M., Lutgendorf, S. K., & Sood, A. K. (2010). Impact of stress on cancer metastasis. *Future Oncology, 6*(12), 1863–81. http://dx.doi.org/10.2217/fon.10.142

Morse, S. A., Ciechanowski, P. S., Katon, W. J., & Hirsch, I. B. (2006). Isn't this just bedtime snacking? The potential adverse effects of night-eating symptoms on treatment adherence and outcomes in patients with diabetes. *Diabetes Care, 29*(8), 1800–4. http://dx.doi.org/10.2337/dc06-0315

Nachmias, M., Gunnar, M. R., Mangelsdorf, S., Parritz, R. H., & Buss, K. (1996). Behavioral inhibition and stress reactivity: The moderating role of attachment security. *Child Development, 67*(2), 508–22. http://dx.doi.org/10.2307/1131829

Nagel, R. W., McGrady, A., Lynch, D. J., & Wahl, E. F. (2003). Patient-physician relationship and service utilization. *Primary Care Companion to the Journal of Clinical Psychiatry, 05*(01), 15–18. http://dx.doi.org/10.4088/PCC.v05n0104

Nelson, E. E., & Panksepp, J. (1998). Brain substrates of infant-mother attachment: Contributions of opioids, oxytocin, and norepinephrine. *Neuroscience and Biobehavioral Reviews, 22*(3), 437–52. http://dx.doi.org/10.1016/S0149-7634(97)00052-3

Nickerson, A. B., & Nagle, R. J. (2005). Parent and peer attachment in late childhood and early adolescence. *Journal of Early Adolescence, 25*(2), 223–49. http://dx.doi.org/10.1177/0272431604274174

Nishime, E. O., Cole, C. R., Blackstone, E. H., Pashkow, F. J., & Lauer, M. S. (2000). Heart rate recovery and treadmill exercise score as predictors of mortality in patients referred for exercise ECG. *Journal of the American*

Medical Association, 284(11), 1392–8. http://dx.doi.org/10.1001/jama.284.11.1392

Nolan, R. P., Reid, G. J., Seidelin, P. H., & Lau, H. K. (2007). C-reactive protein modulates vagal heart rate control in patients with coronary artery disease. *Clinical Science, 112*(8), 449–56. http://dx.doi.org/10.1042/CS20060132

Norris, F. H. (1992). Epidemiology of trauma: Frequency and impact of different potentially traumatic events on different demographic groups. *Journal of Consulting and Clinical Psychology, 60*(3), 409–18. http://dx.doi.org/10.1037/0022-006X.60.3.409

Ong, L. M., de Haes, J. C., Hoos, A. M., & Lammes, F. B. (1995). Doctor-patient communication: A review of the literature. *Social Science & Medicine, 40*(7), 903–18. http://dx.doi.org/10.1016/0277-9536(94)00155-M

Ovens, H. J., & Chan, B. T. (2001). Heavy users of emergency services: A population-based review. *Canadian Medical Association Journal, 165*, 1049–50.

Panksepp, J., & Solms, M. (2008). *The HDRF [Hope for Depression Research Foundation] research strategy in relation to an overview of the current state of depression research.* Unpublished manuscript.

Park, E. W., Tudiver, F., Schultz, J. K., & Campbell, T. (2004). Does enhancing partner support and interaction improve smoking cessation? A meta-analysis. *Annals of Family Medicine, 2*(2), 170–4. http://dx.doi.org/10.1370/afm.64

Pegman, S., Beesley, H., Holcombe, C., Mendick, N., & Salmon, P. (2011). Patients' sense of relationship with breast cancer surgeons: The relative importance of surgeon and patient variability and the influence of patients' attachment style. *Patient Education and Counseling, 83*(1), 125–8. http://dx.doi.org/10.1016/j.pec.2010.04.023

Penninx, B. W., Beekman, A. T., Honig, A., Deeg, D. J., Schoevers, R. A., van Eijk, J. T., & van Tilburg, W. (2001). Depression and cardiac mortality: Results from a community-based longitudinal study. *Archives of General Psychiatry, 58*(3), 221–7. http://dx.doi.org/10.1001/archpsyc.58.3.221

Perner, J., & Wimmer, H. (1985). "John thinks that Mary thinks that ..." Attribution of second-order beliefs by 5- to 10-year-old children. *Journal of Experimental Child Psychology, 39*(3), 437–71. http://dx.doi.org/10.1016/0022-0965(85)90051-7

Petraitis, J., Flay, B. R., & Miller, T. Q. (1995). Reviewing theories of adolescent substance use: Organizing pieces in the puzzle. *Psychological Bulletin, 117*(1), 67–86. http://dx.doi.org/10.1037/0033-2909.117.1.67

Pinquart, M., & Sorensen, S. (2003). Differences between caregivers and noncaregivers in psychological health and physical health: A meta-analysis. *Psychology and Aging, 18*(2), 250–67. http://dx.doi.org/10.1037/0882-7974.18.2.250

Pinquart, M., & Sorensen, S. (2007). Correlates of physical health of informal caregivers: A meta-analysis. *Journals of Gerontology. Series B, Psychological Sciences and Social Sciences, 62*(2), P126–37. http://dx.doi.org/10.1093/geronb/62.2.P126

Pitman, R., & Scharfe, E. (2010). Testing the function of attachment hierarchies during emerging adulthood. *Personal Relationships, 17*(2), 201–16. http://dx.doi.org/10.1111/j.1475-6811.2010.01272.x

Porges, S. W. (2003). The polyvagal theory: Phylogenetic contributions to social behavior. *Physiology & Behavior, 79*(3), 503–13. http://dx.doi.org/10.1016/S0031-9384(03)00156-2

Porter, M. E., & Teisberg, E. O. (2006). *Redefining health care.* Boston MA: Harvard Business Review Press.

Powers, S. I., Pietromonaco, P. R., Gunlicks, M., & Sayer, A. (2006). Dating couples' attachment styles and patterns of cortisol reactivity and recovery in response to a relationship conflict. *Journal of Personality and Social Psychology, 90*(4), 613–28. http://dx.doi.org/10.1037/0022-3514.90.4.613

Puig, J., Englund, M. M., Simpson, J. A., & Collins, W. A. (2013). Predicting adult physical illness from infant attachment: A prospective longitudinal study. *Health Psychology, 32*(4), 409–17. http://dx.doi.org/10.1037/a0028889

Ragozzino, M. E. (2007). The contribution of the medial prefrontal cortex, orbitofrontal cortex, and dorsomedial striatum to behavioral flexibility. *Annals of the New York Academy of Sciences, 1121*(1), 355–75. http://dx.doi.org/10.1196/annals.1401.013

Rappaport, S. M. (2012). Discovering environmental causes of disease. *Journal of Epidemiology and Community Health, 66*(2), 99–102. http://dx.doi.org/10.1136/jech-2011-200726

Ravitz, P., Maunder, R., Hunter, J., Sthankiya, B., & Lancee, W. (2010). Adult attachment measures: A 25-year review. *Journal of Psychosomatic Research, 69*(4), 419–32. http://dx.doi.org/10.1016/j.jpsychores.2009.08.006

Ravitz, P., Maunder, R., & McBride, C. (2008). Attachment, contemporary interpersonal theory and IPT: An integration of theoretical, clinical and empirical perspectives. *Journal of Contemporary Psychotherapy, 38*(1), 11–21. http://dx.doi.org/10.1007/s10879-007-9064-y

Reiner, K., Tibi, L., & Lipsitz, J. D. (2013). Do mindfulness-based interventions reduce pain intensity? A critical review of the literature. *Pain Medicine, 14*(2), 230–42. http://dx.doi.org/10.1111/pme.12006

Rhoades, D. R., McFarland, K. F., Finch, W. H., & Johnson, A. O. (2001). Speaking and interruptions during primary care office visits. *Family Medicine, 33*, 528–32.

Rice, K. G., FitzGerald, D. P., Whaley, T. J., & Gibbs, C. L. (1995). Cross-sectional and longitudinal examination of attachment, separation-individuation, and college student adjustment. *Journal of Counseling and Development, 73*(4), 463–74. http://dx.doi. org/10.1002/j.1556-6676.1995.tb01781.x

Rifkin-Graboi, A. (2008). Attachment status and salivary cortisol in a normal day and during simulated interpersonal stress in young men. *Stress, 11*(3), 210–24. http://dx.doi.org/10.1080/10253890701706670

Robertson, J. (Director). (1952). A two-year-old goes to hospital [DVD]. Available from http://www.childdevelopmentmedia.com

Rodrigues, S. M., Saslow, L. R., Garcia, N., John, O. P., & Keltner, D. (2009). Oxytocin receptor genetic variation relates to empathy and stress reactivity in humans. *Proceedings of the National Academy of Sciences of the United States of America, 106*(50), 21437–41. http://dx.doi.org/10.1073/pnas.0909 579106

Roisman, G. I. (2007). The psychophysiology of adult attachment relationships: Autonomic reactivity in marital and premarital interactions. *Developmental Psychology, 43*(1), 39–53. http://dx.doi. org/10.1037/0012-1649.43.1.39

Rolfe, A., & Burton, C. (2013). Reassurance after diagnostic testing with a low pretest probability of serious disease: Systematic review and meta-analysis. *JAMA Internal Medicine, 173*(6), 407–16. http://dx.doi.org/10.1001/ jamainternmed.2013.2762

Rollnick, S., Miller, W. R., & Butler, C. C. (2008). *Motivational interviewing in health care: Helping patients change behavior.* New York, NY: Guilford Press.

Rosengren, A., Orth-Gomer, K., Wedel, H., & Wilhelmsen, L. (1993). Stressful life events, social support, and mortality in men born in 1933. *BMJ (Clinical Research Ed.), 307*(6912), 1102–5. http://dx.doi.org/10.1136/ bmj.307.6912.1102

Roy, M. P., Steptoe, A., & Kirschbaum, C. (1998). Life events and social support as moderators of individual differences in cardiovascular and cortisol reactivity. *Journal of Personality and Social Psychology, 75*(5), 1273–81. http:// dx.doi.org/10.1037/0022-3514.75.5.1273

Rozanski, A., Blumenthal, J. A., & Kaplan, J. (1999). Impact of psychological factors on the pathogenesis of cardiovascular disease and implications for therapy. *Circulation, 99*(16), 2192–217. http://dx.doi.org/10.1161/01. CIR.99.16.2192

Rusbult, C. E., Kumashiro, M., Kubacka, K. E., & Finkel, E. J. (2009). "The part of me that you bring out": Ideal similarity and the Michelangelo phenomenon. *Journal of Personality and Social Psychology, 96*(1), 61–82. http://dx.doi.org/10.1037/a0014016

Salmon, P., & Young, B. (2009). Dependence and caring in clinical communication: The relevance of attachment and other theories. *Patient*

Education and Counseling, 74(3), 331–8. http://dx.doi.org/10.1016/j.pec.
2008.12.011

Sapolsky, R. (2004). *Why zebras don't get ulcers* (3rd ed.). New York, NY:
Henry Holt.

Sapolsky, R. M. (2005). The influence of social hierarchy on primate health.
Science, 308(5722), 648–652. http://dx.doi.org/10.1126/science.1106477

Sapolsky, R. M., Uno, H., Rebert, C. S., & Finch, C. E. (1990). Hippocampal
damage associated with prolonged glucocorticoid exposure in primates.
Journal of Neuroscience, 10, 2897–902.

Satpute, A. B., & Lieberman, M. D. (2006). Integrating automatic and
controlled processes into neurocognitive models of social cognition.
Brain Research, 1079(1), 86–97. http://dx.doi.org/10.1016/j.brainres.2006.
01.005

Schachner, D. A., & Shaver, P. R. (2004). Attachment dimensions and motives
for sex. *Personal Relationships*, 11, 179–95.

Scharfe, E. (2007). Cause or consequence? Exploring causal links between
attachment and depression. *Journal of Social and Clinical Psychology*, 26(9),
1048–64. http://dx.doi.org/10.1521/jscp.2007.26.9.1048

Schore, A. N. (1994). *Affect regulation and the origin of the self*. Hillsdale, NJ:
Lawrence Erlbaum.

Schore, A. N. (2001). The effects of early relational trauma on right brain
development, affect regulation, and infant mental health. *Infant Mental
Health Journal*, 22(1–2), 201–69. http://dx.doi.org/10.1002/1097-0355
(200101/04)22:1<201::AID-IMHJ8>3.0.CO;2-9

Schore, A. N. (2002). Dysregulation of the right brain: A fundamental
mechanism of traumatic attachment and the psychopathogenesis of
posttraumatic stress disorder. *Australian and New Zealand Journal of
Psychiatry*, 36(1), 9–30. http://dx.doi.org/10.1046/j.1440-1614.2002.00996.x

Scragg, R., Reeder, A. I., Wong, G., Glover, M., & Nosa, V. (2008). Attachment
to parents, parental tobacco smoking and smoking among year 10 students
in the 2005 New Zealand national survey. *Australian and New Zealand Journal
of Public Health*, 32(4), 348–53. http://dx.doi.org/10.1111/j.1753-6405.
2008.00253.x

Seligman, M. E. P., & Maier, S. F. (1967). Failure to escape traumatic shock.
Journal of Experimental Psychology, 74(1), 1–9. http://dx.doi.org/10.1037/
h0024514

Selye, H. (1979). *The stress of my life: A scientist's memoir*. New York, NY: Van
Nostrand.

Sethi, A., Mischel, W., Aber, J. L., Shoda, Y., & Rodriguez, M. L. (2000). The
role of strategic attention deployment in development of self-regulation:

Predicting pre-schooler's delay of gratification from mother-toddler interactions. *Developmental Psychology, 36*(6), 767–77. http://dx.doi.org/10.1037/0012-1649.36.6.767

Sharpe, M., & Carson, A. (2001). "Unexplained" somatic symptoms, functional syndromes, and somatization: Do we need a paradigm shift? *Annals of Internal Medicine, 134*(9_Part_2), 926–30. http://dx.doi.org/10.7326/0003-4819-134-9_Part_2-200105011-00018

Shaver, P., & Hazan, C. (1988). A biased overview of the study of love. *Journal of Social and Personal Relationships, 5*(4), 473–501. http://dx.doi.org/10.1177/0265407588054005

Shaver, P. R., & Mikulincer, M. (2002). Attachment-related psychodynamics. *Attachment & Human Development, 4*(2), 133–61. http://dx.doi.org/10.1080/14616730210154171

Sheps, D. S., Freedland, K. E., Golden, R. N., & McMahon, R. P. (2003). ENRICHD and SADHART: Implications for future biobehavioral intervention efforts. *Psychosomatic Medicine, 65*(1), 1–2. http://dx.doi.org/10.1097/00006842-200301000-00001

Shields, M., & Carroll, M. D. (2011). *Adult obesity prevalence in Canada and the United States* (NCHS Data Brief No. 56). Retrieved from Centers for Disease Control and Prevention website: http://www.cdc.gov/nchs/data/databriefs/db56.pdf

Simon, G., Ormel, J., Vonkorff, M., & Barlow, W. (1995). Health care costs associated with depressive and anxiety disorders in primary care. *American Journal of Psychiatry, 152*(3), 352–7. http://dx.doi.org/10.1176/ajp.152.3.352

Simpson, J. A., Rholes, W. S., Campbell, L., Tran, S., & Wilson, C. L. (2003). Adult attachment, the transition to parenthood, and depressive symptoms. *Journal of Personality and Social Psychology, 84*(6), 1172–87. http://dx.doi.org/10.1037/0022-3514.84.6.1172

Simpson, J. A., Rholes, W. S., & Nelligan, J. S. (1992). Support seeking and support giving within couples in an anxiety provoking situation: The role of attachment styles. *Journal of Personality and Social Psychology, 62*(3), 434–46. http://dx.doi.org/10.1037/0022-3514.62.3.434

Sinha, M. (2012). *Family violence in Canada: A statistical profile, 2010.* Ottawa, Canada: Statistics Canada.

Skinner, W., & Cooper, C. (2013). *Psychotherapy essentials to go: Motivational interviewing for concurrent disorders.* New York, NY: Norton.

Slade, A., Sadler, L., deDios-Kenn, C., Fitzpatrick, S., Webb, D., & Mayes, L. (2005). Minding the baby: The promotion of attachment security and reflective functioning in a nursing/mental health home visiting program. In L. Berlin, Y. Ziv, L. Amaya-Jackson, & M. T. Greenberg (Eds.), *Enhancing early attachments: Theory, research and intervention* (pp. 152–77). New York, NY: Guilford Press.

Sloan, E. P., Maunder, R. G., Hunter, J. J., & Moldofsky, H. (2007). Insecure attachment is associated with the alpha-EEG anomaly during sleep. *BioPsychoSocial Medicine, 1*(1), 20. http://dx.doi.org/10.1186/1751-0759-1-20

Slovic, P. (1987). Perception of risk. *Science, 236*(4799), 280–5. http://dx.doi.org/10.1126/science.3563507

Sockalingam, S., Blank, D., Abdelhamid, N., Abbey, S. E., & Hirschfield, G. M. (2012). Identifying opportunities to improve management of autoimmune hepatitis: Evaluation of drug adherence and psychosocial factors. *Journal of Hepatology, 57*(6), 1299–304. http://dx.doi.org/10.1016/j.jhep.2012.07.032

Sokol-Katz, J., Dunham, R., & Zimmerman, R. (1997). Family structure versus parental attachment in controlling adolescent deviant behavior: A social control model. *Adolescence, 32*, 199–215.

Spurgeon, D. (2001). Rudeness provokes most complaints against doctors in Saskatchewan. *BMJ (Clinical Research Ed.), 323*(7316), 771–2. http://dx.doi.org/10.1136/bmj.323.7316.771a

Sroufe, L. A., & Waters, E. (1977). Heart rate as a convergent measure in clinical and developmental research. *Merrill-Palmer Quarterly, 23*, 3–27.

Statistics Canada. (2008). *Canadian community health survey*. Ottawa, Canada: Author.

Statistics Canada. (2011). *Physical activity during leisure time, by age group and sex*. Retrieved from http://www.statcan.gc.ca/tables-tableaux/sum-som/l01/cst01/health77b-eng.htm

Statistics Canada. (2012). *Canadian community health survey, 2011*. Retrieved from http://www.statcan.gc.ca/daily-quotidien/120619/dq120619b-eng.pdf

Statistics Canada. (2013). *Heavy drinking by age group and sex (percent)*. Retrieved February 4, 2013, from http://www.statcan.gc.ca/tables-tableaux/sum-som/l01/cst01/health79b-eng.htm

Stern, D. N. (1985). *The interpersonal world of the infant*. New York, NY: Basic Books.

Stone, J., Sharpe, M., Rothwell, P. M., & Warlow, C. P. (2003). The 12-year prognosis of unilateral functional weakness and sensory disturbance. *Journal of Neurology, Neurosurgery, and Psychiatry, 74*(5), 591–6. http://dx.doi.org/10.1136/jnnp.74.5.591

Stroebe, W., Stroebe, M., Abakoumkin, G., & Schut, H. (1996). The role of loneliness and social support in adjustment to loss: A test of attachment versus stress theory. *Journal of Personality and Social Psychology, 70*(6), 1241–9. http://dx.doi.org/10.1037/0022-3514.70.6.1241

Sullivan, H. S. (1953). *The interpersonal theory of psychiatry*. New York, NY: Norton.

Suomi, S. J. (1995). Influence of attachment theory on ethological studies of biobehavioral development in nonhuman primates. In S. Goldberg, R. Muir, & J. Kerr (Eds.), *Attachment theory: Social developmental and clinical perspectives* (pp. 185–201). Hillsdale, NJ: Analytic Press.

Suomi, S. J. (2006). Risk, resilience, and gene x environment interactions in rhesus monkeys. *Annals of the New York Academy of Sciences, 1094*(1), 52–62. http://dx.doi.org/10.1196/annals.1376.006

Taylor, R. E., Mann, A. H., White, N. J., & Goldberg, D. P. (2000). Attachment style in patients with unexplained physical complaints. *Psychological Medicine, 30*(4), 931–41. http://dx.doi.org/10.1017/S0033291799002317

Taylor, S. E., Klein, L. C., Lewis, B. P., Gruenewald, T. L., Gurung, R. A., & Updegraff, J. A. (2000). Biobehavioral responses to stress in females: Tend-and-befriend, not fight-or-flight. *Psychological Review, 107*(3), 411–29. http://dx.doi.org/10.1037/0033-295X.107.3.411

Taylor, S. F., Phan, K. L., Decker, L. R., & Liberzon, I. (2003). Subjective rating of emotionally salient stimuli modulates neural activity. *NeuroImage, 18*(3), 650–9. http://dx.doi.org/10.1016/S1053-8119(02)00051-4

Teasdale, J. D., Segal, Z. V., Williams, J. M., Ridgeway, V. A., Soulsby, J. M., & Lau, M. A. (2000). Prevention of relapse/recurrence in major depression by mindfulness-based cognitive therapy. *Journal of Consulting and Clinical Psychology, 68*(4), 615–23. http://dx.doi.org/10.1037/0022-006X.68.4.615

Tennant, C. (1988). Parental loss in childhood: Its effect in adult life. *Archives of General Psychiatry, 45*(11), 1045–50. http://dx.doi.org/10.1001/archpsyc.1988.01800350079012

Tracy, J. L., Shaver, P. R., Albino, A. W., & Cooper, M. L. (2003). Attachment styles and adolescent sexuality. In P. Florsheim (Ed.), *Adolescent romance and sexual behavior: Theory, research and practical implications* (pp. 137–79). Chicago, IL: Aldine.

Trinke, S. J., & Bartholomew, K. (1997). Hierarchies of attachment relationships in young adulthood. *Journal of Social and Personal Relationships, 14*(5), 603–25. http://dx.doi.org/10.1177/0265407597145002

Troxel, W. M., & Germain, A. (2011). Insecure attachment is an independent correlate of objective sleep disturbances in military veterans. *Sleep Medicine, 12*(9), 860–5. http://dx.doi.org/10.1016/j.sleep.2011.07.005

Tulppo, M. P., Hautala, A. J., Makikallio, T. H., Laukkanen, R. T., Nissila, S., Hughson, R. L., & Huikuri, H. V. (2003). Effects of aerobic training on heart rate dynamics in sedentary subjects. *Journal of Applied Physiology, 95*, 364–72.

van der Horst, F. C. P. (2011). *John Bowlby – From psychoanalysis to ethology: Unravelling the roots of attachment theory.* West Sussex, England: Wiley-Blackwell. http://dx.doi.org/10.1002/9781119993100

van der Horst, F. C. P., LeRoy, H. A., & van der Veer, R. (2008). "When strangers meet": John Bowlby and Harry Harlow on attachment behavior. *Integrative Psychological and Behavioral Science, 42*(4), 370–88. http://dx.doi.org/10.1007/s12124-008-9079-2

van Ijzendoorn, M. H., & Sagi-Schwartz, A. (2008). Cross-cultural patterns of attachment: Universal and contextual dimensions. In J. Cassidy & P. R. Shaver (Eds.), *Handbook of attachment: Theory, research and clinical applications* (2nd ed., pp. 880–905). New York, NY: Guilford Press.

Verdecias, R. N., Jean-Louis, G., Zizi, F., Casimir, G. J., & Browne, R. C. (2009). Attachment styles and sleep measures in a community-based sample of older adults. *Sleep Medicine, 10*(6), 664–7. http://dx.doi.org/10.1016/j.sleep.2008.05.011

Vitaliano, P. P., Zhang, J., & Scanlan, J. M. (2003). Is caregiving hazardous to one's physical health? A meta-analysis. *Psychological Bulletin, 129*(6), 946–72. http://dx.doi.org/10.1037/0033-2909.129.6.946

Waller, E., Scheidt, C. E., & Hartmann, A. (2004). Attachment representation and illness behavior in somatoform disorders. *Journal of Nervous and Mental Disease, 192*(3), 200–9. http://dx.doi.org/10.1097/01.nmd.0000116463.17588.07

Ward, A., Ramsay, R., Turnbull, S., Steele, M., Steele, H., & Treasure, J. (2001). Attachment in anorexia nervosa: A transgenerational perspective. *British Journal of Medical Psychology, 74*(4), 497–505. http://dx.doi.org/10.1348/000711201161145

Wartner, U. G., Grossmann, K., Fremmer-Bombik, E., & Suess, G. (1994). Attachment patterns at age six in south Germany: Predictability from infancy and implications for preschool behavior. *Child Development, 65*(4), 1014–27. http://dx.doi.org/10.2307/1131301

Waters, E., Merrick, S., Treboux, D., Crowell, J., & Albersheim, L. (2000). Attachment security in infancy and early adulthood: A twenty-year longitudinal study. *Child Development, 71*(3), 684–9. http://dx.doi.org/10.1111/1467-8624.00176

Wei, M., Mallinckrodt, B., Russell, D. W., & Abraham, W. (2004). Maladaptive perfectionism as a mediator and moderator between adult attachment and depressive mood. *Journal of Counseling Psychology, 51*(2), 201–12. http://dx.doi.org/10.1037/0022-0167.51.2.201

Wei, M., Russell, D. W., & Zakalik, R. A. (2005). Adult attachment, social self-efficacy, self-disclosure, loneliness, and subsequent depression for freshman college students: A longitudinal study. *Journal of Counseling Psychology*, *52*(4), 602–14. http://dx.doi.org/10.1037/0022-0167.52.4.602

Weinfield, N. S., Sroufe, L. A., & Egeland, B. (2000). Attachment from infancy to early adulthood in a high-risk sample: Continuity, discontinuity, and their correlates. *Child Development*, *71*(3), 695–702. http://dx.doi.org/10. 1111/1467-8624.00178

Wells, K. B., Stewart, A., Hays, R. D., Burnam, M. A., Rogers, W., Daniels, M., ... Ware, J. (1989). The functioning and well-being of depressed patients. Results from the medical outcomes study. *Journal of the American Medical Association*, *262*(7), 914–919. http://dx.doi.org/10.1001/jama. 1989.03430070062031

West, M., Livesley, W. J., Reiffer, L., & Sheldon, A. (1986). The place of attachment in the life events model of stress and illness. *Canadian Journal of Psychiatry*, *31*, 202–7.

West, M. L., & Sheldon-Kellor, A. E. (1994). *Patterns of relating: An adult attachment perspective*. New York, NY: Guilford Press.

White, K. L., Williams, T. F., & Greenberg, B. G. (1961). The ecology of medical care. *New England Journal of Medicine*, *265*(18), 885–92. http://dx.doi.org/10. 1056/NEJM196111022651805

Wilkinson, L. L., Rowe, A. C., Bishop, R. J., & Brunstrom, J. M. (2010). Attachment anxiety, disinhibited eating, and body mass index in adulthood. *International Journal of Obesity*, *34*(9), 1442–5. http://dx.doi.org/10.1038/ijo. 2010.72

Williamson, D. F., Thompson, T. J., Anda, R. F., Dietz, W. H., & Felitti, V. (2002). Body weight and obesity in adults and self-reported abuse in childhood. *International Journal of Obesity and Related Metabolic Disorders*, *26*(8), 1075–82. http://dx.doi.org/10.1038/sj.ijo.0802038

Wing, R. R., & Hill, J. O. (2001). Successful weight loss maintenance. *Annual Review of Nutrition*, *21*(1), 323–41. http://dx.doi.org/10.1146/annurev. nutr.21.1.323

Winnicott, D. W. (1957). *The child, the family and the outside world*. London, England: Penguin.

Winnicott, D. W. (1989). Psycho-somatic disorder. In C. Winnicott, R. Shepherd, & M. Davis (Eds.), *Psycho-analytic explorations* (pp. 103–18). Cambridge, MA: Harvard University Press.

World Health Organization. (2009). *2008–2013 Action plan for the global strategy for the prevention and control of noncommunicable diseases*. Geneva, Switzerland: Author.

Writing Committee for the ENRICHD Investigators (2003). Effects of treating depression and low perceived social support on clinical events after myocardial infarction: The enhancing recovery in coronary heart disease patients (ENRICHD) randomized trial. *Journal of the American Medical Association, 289*(23), 3106–16. http://dx.doi.org/10.1001/jama.289.23.3106

Yehuda, R. (2004). Risk and resilience in posttraumatic stress disorder. *Journal of Clinical Psychiatry, 65*(Suppl. 1), 29–36.

Yehuda, R., & Bierer, L. M. (2007). Transgenerational transmission of cortisol and PTSD risk. *Progress in Brain Research, 167*, 121–35. http://dx.doi.org/10.1016/S0079-6123(07)67009-5

Yehuda, R., Teicher, M. H., Seckl, J. R., Grossman, R. A., Morris, A., & Bierer, L. M. (2007). Parental posttraumatic stress disorder as a vulnerability factor for low cortisol trait in offspring of holocaust survivors. *Archives of General Psychiatry, 64*(9), 1040–8. http://dx.doi.org/10.1001/archpsyc.64.9.1040

Zadro, L., Williams, K. D., & Richardson, R. (2004). How low can you go? Ostracism by a computer is sufficient to lower self-reported levels of belonging, control, self-esteem, and meaningful existence. *Journal of Experimental Social Psychology, 40*(4), 560–7. http://dx.doi.org/10.1016/j.jesp.2003.11.006

Zeifman, D., & Hazan, C. (2008). Pair bonds as attachments: Re-evaluating the evidence. In J. Cassidy & P. R. Shaver (Eds.), *Handbook of attachment* (2nd ed., pp. 436–55). New York, NY: Guilford Press.

Zimmermann, P., & Becker-Stoll, F. (2002). Stability of attachment representations during adolescence: The influence of ego-identity status. *Journal of Adolescence, 25*(1), 107–24. http://dx.doi.org/10.1006/jado.2001.0452

Index

The letter f following a page number denotes a figure.

Lightning Source UK Ltd.
Milton Keynes UK
UKOW02f1033040816

279953UK00001B/60/P